HELL-BENT

HELL-BENT

OBSESSION, PAIN,
AND THE SEARCH FOR
SOMETHING LIKE TRANSCENDENCE
IN COMPETITIVE YOGA

BENJAMIN LORR

St. Martin's Press
New York

HELL-BENT. Copyright © 2012 by Benjamin Lorr. All rights reserved. Printed in the United States of America. For information, address St. Martin's Press, 175 Fifth Avenue, New York, N.Y. 10010.

www.stmartins.com

ISBN 978-0-312-67290-4 (hardcover)
ISBN 978-1-250-01752-9 (e-book)

First Edition: November 2012

10 9 8 7 6 5 4 3 2 1

Contents

A Short Note on Folk Singing and
the Space Between Solutions

A folk song is whats wrong and how to fix it or it could be

whose hungry and where their mouth is or

whose out of work and where the job is or

whose broke and where the money is or

whose carrying a gun and where the peace is.

—WOODY GUTHRIE

In many ways, this is the story of a crack-up. It is the year I came to believe that Michael Jackson was a fully realized saint and that fully realized
saints walk among us all the time. It is the year I learned that even the
most beautiful saint is capable of—maybe even driven toward—the greatest
destruction. A year I learned to feel compassion for that arc, not betrayal. It
is a crack-up because I felt the narratives that bound my life together—
atheist, drunk, methodical saver for a methodical retirement—unbuckle
and drift off while, at the same time, I became more certain of the value of
each than ever before. It was the year I convinced myself that I could take
my spinal cord and bend it so severely that I could touch my forehead to
my ass. A year I maintained three jobs while practicing upwards of fourteen hours of yoga a week. Where I started spontaneously wishing for Love
(as an abstract concept) when blowing out birthday candles, flicking eye-
lashes, or performing other obsessive–compulsive cultural rituals of wishing. It is the year I started dating my very close friend's ex-girlfriend and,
not surprisingly, hurt my very close friend's feelings very badly. A year
when I decided to spend one thousand dollars on a stainless steel juicer for

the sole purpose of putting liquid spinach into my diet more regularly. When I met countless well-intentioned, brave liars and got more honest advice from their lies than I could ever hope to repay.

Everyone interviewed in this book knew I was writing a book. My one goal was to accurately try to capture my experience. Those who frequent the mystical section of bookstores are familiar with a concept called karma yoga. It is the yoga of the Bhagavad Gita, the yoga of action. To practice your karma yoga is to practice what you were put on this planet to do. There is no doubt in my mind that Bikram Choudhury's karma yoga is teaching yoga. He has such joy when spreading it. My karma yoga is the practice of writing; just like Bikram, I'm pretty sure I'm going to end up hurting people while I practice.

Prologue: Bombproof?

I am standing at the stage door, peering out through blinding light at blackness. It feels like a high-definition dream. Everyone is here. Assembled in the Grand Ballroom at the Westin Los Angeles in stillness: familiar faces staring straight ahead, this weird collection of antagonism and love, all connected by invisible understandings. The only word that even remotely fits is family. I am shirtless in spandex, staring at them. Above me, a row of klieg lights drops off the ceiling, aimed like compact cannons at the stage. The light shooting from their housing animates the dust in its path; it's the old visual cliché of movie projectors and morning attics, but watching the dust shimmer, I can't help but feel it is stripping open the very fabric of the universe.

At least for this moment, in this room.

In the center, on a stage lit white as a sun, a man holds himself in a perfect handstand. The muscles in his forearm ripple in micromovements.

Behind him there are two billboard-sized screens capturing live projections of his every action. I watch the handstand in triplicate. Slowly, the man raises his chest up and drops his feet forward, arching his back until his heels rest on the top of his head. At that moment, there is a circuit that has been completed: an O that travels from the back of his head up his legs and then around back down his spine to his head again. The thousand-plus people in the audience watch this circuit in absolute stillness. The man holds the O of his body aloft on two arms. He smiles. Then the micro-movements in his arms stop. His breathing disappears. There is a moment that stretches just long enough for my internal instincts to doubt its plausibility, for the hairs on my arm to stand on end, for my senses to consider the unconscious question of whether it is the man who is frozen or the universe around him that has stopped. Then there is a whirr from the burst shutter on a high-res camera, a twitch in the man's forearms, and suddenly we're back. The man returns from the posture the same way he went in. He stands up and bows; the room explodes in applause.

The MC announces a time of two minutes and forty-nine seconds. The audience begins to move. The announcement is repeated for a video camera live-broadcasting the event to the world. My eyes adjust to the glare.

In the front row, Bikram Choudhury, multimillionaire founder of Bikram Yoga, is snapping his fingers calling for a Coke. He is making noises like he is coaxing a monkey with food, "Tht-tht-tht-tht . . . Hey, Balwan, come on, come on, Balwan, come!" When no one scurries up to him, he snorts and looks over his shoulder. He leans into the slender woman sitting next to him, as if to caucus with her about his dilemma, but says nothing. Finally he stands, cutting into the spotlights and turns around, asking the entire room to go find Esak for him.

There is a woman crouching, whose face I know well but whose name I can't remember, who resumes massaging Bikram's thigh when he sits back down.

There is his wife, Rajashree, exactly eight seats away from him. There is Hector, and there is Afton.

There is eighty-three-year-old Emmy Cleaves walking back to her front-row seat in a positively slinky dress. She sits, hair pinned back, shoulders in perfect posture, the grand dame of the entire event. There is Sarah Baughn and her daughter crouched in the back playing patty-cake. There is even Courtney Mace somewhere, invisible, just like she wants to be.

This is the National Yoga Asana Championship, semifinal round. In a moment, I will go onstage to perform a three-minute routine I have spent the last three years learning. My goal is to approximate that man in his handstand. His control, his poise: I want to demonstrate my focus to the room. I want to make at least one hair on one arm stand on end. I will be judged just like an Olympic gymnast, according to the physical nature of the postures—or asanas—I perform. Points will be awarded based on the difficulty of the pose in question and the depth and skill with which I demonstrate it.

There will be other things on display as well. Less measurable, but certainly real. The room is cold, but my armpits are leaking wildly. There is an actual stream of sweat dribbling down my sides. It feels very primitive and glandular, like no sweat I have ever experienced before. It is as if someone turned an internal dial to a slow trickle. I consider wiping the sweat from my torso, but decided against it for fear of getting my hands slippery too. I need my grip. Then all of a sudden, way too soon, my name is called. Mary Jarvis is standing next to me exactly where I need her to be. I grab her hand impulsively and kiss it, almost greedily, like I was trying to eat it. I tell myself my only goal is to share how happy I am to be in here. I tell myself that the only thing Courtney Mace thinks about when she demonstrates is love. Mary wriggles her hand back out of my grasp. Then she uses it to sort of push me out there.

As I walk toward the stage, the room collapses. My legs move but my mind goes blank. Stepping up into the glare, skin sweaty, heart clunking wildly in my chest, in quite possibly the most earnest, hopeful moment of my life to date, I realize that if anything in this room has exploded, it's me.

PART I

It Never Gets Any Easier (If You Are Doing It Right)

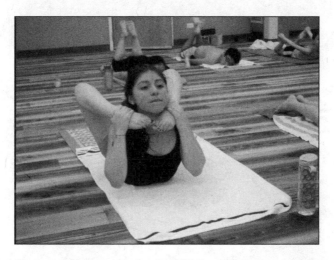

Karla, age 12, preparing for the 2011 Yoga Asana Championship

This story expresses, I think, most completely his philosophy of life. . . . He thought of civilized and morally tolerable human life as a dangerous walk on a thin crust of barely cooled lava which at any moment might break and let the unwary sink into fiery depths. He was very conscious of the various forms of passionate madness to which men are prone, and it was this that gave him such a profound belief in the importance of discipline.

—BERTRAND RUSSELL WRITING ABOUT JOSEPH CONRAD

It Never Gets Any Easier (If You Are Doing It Right)

You adjust to being upside down pretty quickly. Sure the blood starts pressing down on your face, and the floor and all its weird grainy ephemera are a whole lot closer, but in general, your body adjusts. Your breathing relaxes; your brain sort of shrugs. When you look around, things don't appear upside down. They appear as things. That's a woman siting in Lotus, there's a radiator, a row of mirrors, a pair of leopard-print Lycra shorts, someone's irregularly bulging poorly shaven crotch.

At the moment, I'm upside down, marveling at this fact, staring at these things. Across the room from me, Kara is going into her regular seizure. Lauren, two people down, is weeping softly to herself. Michael Jackson is pumping on the sound system. He's telling us "Don't Stop 'Til You Get Enough." I've heard the song my whole life, but right now, belly-button to the sky, and back bent in a shape far closer to a V than the desirable and healthy U I'm aiming for, I decide he's a prophet. A glowing saint. His voice is so fucking pure, so enthusiastic and happy, it's difficult for me to hold it all together listening to him. As I rise out of my back-bend, uncurling to a standing position, I feel a wave of electricity, a shiver up my spine. The room in front of me goes wavy like a reflection in wa-ter; blue and red dots flood my vision. Behind and between these, staring straight back at me from the mirror, is my smile. I watch, amazed at the size of my grin. Then I inhale, stretch to the ceiling, and dive backwards for more.

We're all here—weeping, smiling, twitching on the carpet while expe-riencing profound neurological events—because we are training to become yoga champions. Literally. Not in any elliptical, analogous, or absurdist sense. But actual trophy-wielding champions. This is Backbending Club, a semisecret group of super-yogis who gather together from across the Bikram universe to push one another to the limits of their practice. It's a little like the Justice League, Davos, or TED, only for yoga practice. For two weeks at a time, otherwise dedicated citizens—husbands, shopgirls, bankers—strip out of their pantsuits and ties, shed all civilian attachments, strap on Speedos, and dedicate their lives to asana practice.

Backbenders are not like you and me. These are practitioners for whom two classes a day is an unsatisfactory beginning. Who sneak third sets into regular class. Who stay long after everyone else has left. Who work on pos-tures quietly in the corner until the studio owner gently asks them to put on some clothes and leave. Bodies so finely muscled, so devoid of fat that they're basically breathing anatomical diagrams. Innards so clean, their shit comes out with the same heft, virtue, and scent of a ripe cucumber. Almost every studio has at least one practitioner like this. You know them by their works. By the way you eye them when you are trying not to. By the purely curious way you wonder what skin that tightly upholstered actually feels like. And if your gym, studio, or workplace doesn't have an actual Backbender, it certainly has someone with backbending in her heart. Who desperately wants to go hard-core, if only someone would give her permission.

Backbending Club is what happens when this community of loners crash together. We are here now in Charleston, South Carolina. Local stu-dio owner David Kiser is hosting. To host, David has opened his home and studio to the group for the next two weeks. We take class at his studio, carefully cramming ourselves into the back of the room so as to disturb his regular students as little as possible. In between classes, we practice further. Then we take class again. Then we continue to practice, often not returning to his home until after midnight.

In this respect, Backbending is the antithesis of those glossy lavender-scented *Yoga Journal* retreats. We eat; we do yoga. There are no catered meals, no spacious rooms, no hammock time, no sandy beaches. No refined sugar, no alcohol, no processed foods. No coherent schedule, no personal space, no sarcasm, and no coffee. There are also no fees. Participants pay what they can, when they can.

Right now, surrounded by those hallucinatory red and blue dots, we are wall-walking. For the uninitiated, this means standing with your back to a wall, reaching upward to the ceiling, dropping your head back like a Pez dispenser, and slowly curling your spine backwards. I imagine peeling a banana. To guide yourself as you peel, you walk your hands down the wall. First your head goes past your neck, then your hips, then your knees. Finally, your face ends up on a flat plane with your feet, and your chest is pressed against the wall. It is not a yoga pose. It is an exercise Backbenders practice to increase the range of motion in the spine. By leveraging the pressure of the floor and gravity, each wall-walk pushes the spine into a deeper and deeper backbend.

Michael Jackson is paused. The room goes suddenly silent except for our breathing.

"Everyone look at Karlita."

Twenty-two heads turn. It takes me a second to find her because my internal gyroscope is spinning a lot faster than the room, which it turns out isn't actually spinning. Finally, in the far corner, I find Karla González—a twelve-year-old who flew in from Mexico City. Karla, looking a bit like an insect, is in the logical conclusion of a wall-walk: on her chest, ankles on each side of her ears, feet flat on the floor. She has a sweaty agonized look on her face I usually associate with women giving birth. She does not look like she wants us to be looking at her.

"Now come up slowly. Finish with your arms last."

Keeping her ankles in one place, Karla pushes up from her chest and uncurls to a standing position like a slow-motion pea shoot sprouting from the soil. Suddenly, she is a twelve-year-old girl again. Her face flushes as the entire room applauds. I have the distinct urge to tell her that I love her. Instead, I inhale and try to stabilize the internal gyroscope so as not to puke.

The voice instructing Karla belongs to Esak Garcia. At thirty-four, Esak is a legitimate Bikram Yoga celebrity, the guru's favorite son. His body ripples like a snake when he moves, his torso the keeper of a thousand muscles I have never seen before. Esak attended Bikram's very first teacher training as a teenager—just before heading off to college at Yale—and returns to training every year, twice a year, to, in his words, refresh from the source. More to the point, Esak is also an authentic yoga champion, the first male to have won the international competition, having bent his way to the top in 2005. He is one of the very few Bikramites authorized by the guru to run seminars and is constantly flying around the world giving lectures, demonstrating postures, and gently guiding the spines of the middle-age practitioners willing to pony up his speaking fees.

Backbending Club is a different space. Unlike his seminars, it is an invitation into his personal practice. It is the yoga community he hopes to build. The work here is a refinement of the program he used when training for the championship in 2005. That is the reason for the do-it-yourself mentality, Byzantine dietary restrictions, and the donation-only payment plan. Esak is here to practice; he invites like-minded members of the community to support him.

While we wall-walk, Esak bends along with us but out of time. We go down the wall, he stays up watching, giving corrections. When we come up, we see only his stomach and pelvis arching outward. His eyes have a peripheral vision that brings to mind a frog's tongue zipping out to catch flies. He can be across the room, holding down a conversation, scrutinizing a posture, when suddenly he will yell out a correction in response to your first, tiniest mismovement. A slippage from exhaustion, a momentary cheat. A week into the training, these staccato barks are really the only one-on-one interaction I have had with him.

As we wind down tonight's set of wall-walks, Esak puts Michael on pause once again.

"I know you all are in pain. I know because I can see it in your faces; I know because I am there too. But remember, this is why we are here. Each of us needs to find the painful place and go through it. Do not try to avoid it." He pauses. "The pain is temporary. It is a phantom. But if you avoid it, you will never move past it."

As he speaks, I look around the room. At least three of the women bending on the wall next to me have little blue X's of surgical tape peeking out from below their sport bras. The surgical tape was put there by a chiropractor earlier in the day. The women are doing backbends so severe their ribs are popping out of place. The chiropractor pops them back in and the women return for more backbends. I know this because as one of the only people with a car, I drive them to and from the studio when it happens.

When I drive the women to the chiropractor, I worry about Esak's pain rhetoric. It feels like the worst type of adolescent masochism, Nietzsche filtered through David Blaine. But at the moment, smiley and vibrating with joy, I know exactly what he is talking about. I know because if I let my concentration slip for a second, my whole body will scream in hammer-on-thumb-kick-the-nearest-object-across-the-room rage. Although my ribs are solidly in place, my spinal column feels like someone is driving a knife into it, like it's wrapped in barbed wire. There are precise points that feel black and blue, other places that feel disembodied and almost silly. My fingers are numb. But I find myself backbending easily anyway. Buoyed by my incongruous elation, I find that if I focus on the pain, I can interface with it. It doesn't mean that it stops hurting; it means that the pain shifts and begins to feels like a medium I am moving through. It feels like a melting. When I have melted through, there is another side where I can just breathe.

After the set of wall-walks, we run through postural routines. This is specific training for the Asana Competition. We are drilling seven of the most difficult postures. This is less overtly painful, more just exhausting. Each posture demands muscle contraction, concentration, and then an extended moment of stillness where you inhabit it. In many ways, the routines, with their exacting movements and wild contortions, look like break dance slowed down to a freeze-frame pace.

Esak runs us through them with a stopwatch. At his direction, we repeat the seven postures again and again and again. He pushes us. Then he lies to us. The refrain "this is our last set" begins to signify that maaaaybe it is the fifth or sixth from last. Then he chastises us. Finally without warning, there is an actual last set. Esak announces this by telling us to work on any postures we didn't get to. The room responds by lying still and breathing.

Then he reminds us to finish our chores.

The chores are one of the ways the community gives back to David for hosting us. All the yoga teachers have to donate a class or two to David's studio. That is their chore, so they wipe themselves off the floor and hit the showers early. Those of us who are not yoga teachers have more specific chores. Laundry. Carpet cleaning. Stocking the studio refrigerator. My job is spraying down and wiping the mirrors. The sweat from the day has aerosolized and made them filmy. As everyone else leaves the yoga room, I spray each of the fourteen floor-to-ceiling-length mirrored panels and make circular motions to wipe them clean. It is surprisingly painful work. *Karate Kid* references dance in my brain. For the last few panels, I notice that my left arm is so tired that I have to physically support it with my right one. It feels like a puppy dog arm. Finally, well after midnight, we clamber into cars and drive back to David's house to sleep on his floor.

How I Got to Here:
The Journey of a Skeptic Addict

In 2008, I arrived at Bikram Yoga Brooklyn Heights fat. Fat fat. About six months prior, I separated a rib in one of those ill-advised drinking moments that I used to specialize in. After somewhere between five and twelve vodka sodas at a good-bye party for a friend, I found myself on the iced-over campus of Columbia University, sizing up the relative merits of the campus hedges. And the merits of a hedge after five to twelve vodka sodas refers exclusively to the amount of potential cushion and elasticity it will provide. That I found myself in this scenario was neither an accident nor a drunken inspiration—the good-bye party was for one of my premier drinking buddies, a freshman-year hallmate, and we had returned to our alma mater expressly to engage in a freshman year tradition: bushjumping.

Bushjumping! Just writing it makes my heart leap (and my ribs quiver). The basic idea is self-evident enough: a long running start, a leap, a landing in the hedge. If it went Olympic, points would be allocated for form, difficulty, and volume of scream. But points are beside the point. Lying drunk in a bush, laughing about a new hole in your shirt, and discovering a new zippering scratch the next morning are what really matter.

From an outsider's perspective, all this may seem debatably idiotic for an eighteen-year-old young man, fresh with the taste of freedom from moving out of his parents' house. But the sad fact is that as I stared down this particular bush, on this particularly magic wintry night, I was twenty-nine years old. I had just broken up with my live-in girlfriend. A girl so wonderful and loving that she tolerated almost all my ugly failings so well that I found her intolerable and gradually chased her out of my life. My childhood friend was constantly asleep and living on my couch. I had a meaningful job that I was good at and couldn't stand. Nothing in my life was correct. Anyway, it might make a better story if I separated my rib on that bushjump. But I didn't. My jump that night was a reasonably fine backflip. I landed safely. My friend crashed next to me. We lounged in the hedges and laughed. Then I got up and ran straight ahead into the darkness and dove face-first against the icy ground. I think the idea was something along the lines of a Slip 'n Slide. But it was the dead of winter; there was no water, or ice, or anything except pavement. And so I crashed against the ground belly first, heard an audible crunch, and felt enormous pain before a uniformed officer came over with a flashlight and told me to get lost.

I spent the next six months milking that injury for all it was worth. By milking, I mean using it as an enormous excuse not to do anything physical. These were days spent sitting on my couch reading. Weekends spent at my friend's house sucking up order-in lo mein. The closest I came to athletics was trudging up the stairs to my apartment and collapsing on the couch.

Conveniently, this was one of those marshy New York springs. The rain fell; I watched it from indoors. Soon I started ordering *Diet* Cokes and substituting Sweet'N Low for sugar in my coffee.

It's pretty hard to totally destroy your body with genes like mine. I'm naturally lean. Not muscular-athletic, mind you, but tight-waisted, small-chested, and prototypically pencil-necked. Up to this point, I had led a moderately athletic American life: soccer through high school, occasional jogs to make up for occasional binges, and the standard intermittent commitments to local gyms. This meant the weight, when it came, didn't come on easily or evenly. It took effort and follow-through: imagine a boa constrictor swallowing a sheep, imagine an R. Crumb woman as a man: weird areas of slender breaking into weird areas of sloth.

But determination eventually prevailed, and by month six or so, I was completely transformed. My face looked swollen, my gut smoothed and rotund. Startling things like my socks (!) had stopped fitting, while my new oversized T-shirts simultaneously stretched loose over my stomach yet clung tight to my nipples. Most disturbingly, my ankles started to swell and pulse when I stayed standing too long.

One evening at a party, I overheard a good friend say, "It looks a lot like Ben ate Ben."

I tried glorying in my new physique, especially the belly. I would rub it in mixed company. Use it as a ledge for the remote control on the couch or as a kettledrum when standing above the toilet to pee. On the beach, I became that pregnant-looking fellow, thrusting my stomach forward with a huge grin. But no amount of faux pride could carry me forever. One day I realized I had lost sight of my penis completely.

Yoga wasn't my first choice for getting back in shape. As with everyone who's ever been horrendously out of shape, I spent considerable time fantasizing about the different methods and programs I would use to become fit again. I knew I wanted to change. I knew diet alone wasn't going to be enough. And I knew I needed something low impact. To daydream of jogging was to daydream of stress fractures. Swimming seemed like a strong fit—my well-insulated body was just like a seal's! But the prospect of endless laps bored me before I began. Then there were the martial arts. The

Internet certainly offered lots of commentary on the different styles. Unfortunately, the one class I attended spent most of the time going over techniques for eye-gouging. This felt a bit too pervy for someone close to thirty years old. Finally, there was yoga. I was definitely intrigued; yoga felt like one of those unambiguously good things, right up there with eating more fruit and being kind. But in Brooklyn, where I was living, every third human seemed to walk around with a rolled yoga mat strapped to their back. This type of elvish/archerish behavior didn't inspire.

Probably not unexpectedly, I allowed laziness to make the decision for me. Using Google Maps, I simply made a list of all the exercise studios within fifteen minutes of my house and planned on sampling each of them until I found the proper fit.

The second place on that list—after my brief foray into eye-gouging kung fu—was Bikram Yoga Brooklyn Heights.

I found myself standing in a hot room amid lots of flesh and lots of mirrors.

The men around me were either half-naked (topless with shorts) or upsettingly close to naked (a strap of spandex) while the women, more demure, tended toward sports bras and leggings. I was wearing a baggy oversized blue T-shirt—even though I was warned it was going to be hot—mostly because I wasn't ready to bare my fiercely conical man-breasts to the world. I'm not typically self-conscious, but being around all this radiant flesh reduced my faux-belly-pride to rubble.

Following orders, I stood on my mat and clasped my hands underneath my chin. The thermostat on the wall read 108 degrees.

This was ten thirty on a Saturday morning, and both my brain and mouth felt a little fuzzy from drinking the night before. I had arrived almost a half hour early, one of those measures a hungover man takes to ensure he comes at all. This was my first time inside any yoga studio, but it hit all the clichés I had assembled: rows of shoes by the door, burning sticks of incense in the locker room, scattered chalices and figurines, nothing but the softest colors on the walls.

The studio itself was small, little more than a glorified hallway. When I walked in, a group of chirping skinny women were lounging around the reception area, sipping from stainless steel water bottles. Everyone looked like they had been awake and functional for hours.

In the center of this group, I approached the gorgeous little midget of a woman who was going to be my instructor. She stood just below my breastbone in a colorful unitard, signing students in and handing out rental mats. Nothing in my description so far makes her sound attractive, so I will reiterate: This was a gorgeous little midget of a woman. I don't believe in auras, parapsychology, or even the efficacy of most teeth whiteners, but I do believe this woman seemed to shine.

Our eyes met. She smiled. Then she handed me a waiver of liability to sign. "You'll want a water too. Unless you brought one?"

I stared blankly. I hadn't said a word yet.

"And towels. You'll need at least two towels."

"Just tell me what to do, I'm new."

"Of course." And she laughed.

At this point, gorgeous omniscient yogis were new to me. But if there was Bikram-brand Kool-Aid, I was ready to gulp. More immediately, if there were towels and water bottles to be bought, I was ready to pay. With a credit card swipe, I scampered off to the locker room, excited to learn the secrets this women had clearly mastered.

Ten minutes later, standing in front of the mirror, hands clasped underneath my chin, I eyed myself more suspiciously. Where was I exactly?

I was already sweating and class hadn't begun.

Standing next to me, there was a rail-thin dude in a Speedo smiling manically at himself in the mirror.

And thinking back, signing a medical waiver didn't really jibe with the incense.

Then the beautiful midget opened her mouth and began to speak.

In general, I don't remember much about the first class. I remember at one point thinking, This is tough but by no means impossible. I also remember thinking a little later, Please please please let this end. All I want to do is leave.

I remember finding it hard not to stare at the woman in front of me.

I remember wanting to make her disappear.

I remember lying on my back feeling like a plump roasting turkey.

I remember bright spots of pain as I stretched things that hadn't been stretched in a very long time.

Lastly and very specifically, I remember the force of my blood.

At first, this was more of a curiosity, a refrain in the running monologue going through my head during the class. A certain posture might cause me to lower my head below my waist, and I would feel gravity pull the blood into my face and forehead. The internal monologue would in turn note that this was a novel sensation. But as the class went further, with the poses piling on top of one another and the heat collapsing around me, something fundamental changed. My focus shrank. All that remained was a terrifying awareness of my blood flow. At this point, my heart rate had gone way up and my frame of vision shuddered with each beat. Then suddenly, as a class, we were told to rest. Lying on my stomach, staring at nothing, I could hear the blood gulping through my heart as I recovered; it made an almost squeaky noise as the valves struggled to keep up.

Then the postures continued.

When it was over, I looked up at the mirror in the locker room. The person looking back had clearly just been swimming in his clothes. I was a bit dizzy, so I sat down on a bench for a long while. I didn't feel like I was shining. I felt vaguely wrung out. I was also thirsty. When I started drinking from my water bottle, it locked to my lips like a magnet. I finished the whole thing and refilled it and finished that.

The rest of the locker room was moving at double speed. An old man was singing Sinatra. The rail-thin guy was back at the mirror, shaving. The entire place was flush with the swampy humidity of a steam room, the floor covered with drippings. Pulling dry clothes over wet ones, I hobbled out.

At the door, the beautiful midget instructor stopped me: "You did really well. You must not lead a very toxic lifestyle."

I think I smiled and nodded. So much for all that yogic wisdom I had been attributing to her. Then I stumbled home.

Without changing out of either set of sweaty clothes, I fell asleep on my couch.

I woke up almost ten hours later in the middle of the night. I knew I had to go back to that studio as soon as possible. I felt brand new.

My life had changed.

For the first three months, I thought I had discovered magic. I slept less but felt more energized. I ate constantly but couldn't stop losing weight. My skin glowed. My brain glowed. Muscles started appearing in places I didn't know muscles existed. (Muscles on the ribs? Muscles on the muscles on the thigh?) One day, my pants started fitting again; the next week, I needed to buy a belt to keep them from slipping off. The changes were radical and positive and continuous.

In all, I lost forty-five pounds in those three months, went from being unable to touch my feet at all (my fingers just stretched pathetically about my ankles) to being able to place my palms flat on the floor. I moved from being able to do zero pull-ups to being able to do sets of ten at a time. I realize none of this is strongman-type stuff, but for a nonathlete it felt miraculous. My body had awakened.

This is not to say the changes came easily. If the yoga was magic, it was the snarky kind, the type that comes with an unexpected trade-off from a maybe-whimsical, maybe-cruel sorcerer. Each class itself was grueling. Stupidly painful, stupidly boiling. However much my brain glowed, my body ached more. At one point, my hamstrings turned black and blue from being overstretched. When I walked down a flight of stairs, I threw myself on the banister for support. At work, I would sneak off to a quiet hallway and do back stretches on the floor to relieve the enormous cramps that built up during the day.

One time a coworker, no doubt herself sneaking off for something, found me stretching. "Uh, you all right down there?"

"Yeah, just threw out my back doing yoga."

"Doing yoga?"

"Yeah. Weird yoga," I said, lying on my back in our hallway with my knees tucked to my chest.

"Maybe you shouldn't be doing it."

But when I asked my favorite instructor about it, she just smiled. One of those damned yogic smiles: "It's just your body opening up. Be patient. That pain is almost like a rite of passage. Almost every serious yogi goes through it."

And what I heard: Me? A serious yogi?! And what I saw: New muscles flexing back in the mirror.

So I continued.

I settled into this comfortable dichotomy—a practice that was simultaneously refreshing and crippling me—for another year. Pain would come (say in the shoulder), life would change (no elbows above my ears for a few weeks), my body would "open" and eventually the pain would disappear. Then a new pain would awake, perhaps this time in the soles of my feet, and the process would continue.

Each sequence of pain taught me something new about my body. When our bodies are completely pain free, it's difficult to learn from them. We spring down the steps, letting the muscles and ligaments take care of themselves. Our focus is elsewhere. Pain pulled my inner workings to the forefront. All of a sudden, I could feel the bands of muscle working together or opposing. I could find my edge and learn the consequences of going over it.

The structure of the yoga nurtured these observations. Bikram classes are remarkably static. The same twenty-six posture sequence every time: the same heat, the same humidity, the same drumming instructions coming from the teacher's mouth. Ideally, the studio becomes almost an abstract space, a condition-controlled chamber where you face an identical experience every time you enter. Bending within this repetition feels like a cross between a full-body version of a pianist practicing the scales and an inverted assembly line: you stand still while a procession of postures works on your body and then you do it again and again and again.

It turns out that a body and mind that feel reliably similar day-to-day will react wildly different to the same conditions. Even after months of practice, expectations of performance were not just counterproductive but impossible. I'd walk in eager and strong only to be leveled: dropped like a boxer to one knee after only four postures. The very next day, I'd limp to the studio promising to take it easy and leave elated. My body was dynamic and mysterious. It exceeded anything I thought possible and still managed to abandon me with no notice or rationale. To accept these rhythms—to release from expectations—was to develop compassion: first for the overweight newbie sucking wind next to me, much later for myself.

Beyond this general awakening, however, two important things happened to me during this year. The first is that I met Sarah Baughn.

Back then, Sarah Baughn was a beautiful twenty-one-year-old yoga champion: an all-American yoga queen, part pep squad, part earnest whole-grain intensity, to the point that I immediately had trouble taking her seriously. She was touring the country, giving posture demonstrations to benefit people with chronic disease. And at some point during her tour, she stopped by Bikram Yoga Brooklyn Heights.

Watching her bend, I began to understand one small idea in the yoga universe. Her demonstration began directly after class, the entire studio still crouched over our mats, catching our collective breath, dripping. Most of the postures she chose to perform were from the advanced series, extreme extensions of the regular postures I had been learning. These were backbends so deep her spine looked like it was going to snap; alien forms, part grotesque, part Cirque du Soleil. I had never seen anything like it and I was amazed. Seeing a person with their chest on the floor and their heels on the top of their head challenges your notions of the species. But the more I watched, the more I realized it wasn't the extremity of the postures that was affecting me.

Sarah might do something as simple as sit on her mat, lean forward, and touch her toes—a hammy stretch from soccer practice—but somehow make it totally consuming. She had a concentration that expanded into her entire body. In many ways, it felt like I was watching a waterfall: the same roaring power, the same glassy beauty, with my brain achieving the same hum in its presence. It wasn't difficulty or aesthetics. Most of her postures were the stuff B-list ice skaters would scorn on those terms. It was as if I were watching Sarah perfect herself. Or I was watching a more perfect Sarah. As she poured herself from posture to posture, this woman, standing on a towel on a mat in a slightly stinky room, took on a dimension I had previously associated only with natural phenomena, the stuff of Sierra Club calendars:

rock walls and ice chasms, somehow distilled into the body of a twenty-one-year-old.

After watching Sarah Baughn, I knew that I needed to do more with this yoga than just define my abs. I felt a call. I desperately wanted to do what she just did.

And so a few classes later, I nervously asked my favorite instructor, "What should I do to take my yoga to the next level?"

Again she answered without hesitation: "Enter the tournament. Don't be afraid. I've been watching you."

Nothing about that answer was expected. The tournament? A competition? Watching me? If I thought about it, of course I knew you couldn't have a yoga *champion* like Sarah Baughn without some *championship* event to coronate her. But at the same time, competitions didn't jibe with my understanding of yoga at all.

Still, I had to learn more. I knew there was no way I could win a competition. I wasn't flexible like Sarah Baughn. But then, embodying a rock wall wasn't about winning. Was it?

The second thing that happened that year was my beloved ultra-devoted, ultra-tanned, ultra-Bikram instructor had a stroke.

In all things yoga, Hector was my mentor. Handsome, gracious, modest, muscular, it seemed like he occupied the very pinnacle of health. In many ways, he also represented the very pinnacle of what a Bikram practitioner could be. Hector owned two successful studios, practiced the yoga six days a week, and quoted Bikram liberally in conversation.

To Hector, Bikram was "my guru."

To Hector, who began practicing after an unsatisfactory knee surgery and had used the yoga to heal what his doctors had not, there were no excuses for doing the postures half-assed or incorrectly.

To me, Hector was everything I hoped to get out of the yoga.

Whenever possible, I'd alter my schedule to attend Hector's classes. This was not as easy as it might seem, because the studio had a policy of not revealing when Hector was teaching to prevent overcrowding. In Bikram, all classes are supposed to be identical, and having popular teachers undermines this effect. So I was feeling pretty lucky to find Hector behind the desk checking students in as I bounded into class on this particular day.

"Hector! I was hoping to see you here!"

In response, Hector grimaced back and handed me my usual two towels. For a man who typically walked around with a serene smile, this was unexpected enough to be noteworthy but nothing to dwell on. I grabbed a mat and headed to the locker room; even master yogis were allowed to have off days.

During class, I realized Hector, far from grimacing, was in a great mood: his voice soaring through the posture descriptions, his arms conducting like a maestro. As with all Hector's classes, I pushed myself harder than normal; his enthusiasm was inspiring, his devotion reassuring.

By the middle of class, as usual, I was practically submerged in my own sweat, feeling great. But coming up to my most difficult posture, Tuladandasana, the Balancing Stick, I noticed Hector dropped one of his usual lines. Tuladandasa is a killer posture. Every muscle in your body is tensed and holding you aloft on one leg while the rest of your frame stretches perfectly flat, parallel to the floor. The combination of muscular exertion with the lowered position of your heart is tremendous. Generally, Hector loved quoting Bikram after we finished it and were recovering: "I give you a mini heart attack now, so you don't get the big one later." I'm sure I never would have remembered this absence, except for what he inserted in its place:

"You might notice, I'm having trouble pronouncing the names of several of the postures."

I hadn't.

"That's because I had a stroke recently and lost the use of several muscles in my face."

Say again?

And then he was on to the next posture. No further comment.

I stayed behind. It wasn't that I expected my teachers to be immortal or even flu-resistant. But Hector was a young guy, mid-thirties to my eye. And he was *healthy!* More, there was something about the idea of a stroke. It seemed so . . . so . . . Bikram appropriate. If Hector had bounded into class and shared his battle with leukemia, lockjaw, or multiple sclerosis, I don't think I would have blinked. But a stroke hit me differently. From my very first class, I had wondered about the intensity of the postures: the extreme heat, the pounding in my heart during class, the pain that resulted.

It was easy to write off those aspects if I was making myself healthier. But now I began questioning everything. I had changed a lot from the yoga. But what was the cost? What if the backaches and pulled muscles were warning signs? Had I been so caught up in weight loss and the newly muscled man in the mirror that I was ignoring basic messages my body was sending?

Messages such as, *This yoga hurts. It is bad for you.*

I spent the rest of class limping through the postures, waiting until I could get out and Google the hell out of *stroke* and *Bikram*. Those searches led to more searching, and soon the rabbit hole swallowed me whole. The same stories, testimonials, hysterical warnings, and medical "proofs" were repeated by all manner of experts with no substantiation or evidence. Basic information on the history of the practice or the number of studios operating or the propensity toward atrophied knees was unavailable or hotly contested. The Internet devolved into its clichéd echo chamber, the same arguments spinning around and around like a mad sage chasing his own backbend, like my quick-dry synthetic fabrics at the laundry. It made me dizzy; it made me ill.

At the same time, I couldn't just give up my practice. I loved it.

It might have been the best thing that ever happened to me.

And so I started the process that would lead to this book. I reached out to Esak about joining a Backbending retreat. I contacted sports physiologist Susan Yeargin about the dangers of heat. And finally, I took a long look at the center of the circling information and found one man staring back.

The Man in the Mirror[1]

Sometimes I think I hallucinated Bikram Choudhury. He's too perfect for us, too quick every time I think I have him pinned down. His official

---

[1] Aka What I Learn about Bikram from the Internet

biography reads like a character from a Rushdie novel. By the tender age of
three, when most of us were waddling around, occasionally still crapping
in our diapers, his parents pulled him in from the dusty streets of Calcutta
and began a rigorous course of yogic training. This preschool bending involved meditation, strict dietary controls, and four to six hours of physical
practice every day. To motivate the young master, Bikram was promised a
penny every time he managed to bite his toes without bending his knees.
The guru claims he was never paid.

By five, Bikram was packed off and apprenticed to one of the most famous yogis in all of India, Bishnu Ghosh. A guru himself so powerful that
he would routinely put on demonstrations where he would stop his own
pulse, allow an elephant to walk across his chest, or bend a bar of iron with
his throat. Ghosh demanded total obedience from his disciples, refusing to
train those who didn't follow his dictates exactly, and subjecting those who
did to screaming fits and Brahmanical tantrums until their hair was blown
back and their cheeks covered with spittle. The easily distracted Bikram was
a frequent target of this discipline: when Bikram lost focus, Ghosh burned
the preteen with incense.

Under Ghosh's tutelage, Bikram's powers increased dramatically. By
thirteen, the young, handsome, and mighty Bikram bent his way to the top:
he became the youngest-ever contestant to win the Indian National Yoga
Competition. Bikram held this crown, undefeated, for three years. Fame
quickly followed. Bikram and his guru took to the road, demonstrating
their feats of strength to adoring crowds: part traveling circus, part medici-
nal road show, part evangelical church for the holy temple that is the human
body. Following the direction of his guru, Bikram refused all forms of payment and lived without material possessions.

After his third title, and at the request of head judge and future yoga
legend B. K. S. Iyengar, the fifteen-year-old Bikram retired from the national competition to give other contestants a chance. Iyengar suggested
that instead of competing, Bikram demonstrate the physical powers he had
cultivated. Bikram took him up on it. He ran marathons with no training.
He became a competitive weight lifter and broke records. He continued
public exhibitions, drawing larger and larger crowds: stretching out over a

bed of nails, dragging automobiles up and down Calcutta's streets, and slowing his heart rate until he could be buried alive.

Around this time, Bikram learned he didn't need to sleep.

From here things get weird. At age seventeen, during a routine training session, Bikram slipped and dropped a 380-pound weight on his knee, crushing his patella like a seashell. Doctors who were rushed to the side of the young celebrity declared he'd never walk again. Bikram knew better. He turned to yoga, to his guru, and together they designed an especially powerful posture sequence that healed Bikram fit as a sitar in just under six months. He not only walked, he returned stronger. Following a directive from Ghosh, Bikram moved to Mumbai to open shop as a healer and share his training. With the miracle knee proof of his yoga's efficacy, his fame exploded; soon he was known as the Yogiraj, Guru of Mumbai.

Then, at the height of his fame in India, at what turned out to be his guru's dying request—for yes, at just about this time, Bishnu Charan Ghosh, leading light of early twentieth-century physiculture, one of the few universally acclaimed masters in the yogic world, decided to take leave of his mortal coil and induce a heart attack in himself at the age of sixty-nine (he had previously declared that a heart attack was the least painful way to go)—at this crucial juncture, Ghosh made Bikram swear an oath:

> My guru took my hand and told me something, in English, which he never spoke. "Promise me you will complete my incomplete job," he said. He meant bringing yoga to the rest of the world, to the West and America. And I replied, "Yes, I promise. I will."

And thus, at age twenty-four, Bikram left India to bring yoga to the world.

(A man given to few regrets, Bikram does have one regarding this particular sequence in his life: "Looking back, I can't help feeling sad, mostly because I miss him every second of every day with every ounce of my heart. But I'm also sad because I forgot to ask him how long I am supposed to continue teaching hatha yoga to fulfill my karma yoga! Do I have to keep doing this for my entire life?")

The first brief stop in this process was Japan. There, in the wealthy Shin-juku district, Bikram attracted the attention of a group of researchers from the University of Tokyo who were studying tissue regeneration. These scientists applied their clipboards, lab coats, and evidence-based minds to the knee-healing sequence Bikram and Ghosh had developed. Recognizing its promise as a therapy, the scientists agreed to help Bikram prove its benefits if he would let them conduct research on its mechanics. Two noteworthy developments resulted. First, inspired by the saunas the Japanese scientists took on their lunch breaks and worried about new nagging injuries developing in his Japanese students, Bikram started dabbling with external heaters to re-create the heat of Calcutta (average temperature 88.7 degrees F). Second, to help the lazy urbanite mind focus on posture alignments, mirrors were added so practitioners could correctly adjust themselves as they practiced. This was an old technique his guru had used when training weight lifters, and Bikram saw no reason why yoga practitioners couldn't benefit as well.

Unfortunately, before this groundbreaking collaboration could fully realize its potential, fate intervened. Richard Nixon, America's own dark magician, was touring Southeast Asia publicly checking in on United States military bases, privately scouring the locals for remedies for his chronic phlebitis.

When word reached the president about the young yoga master and his miracle system, he summoned the guru immediately and demanded a session. Bikram agreed. Clothed in nothing but athletic shorts and jowls, the president bent before him. The experience shattered Nixon's expectations. His phlebitis was cured! Overjoyed by the results and overwhelmed by the guru's expertise, the president issued an open invitation to Bikram: Come to America, bring your yoga, live in my country!

Not one to reject the ebullience of a sitting president, Bikram flew to America at once. He arrived on a chartered plane—without visa or bank account—and was welcomed on the runway by a phalanx of high-ranking administration officials. After asking around to determine who in his new nation was most in need of his healing yoga, Bikram flew to Beverly Hills to open a studio.

The rest was easy. It turned out that in addition to healing knees, Bikram's yoga was fairly miraculous at burning fat and toning muscles. Few places on the planet were as well equipped as Beverly Hills to recognize and deal with such an advance. Word spread fast. Students flocked to his classes, and Bikram packed them in until every inch of his small studio's floor space was lined with bending humans.

What he saw during these classes brought joy to his heart, for it reminded him once again of his guru's infinite wisdom. America needed his yoga more than any place he could conceive. His students were soft, lazy creatures: giant children, ruined by material riches and corrupted by an abundance of easy choices. Every spine he saw was crooked; every joint he bent was stiff. This was great news! In India, gurus prescribed individualized posture sequences for their clients. But that wouldn't be necessary here. The "Xerox copies" he found in Beverly Hills could do a basic sequence for years and still receive benefits.

Instead of offering altered posture sequences for his American students, Bikram altered his approach to teaching: supplying more detailed descriptions of the postures to guide their bodies, strict discipline to control their minds, and bright pain to humble their egos. "You all grew up in California on a king-size water bed, I grew up on a bed of nails," he'd explain when asked about this approach. "If you feel dizzy, nauseous, you must be happy."

In this context, the added heat he had discovered in Japan seemed like a second miracle. It operated like a shortcut for the American disaster. Not only did it allow the rigid to deepen their postures—softening cartilage, loosening joints, expanding constricted blood vessels to feed their muscles—but more important, with the thermostat cranked high enough, even the richest, most fabulous client could be melted into a haggard mess. The more Bikram came to appreciate the miracle of the heat, the more the thermostat in his studio started sliding up: from 85 degrees F to 95 degrees F one week, to 100 degrees F the next, ultimately climaxing at a scalding 110 degrees F.

With those quick turns of the dial, the deal was sealed. Adding heat meant subtracting clothes. This exposed flesh, combined with the requirement of staring at full-length mirrors during class, combined with the startling results, combined with jam-packed classes, proved too much for the Beverly Hills mind. Fever broke out. By 1980, classes were filled to capacity. Newspapers were filled with bad puns about the hot new craze. And then the Hollywood elite got in on the act. By age thirty, Bikram was ringleader of a full blown six-ring celebrity circus: The Beatles, Raquel Welch, Barbra Streisand, Michael Jackson, Ted Kennedy, Madonna, and Quincy Jones all showed up to suffer at his direction (and then pose patiently for a picture after class).[2]

The only limitation was that there was only one Bikram, who, for all his feats of strength, could teach only one class at a time. Complicating this, Bikram's growing fame in Beverly Hills coincided with a more general yoga upwelling. All manner of shaggy, tubby, druggy seekers were running around town calling themselves yoga teachers. This was trouble. If Bikram was going to deal with the new influx of students, he needed more teachers. But looking around, it wasn't easy to find instructors he could entrust with the power of his yoga.

Luckily a solution appeared. After a particularly agonizing class, Shirley MacLaine took the guru aside and explained that he should really be charging for his classes. Charge? Bikram eyed her suspiciously. Up until this point, Bikram had followed the Indian convention and kept his classes free, accepting donations from his more generous clients. But as Shirley pointed out, he was in America now. And Americans didn't respect things that were given away free. This yoga was special, and he needed to protect it.

The need for quality control and Shirley's American Way combined in Bikram's mind, forming a perfect marriage: discipline and capitalism, cash and control. After hiring a manager, an accountant, and a lawyer, Bikram

---

[2]Speaking for them all on the mid-1980s TV show the *New Age Connection,* we have the young Charlie Sheen. Bikram is his "mentor, guru, teacher, and friend," says Sheen. The yoga not only provides calm and focus, which help with his baseball, but Bikram is also beginning to teach him something more intangible and elemental. "He puts a mirror in front of us. . . . He teaches us god realization . . . or how to be human."

began the process of expanding. For his teachers, he chose the best of the giant children: the most flexible ones, containing the best spines. But he never let himself forget they were children. In addition to demanding that they teach only his yoga, in exactly the sequence he had developed, Bikram recorded himself leading a class. He then used the recording to write up a script—he called it his dialogue—which all teachers would have to memorize and recite during class. Practicing at a Bikram studio, he decided, would be like practicing with Bikram himself, only with the direction uttered through someone else's lips.

By forty, Bikram controlled a growing network of studios and let a motorcycle ride over his chest on the evening news. By forty-five, he had saved Kareem Abdul-Jabbar's NBA career, rejuvenated John McEnroe's tennis game, collaborated with NASA to bring yoga to astronauts, and massaged a pope. By fifty, he had discovered diamonds and fedoras. By sixty, Bikram was sitting firmly on top of a yoga empire, operating in thirty-seven countries worldwide, showing up to teach his classes in only a Rolex and a Speedo. In the intervening years, he married an Indian yoga champion half his age (she won the national competition five times to Bikram's three), bought a ten-thousand-square-foot house in the Hollywood Hills, stashed close to forty Rolls-Royces in its garage, and fathered a pair of beautiful children.

But what never changed over all those years, what couldn't change, was his devotion to his mission, to his karma yoga. And so, millionaire many times over, Bikram is still right there today, teaching class himself, on a dais in his headquarters in Beverly Hills: hips wrapped tight in leopard print, chest freshly waxed, demanding perfection through his headset microphone to a room of hundreds, smiling as his students compete to feel pain in front of him.

Sometimes I think if he didn't exist, someone would have to invent him.

But then sometimes I think that's exactly what happened. That it was Bikram who hallucinated Bikram, that he's his own Rushdie. After all, all the information above comes from one of his official biographies or from an interview with a senior teacher. Much is unverifiable. And the details shift constantly. In some accounts he started training at three, sometimes at six; other times he won the championship at eleven, twelve, or thirteen. And his famous yoga sequence, the very core of Bikram Yoga, was actually not so much developed or designed by Bikram, but largely excerpted with only the slightest of changes from a longer series of ninety-one postures that have been firmly in the public domain for the last hundred years.

Other Bikram claims are not so much vague as completely unknowable. Nixon, currently frolicking among the immortal sages, will be forever unavailable to confirm or deny his Bikram moment. (Of course, this hasn't stopped the president's library from expressing extreme skepticism that the two ever met.) Likewise, Bikram Yoga Headquarters has repeatedly rejected requests for citations, references, or copies of the Japanese medical research central to Bikram's original health claims. And NASA has been unable to locate even the hint of a relationship with Choudhury or anyone else on a project involving yoga. The extent of Bikram's own weight lifting injury is, of course, lost to time along with his medical records.

We do have the celebrities, of course. Bikram's studio is lined like a Manhattan diner with their framed autographed pictures. But even here things get tricky. For every Jim Carrey, who has repeatedly and publicly thanked Bikram for his girlfriend's butt, there is a Madonna. Here is Madonna talking about her yoga workouts with morning-radio host Johnjay on his nationally syndicated show.

> **Johnjay:**   You ever do Bikram?
> **Madonna:** Uh, yeah. I mean that's like turn the heat up so hot, you don't have to do anything 'cause you just sweat?
> **Johnjay:**   Yeah, it's like 110 degrees and 50 percent humidity. . . .
> **Madonna:** Do you like that?

As for the Beatles, Bikram told the BBC he treated them in 1959—before they had formed as a group.

Finally, there are the claims that have simply melted away over the years. It was once common knowledge among students that Bikram won an Olympic gold medal. He bragged constantly during the pre-Internet

1970s about the world records he set in weightlifting. Or that Nixon greeted him on the runway when he arrived in America. Nobody in the Bikram world mentions these anymore.

But then, just when you've decided the man is an unending charlatan, a self-promoting boob, a yogic version of a spoiled American child actor grown old (to say nothing of his back spasms, his death threats, and the legions of patent lawyers at his beck and call), he will reinvent himself before you. He will unnerve you. You'll walk into his studio in Beverly Hills and find him singing sweet lullabies to his students during class. You'll watch him talk to an elderly student, in his leopard-print and Rolex, with the heartbreaking compassion of a master healer. You'll find him listening to a woman in tears describing her son with cystic fibrosis. And you will watch as Bikram ushers her back to his office to design an individualized posture sequence to help alleviate his symptoms. You'll read glowing unsolicited testimonials from professional athletes and supermodels, the two classes of professionals who probably know most about maintaining the body.[3] You'll learn that those forty-something Rolls-Royces in his garage are used cars he bought as wrecks, and that he repaired them with his own hands. Late at night, while he wasn't sleeping. Vocation: fixing junk bodies. Avocation: fixing junk cars.

You'll look at his shirtless, hairless chest and realize that at sixty, his type of health can't be faked.

You'll talk to him and realize that his manic conversational energy is exactly what you'd expect from a man who hasn't slept in forty-six years.

And whatever you ultimately decide, what's not in dispute, what's clearly

---

[3] A brief sampling of a much lengthier list: Hall of Fame basketball player Kareem Abdul-Jabbar ("I practice Bikram Yoga. . . . There is no way I could have played as long as I did without it"), ultra-endurance runner Dean Karnazes ("I must admit, it's amazing how something so torturous can leave you feeling so good"), tennis player Andy Murray, currently ranked number three in the world ("It has helped me a lot with my fitness and mental strength"), *NBC News* Chief Medical Correspondent Dr. Bob Arnot ("I was taking twelve to sixteen Advil a day for pain. Almost by accident I tried Bikram Yoga. . . . I have been virtually pain-free for two years"), Jennifer Aniston ("My legs got leaner. My arms got strong. I've maybe even grown a half inch from aligning my spine"), Elle Macpherson ("Bikram is great for detoxification and circulation"), and Jenny McCarthy, who decided to satisfy her Bikram needs by building a studio in her garage.

not a hallucination is that right now in America there are just over 1.1 million men, women, and children who regularly come together for ninety-minute doses of his healing. That at his command, legions of grown men will don spandex and roll around on a mildewy carpet trying to bite their toes without bending their knees. That twice a year as a guru, he charges just under eleven thousand dollars for the privilege of bending in his presence and receiving his training. That there are 1,700 studios open worldwide, filled with more than eight thousand instructors willing to devote their adult lives to reciting his words from a script. That many of them adopt a faux Indian accent when doing so.

It's dizzying. The Freudian concept of ambivalence goes beyond uncertainty and mixed emotions. True ambivalence, Freud insisted, is a condition where we contain opposite emotions inside us, simultaneously exploding out in completely opposite directions. This is Bikram.

Heat

Dr. Yeargin is a sweat scientist. A professor in the Department of Applied Medicine and Rehabilitation at Indiana State University, she has spent a career investigating the complex physiological interactions between heat, hydration, and athletic performance. She has consulted with professional football teams, enthusiastically sampled drippings from marathon runners, and applied rectal body temperature probes to hulking jocks. Given that intense heat is the sine qua non of my Bikram experience, she feels like the perfect person to talk with. Also given the logistics of rectal probes, I'm guessing she is pretty charismatic.

When I talk with her, she is about to run fieldwork with firefighters, investigating the effectiveness of head-cooling helmets. The firefighters, dressed in full Vader-like protective gear, will run through training exercises designed to mimic real-life rescue operations while Dr. Yeargin attends to their physiology: capturing their core body temperature, heart rate, skin temperature, and sweat rate in action. The whole scene seems like the intersection of hard science and a romantic comedy, with the brainy, diminutive

Dr. Yeargin on her tiptoes adjusting the placement of sensors while the fire-fighters lounge between training sessions, crack jokes, and prepare to rush back into danger.

The data she collects will be analyzed backed at her lab. She hopes the results will be used to design better cooling systems for helmets—or perhaps to move away from head cooling completely.

"I do a lot of work with children too," she said. "And children are reasonable. When a child gets hot and verges on heat illness, they get grumpy and whiny and quit. Adults, on the other hand, tend to think they can push through anything.

"One of the dangers of a head-cooling device might be that it encourages that mentality. It doesn't help anyone if we have firefighters that think they are perfectly fine but are actually on the verge of collapse."

Understanding the mechanisms behind that collapse is what led Dr. Yeargin to study heat in the first place. In the summer of 2001, just as she was entering a master's program in exercise science, she watched three consecutive heat stroke deaths ripple through the sporting world: one each at the high school, college, and pro level. The deaths were senseless and mysterious. One occurred at 88 degrees and 60 percent humidity, a typical Florida summer day. One occurred surrounded by coaches, trainers, and elite medical facilities. All involved athletes in prime physical condition who, after completing their workout for the day, simply fell into comas and died. The more she investigated, the more interested she became in the physiological mechanisms that triggered these deaths. She switched the focus of her master's. When she was finished, she switched the focus of her career and began work on a Ph.D.

From her office, Dr. Yeargin gives me a crash course in the physiology of exercise during extreme heat. "Your body is battling two sources of heat coming at it from two directions," she explains. "First, inside the body, your muscles are producing heat through metabolism. Second, and more importantly, heat from the outside world is penetrating inward." Combating these forces is absolutely essential to survival. The body has a critical core temperature just north of 105 degrees, after which the brain begins to shut down and organs start to fail.

To exercise in heat is to create a series of dilemmas: the body must negotiate the urgent need for cooling with the desire to continue exercising.

This begins with the body's normal response to heat, shunting blood from the core to the skin. As blood cycles to the surface, it dissipates heat into the atmosphere and then cycles back to cool the entire system. During exertion, however, the muscles of the body require increases in blood to function. In response to the two separate needs, the body shunts blood in two directions: into the muscles to feed performance and out to the skin to cool. This fork, however, leaves a gap: the major organs of the body—especially the gut, liver, kidneys, and brain—can be underserved and undernourished.

Compounding this rerouting is a massive relaxation of the vessels holding the circulating blood. Heat stimulates a reflex, dilating the size of the blood vessels. In the form of a heat pack on a tight muscle, this expansion can be wonderful, increasing circulation, allowing deeper flow into the muscle. When applied bodywide however, the sudden increase in the size of the vessels decreases the pressure in the system (think of the difference in pressure between water running through a tiny nozzle or a wide tunnel). The reduction in pressure forces the heart to pump harder to push blood the same distance, further straining the system and reducing blood available to other organs.

Finally, of course, there is sweat. Lots of it. Pumping fluid to the skin allows evaporation to release unwanted heat. The hotter it gets, the more the body sweats; the more sweat, the more evaporation cools.[4] The flipside to this process is a decrease in blood volume. The sweat sliding down your back is no longer circulating in your body. As the plasma volume decreases, there is a cascading effect, compounding all previous reactions. The heart must work even harder still. The organs receive even less blood. Less blood

---

[4]And as anyone who has ever experienced the growing trapped anxiety of soaking through their undershirt during a meeting can attest, sweat is effective only if it is evaporated. In conditions where evaporation is precluded, such as a wool suit jacket or a rainy day—or an artificially humid room—the sweat has a much more blunted effect. In these conditions, the body continues to increase its rate of sweat in the hope of cooling, but instead of reducing temperature merely loses more fluid.

flow means less cooling at the skin. Core temperature escalates and the body comes ever closer to shutdown.

All of which is why exercise in high heat feels harder: The muscles are starved for energy. The brain isn't receiving enough blood and starts sending freakout feedback messages. The heart physically can't beat hard enough to pump blood to all the places it is needed. The result is the common demoralizing effect where a relatively easy workout can suddenly feel incapacitating.

"The brain is especially sensitive to these changes," Dr. Yeargin explains. "It is a princess. It wants the perfect temperature, perfect electrolyte balance, perfect sugar levels. . . . If it doesn't get it, you see confusion, disorientation, irritability, grumpiness."

Hallucinations?

"Hallucinations and fainting and seizures and coma." When you faint, your body is essentially commanding you to lie down fast. The new orientation makes it easier to get blood to the brain.

I think of classes where I have been ruthlessly and suddenly dropped to one knee.

When I tell her about the yoga, she is skeptical. "Most of my work is telling people to avoid exercising in exactly that type of situation. . . . When I study heat stroke, I put people into a room that is about one hundred four degrees to purposely stress their bodies.

"That type of situation can be devastating if core temperature rises to a dangerous level. . . . Rapid deterioration of organs, coma, death." There is a loss of control as the brain shuts down: internal feedback mechanisms fail, toxic substances flood from the gut, cells starve, a bad situation becomes much worse. Even if a heat stroke victim survives the initial event, there is often long-term damage to the brain, kidneys, and liver.

Listening to her talk, I can't help but nod my head in agreement. I wonder how anyone ever manages to make it through class alive, much less return and claim it's healthy. Not only is it hot, but many studios artificially raise humidity, making it even more miserable and destroying whatever cooling effect comes from sweat. Not only are the exercises intense, but many are designed specifically to cut off and stress blood flow. It's crazy making. But what's especially crazy making is that it feels great. I emerge from class feeling reborn.

And so somewhat reluctantly, I find myself explaining the benefits to Dr. Yeargin, hoping that I don't sound like a New Age crank. I tell her about my weight loss. My gains in strength. The feeling that my concentration, clarity, memory, and reaction time have all improved. The extreme energy. The elation that carries throughout my day, lasting beyond any postexercise runner's high. My voice swells, and I tell her I think it makes me a better person.

She considers. She is kind. "To be honest, it's an unstudied area. I'm almost positive there is nothing in the scientific literature on that. . . . There are acclimatization effects, however. That's why you can handle it day in and day out. Maybe there is something there."

Dr. Yeargin explains that in response to the stress of exercise in a hot environment, the body adapts. It becomes radically more efficient. After seven to fourteen days of exercise in the heat, people undergo a series of physiological changes known collectively as acclimatization. Some of those changes, like a lower temperature at the onset of sweating, feel obvious and banal. Others, such as increased oxygen consumption and increased exercise efficiency, hint at something more surprising. Muscles in acclimatized athletes show reduced glycogen utilization and diminished postexercise lactate concentration, meaning they use less food to accomplish the same effort and give off less waste during the process. Livers in these athletes begin producing additional proteins to increase blood plasma volume, causing in turn, a decrease in the strain on their hearts. Blood cortisol levels—a measure of stress—fall in these athletes during intense exercise, meaning they are less stressed by events that strain nonacclimatized athletes. Nobody knows how these benefits carry over to life outside of the heat—it's unstudied—but what is clear is that sustained exercise in heat activates some primal mechanism that causes the body to increase its efficiency.

"Acclimatization is great," Dr. Yeargin emphasizes. "But it doesn't eliminate the risks. No matter what, staying hydrated is crucial. Water, water, water. It doesn't matter how adapted your body has become, dehydration is terrible. It puts a huge strain on your heart and wreaks havoc with your organs."

They are such sweet, sensible parting words that when I get an email from Esak later, it almost feels necessary. The cognitive dissonance must be restored. "Hi Family," he writes to all us prospective Backbenders. "When we practice together it will be with no water. If you have never done a class with no water before, you may want to eliminate it now. It may seem like a hard thing to do, but it's really not that big a deal. We'll talk more about why when you get here."

Chad

Heat is not new to yoga. In Indian mythology, the world itself is created by the god Prajapati "heating himself to an extreme degree." Spiritual work is repeatedly compared to work in the forge. Scholar Georg Feurstein notes that "the earliest term for yogalike endeavors in India is *tapas*. This ancient Sanskrit word means literally 'heat' derived from the verbal root *tap,* meaning 'to burn' or 'to glow.'" Practicing *tapas* gave the gods their immortality. Likewise, it is through heat the ascetic becomes clairvoyant, the sacrificer becomes pure, and the sage becomes realized. To generate meditative powers, worshippers turn to Agni, the god of fire, hoping to internalize his flame.

Nor is this obsession with heat abstract. Methods for internalizing and generating heat are endlessly discussed and recommended in the holy literature: fasting, withholding respiration, intense concentration, and—in a direct wormhole to Bikram and his space heaters—vigils in front of fire. Again and again, the ancients describe "cooking the body in the fire of yoga" to make the body pure.

Of course, provisos to cook the body or take vigil before a bonfire were written centuries before the invention of the modern furnace, and so I decide I need to know a little more about heat as it is applied to yoga studios. To do this, I go straight to the master.

Chad Clark is a heat artisan. He has designed, built, rebuilt, or performed emergency resuscitation on more than five hundred hot yoga studios from Alaska to Australia. For years, he would drive cross-country from studio to studio in a truck jammed full of everything needed to keep a hot yoga studio hot. Now his business has grown to the point where he primarily consults over the phone for breakdowns, or flies out to participate in the design process directly. His reputation is not just behind the scenes. There are Bikram practitioners who know exactly which studios Chad has built and will detour out of their way to take classes at them. He has designed yoga studios in celebrities' homes and worked for years at Bikram's International Headquarters in Los Angeles.

Chad is not *Yoga Journal.* He looks and drinks like a hero from a Richard Russo novel. His body has the approximate proportions of a boiler. Face with slight scruff, receding crew cut hairline, and the blue-collar smile of a goofball who also knows he's tougher than you are: he hails from Scranton, Pennsylvania, and grew up in a family dominated by a family-run construction business. In his teens, when he used to bounce for clubs in New York City, people would ask for his autograph because they assumed he played football for the Jets. Nowadays, Chad's got the type of thick fingers that look well adapted to casually twirling off lug nuts that most of us wouldn't even consider loosened. When he wears button-up shirts, he tucks them in too tight, revealing a nice overhanging gut. His pants have smudges indicating exactly where he wiped his fingers when working. All of which is to say, in appearance, Chad is exactly what you'd expect from a guy who can disassemble and rebuild a furnace from memory, but not at all what you'd expect from a guy who has devoted his adult life to hot yoga.

"I got into this full-time because I couldn't afford the phone bills," Chad is telling me, hunched over a beer. "Studio owners would call at all hours of the night with these emergencies. If you are selling hot yoga and your heater breaks, it's bad for business. I wanted to offer advice, but I literally couldn't afford my own phone bills.

"Of course, long before that, I got into this because the yoga works. I had the type of back pain that shuts your life down." Chad graduated from school with degrees in electrical and mechanical engineering, and he parlayed his general intelligence into a job as an investment banker on Wall

Street. But his passion has always been working with things—ripping out insulation, throwing up drywall, rebuilding machines of all sorts and complexities. A lifetime spent crouched while his fingers were tinkering left him with an angry lower back. When he was knocked around in an otherwise minor car accident, the pain grew unbearable. He tried to rehab it. When that didn't work, he walked into a Bikram studio. "And within my first few months, I had my life back. . . . No one believes in the yoga more than I do."

A Chad Clark studio is different because of the control a studio owner has over the environment. "When I first started, it was 'How can I get this thing hotter?' Studio owners were just trying to take conventional furnaces and use them to heat commercial spaces." It was very much a do-it-yourself community of isolated practitioners, all excited to experiment with a new innovation, but with little practical experience. Bikram had brought a fundamental new idea to both exercise and physical therapy. By providing a shortcut to raising heart rate, the heat allows relatively simple movements—which almost everyone can engage in—to have much more potent cardiac benefits.[5] Just as important, it allows muscles to relax in a deeper stretch, leading to more penetrating blood flow. From a rehabilitative standpoint, heat also induces a temporary analgesic effect. This allows people with chronic pain to exercise—often for the first time in years—the areas of their body that cause them pain. Which in turn, allows them to strengthen atrophied muscles whose atrophy is often directly related to their chronic pain in the first place. It stops a vicious convalescent cycle.

As an engineer, Chad can deliver heat any way an owner wants it: dry,

---

[5] Reference points from my own practice: During the most strenuous postures, my heart rate rises to 90 to 95 percent of maximum heart rate (around 175 beats per minute). Just as with the much newer exercise fad/phenom of high-intensity interval training, maximum effort is sustained for brief periods (ten seconds to one minute, depending on the specific posture) and then completely released for an equivalent period of rest. My average heart rate for the ninety-minute class is roughly 60 to 70 percent maximum heart rate (130 bpm): or exactly in the sweet spot known as "Fat Burn" on elliptical machines across America. It is important to note that doing the exact same series of postures without external heat produces, for me, an average heart rate of only 45 to 50 percent and spikes that reach 65 to 70 percent, thus significantly reducing the cardiac benefits and eliminating the benefits of high-intensity training.

humid, filtered, oxygenated, static, or with flow. Depending on those variables, exercise in heat can feel extremely different while offering similar therapeutic benefits. For instance, the decision to recycle warm air or pump in fresh (oxygen-rich) air from the outside will have a large impact on the practitioners' comfort but almost no difference on the degree to which their blood vessels expand. Chad's insistence on building studios that pipe in fresh air is one reason I hear of practitioners detouring to his studios.

But when I ask him to explain how the heat is actually delivered in most studios, there is little complexity in his response. "Most of the yoga studios I work for, they just want the room as hot as possible—period. Half of them get to me in the first place because they've destroyed their system by pushing it past capacity or by trying to circumvent an automatic shutoff.

"Everyone will say they use the heat for therapy," he says. "Which, of course, is true to an extent. But I know the engineering and I know the personalities. You don't need it to be 110 degrees for blood vessels to expand or to get a cardiac benefit." Vasodilation is a reflex reaction, not a progressive effect that continues the hotter it gets. Similarly the analgesic effect occurs with ambient temperatures well below the debilitating. "Heat makes things hard. Point-blank. Studio owners want to use the heat to push people."

Referring to one of Bikram's most senior teachers, he says, "Jim Kallet wants his regulars on their knees. That's a direct quote. . . . It's a special type of madness. But of course, once you get sucked into that world, it's all madness."

That world?

"The world near Bikram . . . Once he discovered me, Bikram wanted me to do everything. I was his 'superintendent' at his Los Angeles studios. I drove him around like a personal valet. I used to carry this crazy wallet for him that was stuffed with cash. I would come out and do personal repairs at his house."

Chad flashes me his goofy grin and slams the rest of his beer. "Let me promise you one thing. You have never been in a place with more mirrors.

You absolutely have to see it to believe it. His house is a satire. Red leather sofas, white leather sofas, these huge dripping chandeliers in every fucking room. . . ."

I ask him what type of work he did there, but Chad stays put for a moment.

"I mean can you imagine the mind that lives there? Gold. Fake gold. Platinum. Giant stone tables. Insane thrones scattered around. And everywhere, everywhere mirrors."

Lost in the Present Moment

I arrive for the first day of Backbending a little after midnight.

Driving up to David's house, I say a silent prayer for my phone's GPS. David lives in one of those vaguely jingoistic, embarrassingly American gated communities—literally just off Rifle Range Road, down the block from Boston Grill Road—complete with a series of identical dark green lagoons, endless cul-de-sacs, and motion sensor lights that tick on, house after house, if you are one of the few who walks rather than drives past them. It is a neighborhood for the newly but truly rich. You can actually smell the homeowner restrictions in the form of the bagged grass clippings tied up neatly on the front right corner of everyone's identical white cement driveway.

It's obvious when I roll up to David's address. His eight-car garage is wide open and overflowing with cars, yellow light spilling on the street.

The rest of the house looks quiet, however. I decide it's too late to ring the doorbell politely. I didn't call, and at this hour, David may or may not be expecting me. Instead I knock meekly a few times. I curse my small bladder. I curse my many rest stops. I knock again; I jiggle the handle. I Google a hotel on my phone. I jiggle the handle again.

And with a classic horror-movie groan, it swings open.

Peering in, backpack on my shoulder, I find every light on, but nobody around. The floor is littered with Whole Foods bags and bedding materials.

In the background, I can hear gunfire from a TV. A lone head of broccoli lies on the floor, ready to roll through the scene like tumbleweed.

As I step inside and clear my throat, looking for someone to greet, a leggy woman chewing on a rib of celery bounds downstairs in her boxers.

"Hey!" she says smiling, before zooming past me.

"Hey," I say to myself and slip off my shoes.

As I plunge deeper into the house, the wreckage only grows. Water bottles stuffed with cut limes line bookshelves with no books. Drying sports bras and athletic pants drape over door handles. A coffee table is littered with value-sized bottles of electrolyte replacements. Everywhere clothes, bedding, and salad greens.

By the living room, I have found the yogis. I introduce myself, asking for David, our host, or Esak, the organizer. It is quickly apparent that nobody knows anything. The yogis, about twenty or so, are milling, typing on laptops, chatting about studios, exuding the same vulnerable feeling of freshman orientation. Which makes me feel a lot better. Esak hasn't arrived yet, and as I make my way around the house, everyone tells me, "David's around," but nobody seems to particularly care where.

When I find him, now close to 1 A.M., David is making an avocado sandwich in the kitchen. He is tanned and trimmed and bearing a bright white band of teeth that wouldn't look out of place on daytime TV. We shake hands, and I thank him profusely for giving up his house for the next two weeks. He looks slightly surprised by this expression of gratitude, like no one would think twice about letting a small community of complete strangers camp in their living room. Then he whips out a bottle of spray butter and dusts it over his avocado. So maybe David and I approach the world differently on multiple levels.

When I ask him about sleeping arrangements, he looks surprised again.

"Anywhere! Just poke around. I think most of the good spots have been taken. Maybe some carpeted floor upstairs."

I scrounge and make introductions. By 2 A.M., I am spread out in a sleeping bag on a small uncarpeted section of the main hallway. I fall asleep with the lights on, giggling conversation down the hall still constant.

. . .

I wake up the next morning before my alarm goes off. Approximately twenty-five times. First there are the feet stepping over me. Then there are the coffee grinders being used to puree various nuts, spices, and supplements. Then the collisions at the bathroom—the frantic result of a house filled with individuals hell-bent on maximizing their hydration—the eruptions of the teakettle, the laughter, and the crotchety grumblings of freakishly athletic yogis complaining about their sore backs.

Somehow, however, by the time I actually scrape myself off the floor, the house is empty.

The wreckage from last night has been pulled into little pods. What once looked like a weird vegan tent city has been raked into order. Bedding materials are neatly folded, backpacks bulging but zipped, and those loose rolling veggies lassoed together and placed into their appropriate Whole Foods bags.

I triple-check my watch to make sure I'm not late. We still have an hour to get to a yoga studio located about five minutes away. But perhaps the schedule changed. I still haven't seen Esak. Regardless, I decide I need food, and so closing the front door behind me with no way of locking it, I pick up a protein shake from a gas station and head to the studio.

At 10 A.M., we take our first class of the day. From that point on, we never really stop practicing for the next two weeks. The delirium of a single class becomes compounded by repetition until the entire experience expands into one long waking dream.

I learn that puking can feel euphoric when I disgorge the protein shake into the studio toilet around noon.

I learn a tiny blond woman covered in upbeat cheerful tattoos—a tiny rainbow, the outline of a star—can effortlessly balance her entire weight on one arm.

I learn that Esak goes into full-body convulsions on occasion when he backbends. And that Kara, a financier from Chicago, goes into full-body convulsions *every time* she attempts her first backbend of the day.

I learn that the only reason either of them care about those seizures is that they can be slightly embarrassing and off-putting to strangers.

I listen when Brett, a lanky yoga instructor from Kansas, declares he doesn't have the strength to eat the single thumb-sized nub of carrot he is holding. I learn he is being sincere when he drops the carrot and curls into the ground to go to sleep.

I learn the phrase "the beatings will continue until morale improves" has a completely nonsarcastic application.

I learn that even Esak can be unenthusiastic about training. But even more quickly I learn that it marks a difference between us. Where I start excited but grow tired from our endless sets, his energy increases the more we do. After a vicious set of lunges, promised as our last before lunch, I catch him looking around eagerly, desperate to squeeze something more in.

I learn that the face of someone crying is completely indistinguishable from the customary ruddy agony produced by backbending, but that the refusal to pause or make eye contact is a dead giveaway.

I learn that sometimes when given a forty-minute break, the smartest thing to do is just to lie still in your own sweat the entire time.

When it is over, after approximately fourteen hours of yoga-related activity, I find myself at a late-night supermarket. It is just before 1 A.M. My body feels limp and slightly beaten. My brain feels something like pavement right after a rainstorm. Thinking about repeating the process tomorrow is un-imaginable, so I make a rule that I won't. The trip to the supermarket is a necessity after the white protein shake I expelled earlier; and when I an-nounced my intention, a number of other Backbenders enthusiastically jumped in my car at the opportunity.

As the rest of the group disperses into the empty grocery store, I sit down on the floor in the front, my back eased against a stacked display of beer. There is only one register open at this time of night, and the sad-looking man at the far end of the conveyor belt doesn't even glance at us. I am sure we look utterly banal. But the abundance of food, color, and cold air feels overwhelming and dreamlike to me. I sit for I don't know how long, taking it in. Eventually, Lauren, the weeper, bounces over to me, giddy. She is carrying a two-liter of seltzer water, a giant jug of no-sugar-added grapefruit juice, and a single Styrofoam cup. She announces they are ingredients for a magic potion that will get her through the week. Then she sits down next to me and proceeds to mix them in equal parts.

Moments later, Brett walks over with an ice cream sandwich and offers me a bite. I want to cry with gratitude. Not for the ice cream, which I somewhat insanely decline, opting instead for raw bok choy, but because I feel an overwhelming biological sensation of brotherhood. A similar emotion pours out triplefold when Fiona, from Ireland, skips down the aisle holding a can of Coke. She is agonizing over whether or not to buy it.

"Esak would killlll me if he found out," she says, and then laughs and laughs at her own completely unfunny non-joke. "Wouldn't he? He would killlll me."

I have no idea what Esak would think, but I am feeling so good and so bad at the same time that it occurs to me his judgment couldn't possibly matter. It's so much less complicated, so much less interesting. In fact, surrounded by a woman guzzling grapefruit juice so recklessly the front of her shirt has become a dark bib from the overflow, a grown man eating a contraband piece of ice cream, and can of Coke that is causing existential breakdown-style laughter in a woman who flew halfway across the world for the experience, the moment on the grocery-store floor begins to feel so distended and out of place from my normal existence, I decide that I must be having one last hallucination of the day.

Change Your Mind

Hallucinations are not a trivial part of Backbending. As a purely physical exercise, wall-walking is worthy of inclusion in any fitness routine. I arrived at Backbending both scrawny and muscular, with the oversized thighs and undersized chest that I am beginning to recognize as a body by Bikram. After just a few days of wall-walking however, I can already see new musculature rising up against my skin, almost like lost continents surfacing from the ocean. But the physical aspect of wall-walking is not where the real effort lies. Backbending is training for the mind: both the deep primitive areas governing pain and the more socially important limbic channels responsible for emotions and fear. Hallucinations, waves of tears, anger, and pulsing headaches are just a few of the many releases that occur as you work.

Esak instills this idea in us on the second day. After a class, he pulls us into a circle. "The first rule about Backbending is we don't talk about Backbending. It's just like Fight Club. If someone asks, tell them you went away to train for competition. If they ask what you did, tell them to come and find out. Backbending can't really be told. People need to come and experience it for themselves." He pauses. "The second rule is we have to stop calling this Backbending Club. It gives people completely the wrong idea."

The reason it gives people the wrong idea is the words do not do justice to the experience. Backbending is awesome. Not awesome in the teenage sense of the word, awesome in the literal sense: It echoes with grandeur. Your chest blows out, your heart floods with blood, and your brain vibrates. Every human has a half-inch-thick cord of nerves running down the center of his or her vertebrae. These nerves extend down from the brain stem along the entire length of the spine until finally billowing out to the rest of the body. When you radically bend the spine, building and flexing the muscles that line and guide the vertebrae, those nerves are being toyed with: physically moved, rubbed, tweaked, and teased.

The red and blue spots, the wavy rippling room, the uncontrollable weeping, and the occasional seizure are phenomena that result from this manipulation. Backbenders call it Third-Eye Blowout. It's neither desirable nor to be avoided. It just happens. I've wall-walked until time slowed down, until I've heard a deep roaring white noise all around me, until I've felt heat shoot through my arms like I was an X-Man. I've heard other stories of backbending blackouts, of practitioners seeing blue sparks shoot from their fingers, and of full-blown narrative-length hallucinations. To be sure, far more often, I've felt nothing, broken a mild sweat, and called it a day.

If you've never done an extreme backbend, you'll have to take these reactions on faith. But they're real—repeatable, predictable, and remarkably consistent between practitioners. If you'd like to try, by all means find the nearest wall. Every back can bend in this manner. Maybe not so deep at first, but whether you're five or fifty-five, former athlete or former invalid, your vertebral column is more than equipped for both forward and backward bending. It is part of a human's natural range of motion. No bones chip off, no tendons snap. I've seen people with rods in their spine backbend. You can actually see the metal poking up against the skin.

But there is a reason why people from five to fifty-five avoid backbends. They hurt. If you backbend sincerely—peeling yourself into an arch that is just beyond your comfort zone—you will feel pain. And if you do it repeatedly, the pain will grow: hot, unambiguous, and very, very insistent.

Most people stop at the first whisper of the pain. Actually, most people stop at the prewhisper, at some instinctual trigger point ten miles before the sensation has even walked over the horizon. That is their practice: satisfied just to be bending something, oblivious to the pain beyond. On the rare day they get to the whisper, they typically back off, rub their back a lot in the locker room, and talk about pushing their edge. And that's sensible. But that's not Backbending Club. To really backbend, you have to become intimate with pain, not as an informational entity that raises awareness, not as a warning, but as a phenomenon, a presence you can dialogue with. You have to engage the phenomenon every time it comes up, and ultimately move through it while it screams in your face.

To put this in perspective, before I had ever heard of yoga competitions or Backbending Club, but while I was still quite serious about yoga practice, I used to do exactly three wall-walks a week. These came every Tuesday during the advanced class offered at my home studio. And those three were a feared highlight of the whole three-hour class. Actually, I feared them all week. The minute and a half it took to complete them would grow all out of proportion in my mind. Often, I would stall out in class just before we got to them, lie on my side, watching other people move on toward them. Other times, I would complete one, then lie down dizzy and decide that this week, I'd save my energy for the postures that came later. One wall-walk was enough.

At Backbending, we never do fewer than sixty a day. Learning to manage, breathe through, and control the sensations that come up is an essential part of the work. It is a combination of managing fear, managing pain, and detaching from sensory perception. As Esak explains: "When you do a posture, you must choose to remain in it. You must choose to ignore the pain, choose to continue to explore your body. The pain is a phantom; ignoring it is a choice. Yoga makes us confront that choice. It makes us free to choose."

The ultimate extension of this training in choice is learning to control your imagination. At their most extreme, backbends look bizarre, completely improbable. People stare at them with the same weirded curiosity usually reserved for the edges of the animal kingdom: puffed-out marine creatures, the yawning dislocated jaws of snakes. It's not that backbends are ugly exactly—they're just anti-human. Staring at a reversible spine is a double-take moment, an instance where the eyes legitimately can't believe what they see.

To inhabit these postures requires changing your belief system. A middle-aged man walks into a yoga studio convinced he can never touch his toes again. To transform himself into the asana of Standing Bow—a posture where in ultimate extension, he is not just touching his toes, but fully in the standing splits, one arm stretching forward like an arrow, the other stretching upward to grab his extended foot—he must learn to do the impossible. He must enlarge the boundaries of his imagination. He must know that at fifty-one, body banged up by age, brain occluded by expectations, he can choose to embody Standing Bow. The postures are both a metaphor and a means for that process. They are tools for creating a connection between the imagination and the physical world. Realizing this connection—this union between body and mind—could be called yoga.

Of course, it also could not.

If you were raised like me, yoga probably conjures up a healthy set of associations: the YMCA; leggings; practitioners with a little paunch; gurus with visible ribs; closed eyes; crossed legs—a big, calm, relaxing pretzel. If you have a little more experience than I ever had, maybe it also conjures up ideas of nonattachment, nonjudgment, Himalayan caves, internal heat, and righteous breathing. And if you've actually picked up some texts and studied, maybe you can recite some dos and don'ts, point to the appropriate glands that correspond to the various chakras, and explain to bored, trapped people at cocktail parties why what the people in leggings at the YMCA do is just one small piece of the big yoga pie.

All of which is why I'm sure there are plenty of people reading my description of Backbending and yoga champions with a steadily escalating sense of outrage. Outrage like: What is going on here? What type of insane corruption am I reading about? Doesn't this asshole know pain has nothing to do with real yoga! And as much as I empathize with those reactions, their outrage will always be misplaced. Yoga is simply one of those things impervious to certainty, as incapable of corruption as it is of authenticity. And no amount of bossy, possessive attempts to claim a "real yoga" will make it otherwise.

Imagine for a moment if a group of people decided to fetishize the English word *craft*. As in:

"I practice craft."

"I'm a crafter."

"Oh, macramé—that is totally an invention of the 1950s. I mean, *sure,* it feels good, but honestly, plastic has no part in craft."

"I only Bead and Weave, because those represent the true spirit of craft."

"Macaroni Art? Farce! How could you have Macaroni Art before Arturo Boolini invented the mechanized pasta press in 1853? Which he did, by the way, *in Chicago.* Talk about cultural fusion, or should I say *confusion.*"

You would not like those people very much. An abstract noun like *craft* has no single pure meaning. And these craft-fascists would be profoundly unhelpful if you had a genuine interest in actually learning something. Figuring out the most authentic form of craft wouldn't let you know where the most aesthetically pleasing crafts came from, and it wouldn't tell you which crafting discipline would be the most personally fulfilling. Moreover, crafting techniques that were used one thousand years ago would be valuable only if they were still relevant today. Who wants to weave baskets out of grass in a world where nobody really uses baskets anymore?

In his book *Yoga in Modern India*, Joseph Alter makes a similar point by pulling out the Webster's of India: *Bhargava's Standard Illustrated Dictionary:*

> *Yoga:* n. mas. *One of the six schools of Hindu philosophy, a union with the Universal Soul by means of contemplation, means of salvation, the 27th part of a circle, a sum, a total, profound meditation to earn and enhance wealth, unity, conjunction, union, combination, mixture, contact, fitness, property, an auspicious moment, a plan, device, recipe, connection, love, trick, deception, as a suffix used in the sense of "capable, fit for."*

If read with our YMCA expectations, this definition makes no sense. I mean, "a union with the Universal Soul" sounds familiar, but "a profound meditation to earn and enhance wealth" sounds like irony. *A property? A recipe? A trick?* Are you kidding?

If there is a joke, it's on us. Yoga is a vast history: it can be contemplation; it can also be a postejaculatory man attempting to suck his semen back up his penis like a straw.[6] It can be sticky mats and creepy Muzak-laced trance music; or it can be an extended fifth-grade fantasy to acquire magic powers and evade mortality. (The third book of Pantajali's *Yoga Sutras* is entirely devoted to detailing the magic powers or *siddhis* available to an adept.) It is big tent, and the only thing for certain is the more certain someone gets about yoga, the wronger it goes.

Given this multiplicity of meaning, and in order to put the modern

---

[6] This penile-straw being *vajroli mudra*. A practice that the bible of hatha yoga, the *Hatha Yoga Pradipika*, introduces by explaining, "the yogi who knows *vajroli mudra* attains success in yoga even if he acts without following any other injunctions laid down in this text." An emphasis that makes *vajroli mudra* seem far more important than, say, assuming postures or practicing breathing exercises. In *vajroli mudra*, "the fluid poured from the pelvic region should be raised by practice . . . saved by exerting an upward pull." Lest anyone be confused about what is being suggested, the text continues suggesting that a tube be inserted into the urethra to widen the hole and help the yogi acquire appropriate skill. Most modern translations of the *Pradipika* either omit those verses entirely or fail to translate them, claiming they are uninteresting to the modern practitioner.

yoga experience in context, it is helpful to go back to first principles and look at the intellectual cauldron where yogic ideas first evolved.

Yoga, the word, first bounced off the tongues of nomads on the wagon trail. The Sanskrit verb *yuj,* from which our noun *yoga* derives, refers to the act of hitching or joining "a wheeled conveyance to a draft animal," analogous in sound and meaning to English word *yoke.* Yoga, in this practical sense, was integral to their civilization. These proto-Sanskrit speakers were in the midst of a several-century migration down from Russia, navigating their oxen-drawn carts over the foothills of the Himalayas into the Indian sub-continent. Most of what we know about them comes from their early religious texts, the Vedas. The earliest of these, the Rig Veda (circa 1500 B.C.E.), depicts a yoga largely practiced by warriors either prior to charging off into battle (as they hitched up horses to their chariots), or more metaphorically, at death (when driving the horses on a holy chariot "upward through the barrier of the sun").

This emphasis on the practical yoke behind our esoteric yoga is not to belittle it. The ability to control a horse, an animal then only a few generations away from wild, was a radical technological advance. To practice yoga was an act that invoked the snort and bristle of breaking an animal, as well as dominance over a powerful other. When the wagoneering proto-Sanskrit invaders rolled into the Indus Valley, they confronted a civilization more advanced than anything they had encountered before. The people of the Indus Valley were urbanites: They lived in dense cities; they appreciated sculpture; they cleaned themselves using an aquaduct-driven bathing system of a sophistication that wouldn't resurface until the Romans. But they had no horses, they had no chariots, and they had no agricultural draft. And thus as the proto-yogi, master of his vehicle, lord of his chariot, rolled into town, it was with reverence, terror, and respect that they greeted his arrival.

In the same way the neuroscientific sages of our day draw on the language of the computer to describe their findings, the ancient philosophers borrowed from the radical new technology of their day, the yoke and chariot. The *yuj/yoga/yoke* conglomeration appears often in their writings in a wide variety of allusions: the connection between words in a couplet, the link between a visionary thinker and his vision, a union at death with the divine. At the same time these images were creeping into scripture, the merger between the Sanskrit and Indus Valley civilizations initiated a metaphysical renaissance. The primordial verses of the Vedas were reinterpreted, their stories translated into teachings or Upanishads that began to systematically address the major stargazing themes that make up man's quest for knowledge. The limits of the universe. The nature of perception. The origins of life. And most obsessively, the fabric of ultimate reality.

While contemplative meditative states have probably been around as long as humans have been taking idle walks, the Upanishads began detailing techniques for inducing and cultivating this awareness. When practiced, these techniques—such as breath control, appetite control, and sustained focus on objects, ideas, and vibratory sounds—allowed a person to strengthen control of their mind, in ambition, not unlike the crossword puzzling of today's seniors. The Upanishadic philosophers believed that acquiring a heightened mental focus was a necessary first step to accurately contemplating the larger questions of existence.

Exactly how and when these practices became linked with a system of thought called yoga is currently the subject of tens of thousands of pages of academic debate. I wouldn't dare delve into it even I could. It is the stuff that instantly slams me into the meditative state of a nap. However, what pretty much everyone can agree upon is that over the course of approximately one thousand years—from, say, 1500 to 500 B.C.E.—these philosophic ideas evolved while the imagery coalesced. Until, finally, during a discussion on the possibility of immortality, a text known as the *Katha Upanishad* bursts forth with the first mention of yoga as a spiritual discipline.

In the *Katha Upanishad,* a young boy asks the Lord of Death, Yama, the type of innocent question that only young boys can ask Lords of Death:

What happens to people when they die? Instead of answering directly, the god decides that in order to reveal the secrets of immortality, he must first instruct the boy in the practice of something called Yoga.

To impart this knowledge, the Lord of Death relates the following metaphor:

Know thy Self as the lord of the chariot
The body as the chariot.
Know the intellect as the chariot-driver
And the mind as the reins.

The senses of perception are the unruly horses
The objects of sense, the terrain they range over

He who has understanding
Whose mind is constantly held firm
His senses under-control
Like the good horses of a chariot-driver (KU 3:3–6)

This they consider Yoga
The firm holding back of the senses (KU 6:11)

And there, looking suspiciously like an LSAT question is the essential yogic metaphor, containing the first principles needed to undertake the spiritual discipline. Mind, body, sensory perception are all aspects of the self—represented here as the chariot driver, chariot, and unruly horses. A person who can control their sensory perception, who is not misled by its illusions, by its false demands, by its nagging aches and possessive jealousies—is unified. Such a person has control over not only their own body, but also how they interact with the worldly sense-objects they come into contact with.

The yoga in this metaphor uses stillness and control to examine sensory inputs and the motor outputs. Practitioners learn to observe sensations, detach from them, and choose instead to yoke their awareness to themselves as a whole or the universe beyond.[7] To practice yoga is to cultivate that connection.

Yama proceeds to elaborate on this metaphor over the sixty-three verses that follow its introduction. However, it is only with his final instruction to the youth that the god ties this knowledge together, explaining its link to immortality and putting a purpose to the techniques described above. In this final instruction, he reveals perhaps the single greatest spiritual insight of Upanshadic thought: the fruit of yoga and promise of successful practice.

Speaking to the youth, Yama explains this insight thus:

> *There is a Self within the self*
> *Eternally ensconced in the hearts of every living creature.*
> *One should, with one's intelligence, strip him out of one's body*
> *One should know him as the shining, pure immortal one. (KU 6:17)*

Yama is suggesting that beyond our reflexive understanding of identity, there lurks within us an authentic self, a self within the self. By using our intelligence and mental control, we can strip out and identify this authentic self. And when we do, we will know him—we will know ourselves—as nothing more and nothing less than gods: immortal, pure, infinite, and connected to all beings.

There is something resonant about the idea of turning inward for salvation. As ethnographer Mircea Eliade points out, this concept of transcendence is the exact opposite of the Christian concept of ecstasy, which from the Greek root *ex-* means "to go outward." Instead, yoga postulates an "instasy," a journey into ourselves, whereby we discover and come to fully realize that we are made of the same material that pervades all existence: call it atoms, quanta, strings, or spirit. Once we identify ourselves in this fundamental manner, we become connected to the entire universe—not unlike

---

[7] Or in specific application to postural yoga, Esak would say, "We use the posture as a playground to explore the fundamental unity of our body and mind. The body becomes a medium to learn how to control the mind."

the individual unique drops of water creating and subsumed within a vast ocean. Separate and yet inseparable; fragile yet impossible to destroy. It is a vision that is simultaneously mystic and purely materialistic, open to dreamer and cynic alike.

In this sense, yoga is a case of mistaken identity, the story of a cognitive error. By identifying ourselves with something that inadequately describes us (our body, our brain, our sensory perceptions) we are prevented from seeing what we actually are (the indestructible matter/energy that makes up the universe). The techniques, the tools of yoga, are simply the somewhat strenuous activities taken to correct this misapprehension. At heart, this is a yoga of recognition: If consciousness, creativity, memory, emotion are properties that arise from the periodic building blocks of the universe, then there is, at the very least, a possibility that the universe as a whole is animated with those same qualities. We are energy surrounded by energy. Realizing that union—on a primary, experiential, and nonintellectual level—is what I call the practice of yoga.

The difficulty with the *Katha Upanishad* and almost all other ancient references to yoga is that while rich in purpose and allusion, they are impoverished in detail. The *Katha* does a good job of explaining what this yoga-tool is capable of, as well as the basic mechanisms it operates with, but it gives almost no help in implementation. As with any tool, a how-to guide is critical. Understanding the endpoint of yoga in the *Katha Upanishad* isn't going to help you arrive there any more than reading a description of a cowboy riding on the trail will teach you how to throw a saddle over a horse, shove a bit in its mouth, and break it under your control.

The absence of this guidebook—the most important step from a practitioner's standpoint—is where we enter obscurity. It is where a thousand gurus bloom. It is why for all its promises of authenticity, yoga will never have certainty.

In an early attempt to clarify this tangle, Patanjali, a sage of the second century—alternately identified as a grammarian or thousand-headed ruler of the serpent race—took it upon himself to organize the many disparate yoga schools of his day into a cohesive system. Anticipating his placement on the self-help shelf of today, and inspired by the Buddha's EightFold Path, Patanjali compiled a step-by-step guide to liberation: an eight-limbed—or Ashtanga—yoga system.

Patanjali organized yoga practices into a stepladder, with each of the eight limbs built atop the proceeding one so that a practitioner could start at the basics and ascend to the heights promised by the *Katha Upanishad*. Beginning with simple and fundamental ethical prescriptions, not unlike the Ten Commandments, Patanjali instructed his yogis to master progressively more difficult techniques: first for sitting in contemplation, then for linking breath to contemplation, then on withdrawing the senses, then on focusing the senses, and finally, the ultimate step, samadhi, yoking to the divine. It is a gentle stepladder, largely focused on contemplation and internal meditation.

Approximately one thousand years later, a wholly different yoga emerges from the jungle. This yoga, hatha yoga, translated literally as "the yoga of violence or force," arose in dialectal response to Patanjali's abstract approach. Like all great revival movements, hatha emphasized personal experience in the place of formal doctrine. It literalized concepts like transcendence and union, applying them directly to physiological responses in the human body. This new approach was the work of the Naths, a split-eared sect of Shiva-worshipping yogis driven into northern jungles of India by waves of Muslim migrations. Drawing on Buddhism, Tantrism, indigenous alchemy, and an obsession with physical health demanded by their wet, pestilent home, the Naths created hatha: a yoga to align with the great tantra proverb: "One cannot venerate a god unless one is a god oneself."

In hatha, yoking to the universal is a by-product of proper physiological alignment, the body fined-tuned like an old-fashioned antenna to get a clearer broadcast signal. By removing impurities, strengthening the physical core, and controlling the literal gateway to spirit that is breath, the hatha body is perfected into a sort of divine lightning rod: a *vajra deha* or diamond body, an awakened channel for conducting the universe's energies.

The violence of the Violent Yoga comes primarily from the method used to achieve these results: the forceful fusing of opposites. It's an ideal embodied in the Sanskrit name *Ha-Tha* (where *Ha* stands for the solar, masculine energies and *Tha* for the lunar, feminine forces) and reiterated throughout all hatha practice; but it is perhaps best appreciated by the Naths' principal innovation: postures or bending the body into forms.

Prior to the medieval rise of hatha yoga, standing contortive postures simply did not exist in yoga. The word *asana* was present, however it was used almost exclusively in the etymological sense, as "seat" or "throne." The asana practices described in pre-hatha yogic literature were meditative postures: firm and stable positions, thrones from which to contemplate existence.

In hatha, asanas serve an entirely different purpose. The body is used as a stage: held in stillness while internally exploding with exertion; limbs stretched while muscles are contracted; tension explored until its duality resolved. Vyasa the sage says that perfection of posture occurs "when effort disappears . . . when the mind is transformed into infinity." Mircea Eliade the ethnographer says, "refusal to move, to let one be carried along in the rushing stream of states of consciousness . . . is to abolish (or to transcend) the human condition by refusal to conform to the most elementary human inclination."[8] Holding an asana embodies the chaos of existence framed within the stability of the universal.

If yoga is a science, then the hatha yogis of the jungle were its madmen, hair forever frizzled, face smeared with ritual ash, wide-eyed and forever ready to the throw the Frankensteinian switch. Their early texts alternate between being refreshing and frightening in their vulgar specificity: nasal passages are cleaned with water (neti!), water is sucked in through the anus in self-enema (basti!), the rectum and intestines are pushed out and washed by hand in water (bahiskrita dhauti!?). Coordinate with the Vedic belief that all perception is illusion, in hatha the natural world is present to be subverted. However, unlike the comforting liberation promised in the ancient texts, hatha techniques read like a string of cocky Faustian bargains. Each practice comes equipped with a long string of impossibly oversold

---

[8] Mary Jarvis, Esak's coach and mentor, says, "Maintaining stillness in the struggle of a posture is a route into the present moment."

benefits: Drinking the middle third of your urine stream will, for instance, destroy diseases of the eyes, grant you clairvoyance, purify the blood, and give insight into the divine.[9]

This simultaneous propensity toward magic, sex, and the vulgarities of the human body did not make the hatha yogis particularly popular. Within India, their claims were greeted with skepticism, their personal habits, disgust, even as their knowledge of the human condition afforded respect. They lived on the peripheries of society in dung-smeared huts. They proved their transcendence through bizarre austerities (remaining chained to a single spot of ground for days) and masochistic feats of strength (a bed of sharp nails for the back). They were often called in to help barren women conceive and cure ailing children. In fables, hatha yogis are portrayed as powerful but potentially evil meddlers, resources of last resort, analogous to the witches and sorcerers found in Western fairy tales.

With the arrival of the Colonial British, the Naths became outlawed people—in the grand shameful tradition of indigenous groups who are not easily assimilated. Labeled as "Miscellaneous and Disreputable Vagrants," their traditional costume and outfits were banned. This shift into persecution drove many hatha yogis into petty crime and street performance. Once-sacred demonstrations of divine power became fixtures of the carnival, the desperate schemes of the beggar.

When yoga jumped to America, its different traditions were packaged together for export, presented to eager audiences as a cohesive whole. The first great yogic ambassadors were practical-minded reformers: intellectuals eager to modernize Hinduism by infusing it with enlightenment thought and Christian imagery, fund-raisers looking to use Western money to help India's poorest. Hatha, with its vulgar preoccupation with the body, its culture of superstition, and its associations with the street, served none of their purposes. Instead its "queer breathing exercises" and "gymnastics" were neatly

---

[9] This being *amaroli,* another gem left untranslated in many modern versions of the *Pradapika.* Modern practitioners tell me the urine is "an acquired taste, like beer."

snipped off and grafted onto Patanjali's third and forth limb, presented as a subsidiary of that rather more ancient, more cerebral, and more Christ-friendly tradition.

This unnatural grafting has resulted in an odd sort of legacy. For the most part, the false grafting did not take. But instead of wilting away, posture has flourished in isolation: devoid of connection with its historical background, subject to incredible but hidden innovation. Hence the truly secular America yogacizing gym class, ripe with asanas that didn't exist one hundred, much less one thousand, years ago. To fill this void, the postures connected with exercise and therapy, with the Human Potential Movement and nutritional claims, with altruism and vacation getaways—each providing new American soil for the snipped appendages of hatha to root.

And when the medieval spirit of hatha does seep through and assert itself, which of course it does now and then, everyone gets a little weirded out and wonders how this inauthentic, almost martial, more magical than mystical, explicitly narcissistic crap got associated with their "real yoga."

To a practitioner, all this uncertainty can feel really uncomfortable. When I first started practicing, I got tremendous satisfaction from the fact that the postures I was doing were thousands of years old. Not only is there something innately cool about heritage and tradition, but on a purely physical level, it helped. I was confident: Of course the postures wouldn't hurt me—all the kinks had been ironed out centuries ago. What was being transmitted to me by my lovely bouncy teacher in her leotard was clarified, reified, time tested, and approved by an unending succession of gurus (all wizened, bearded, and scrawny with dancing eyes) stretching back to the time when sages sat lonely in caves.

But in reality, yoga just ain't that type of enterprise. It is ten thousand rain droplets rather than one holy spring. The yogic literature is too vast, too muddled, and ultimately too limited by the fact that it is only literature in a tradition that has passed its most vital secrets orally. The postures are being innovated. The ideas reorganized, reinterpreted, and reimagined. And there is a long, hearty history where lone individuals have appointed themselves all-knowing gurus and deliberately twisted facts to their own satisfaction and cosmology. So throw your ideas of authenticity out the window, and when I bring up practices like the competition, backbending, and hallucinations, try to do something yogic (wink) for a change: Let people claim yoga as they always will, but this time, detach, observe, and make no judgments.

Portrait of a Guru as a Young Man

For Esak, detaching and observing came through competition. Hoisting a trophy didn't hurt either.

"Yoga is union," he says. "It is resolving duality, realizing the oneness we are a part of. You don't need to push yourself to extreme depths to realize that. . . . I would never tell anyone that backbending or competition are necessary. I would never even recommend it to them if they weren't already interested, but for me, they acted like a switch.

"It makes some people in the yoga community incredibly angry, but for me, competing, preparing to compete gave me an excuse to practice all day long. . . . And the extremity opened me. It deepened my practice; it changed my understanding.

"Even if I wished it away, never competed again, it's part of me right now. It's part of who I am. Which means it's part of my yoga. Maybe someday I'll move past it, maybe someday the whole community will move past it, but until then, competition only reflects what is already part of us."

Given his pedigree, competition was an unexpected route to self-realization. Esak was practically born in posture. When his mother was twenty, she ran away from her childhood in Milwaukee to follow a Sufi mystic. A yoga class followed, and unlike the mysticism, it stuck. She continued practicing through her pregnancy. There is a lovely picture of her in a headstand with an embryonic Esak in her belly. When he was born, she began teaching at local health clubs, eventually holding classes in their home.

"But growing up, I never thought about it," Esak says. "My mother never invited me to a class, never pressured me once. It didn't enter my life."

Instead he gravitated to American sports, especially football and baseball. The first time he heard the term *enlightenment* was from a girlfriend whose parents were Buddhist. When he describes high school, it hits the wholesome trinity of varsity athletics, studious academics, and weekend beers. Never yoga.

When he was seventeen, that changed. His mother met Bikram at a seminar and was smitten. Very soon after, she flew off to attend Bikram's teacher training in Los Angeles. For the first time, she pushed her son to join her. It was Bikram's first training, tiny and intimate. "She was very insistent—she knew it would be powerful and really wanted to involve me." Esak flew out during his spring break and took classes with the trainees. His mother made a point of introducing him to Bikram.

He loved it and reveled in the ways it would improve his baseball.

At Yale, the yoga became a refuge but never the main attraction. "Freshman year, I had a dorm with an incredibly hot furnace, and I had a tape of Bikram teaching a class." When he got stressed, Esak would slide the cassette tape into the machine, punch the buttons, and bend. It was an escape. "I wasn't even thinking about yoga as yoga," he says. "It just helped keep me balanced. I'd be sitting in a cubby studying all day and needed it to stretch out." His roommates were fascinated, and when his mother visited, she organized a class in the basement.

But those moments weren't the norm. The academic environment of New Haven left him disenchanted. "I was working incredibly hard, on one level very successfully, but I didn't see where the work would take me," he says. "My peers were either going into academia, law, politics, and I didn't connect with that."

In response, he began sneaking off four nights a week to a local capoeira studio. The martial art spoke to him. Soon he had convinced the political philosophy department to give him a fellowship to travel to Brazil. He stayed for three years. The yoga came with him, but still as a sideshow. "People were getting injured all the time, everyone was curious, so I taught informally. The yoga had its place, but in Brazil it was always secondary to capoeira."

When he returned, yoga began taking on a progressively larger role in his life. In 2001, he went to teacher training a second time, spending the full nine weeks immersed with Bikram. By 2002, he was making a living teaching in the San Francisco Bay area.

In 2003, he decided to compete. And almost immediately the switch was thrown.

"It is difficult to describe. I came from a capoeira background, which is very much about ritual and celebratory energy. Yoga is different. It is internal. . . . I can tell you that externally my body changed dramatically. Capoeira requires a lot more bulk, and aesthetically I liked that. It was good for the beach. With yoga, my body tightened. . . . I felt like I looked emaciated. But the energy pulsating through my body was amazing—there was an incredible vibrancy.

"It's hard to communicate. I look at the champions today and I think, he looks too skinny, that guy doesn't have the muscle. . . . But the energy they are carrying around is not visible; it is not in the muscle."

In many ways, Esak feels like a shining example of the promise of yoga. He rarely sleeps, yet he never seems tired. His body simultaneously brings to mind metaphors involving chlorophyll and robotics. When faced with a problem, his reasoning always begins with the communal. During discussions, he will take long, socially awkward seconds to pause and digest questions before answering them. He does not appear to give compliments. His insistence on rigor can feel assaultive, his casual honesty like an unexpected jab.

When I ask him about Bikram and Richard Nixon, he looks at me and smirks.

"Look at yourself here backbending and ask whether it matters. Will it help your Standing Head to Knee posture? Look, I want the stories to be true. I do. But ultimately, I don't think it matters at all."

Esak embodies the cultural stereotypes of a yogi as well. He fasts on Mondays. Invites us to meditate with him every morning. His diet is primarily raw and green. Bikram—who advocates eating whatever you feel like, especially fast food—calls him a goat and teases him by *baaaah*-ing when they eat together.

He is also ambitious. Esak is a free market, Julian Simon yogi. It may be his most Bikram-like characteristic. He hears an idea he likes, and you can actually feel the neural gears shifting as he figures out how to actualize it. He is a believer that spreading two goods—yoga and his own interests— must necessarily intersect. He collects sponsorship and endorsement deals.[10]

Three days ago, a woman at Backbending revealed, in addition to a day job, she owned a business selling bottled oxygen to Target and Walmart. The oxygen comes in little canisters with a padded face mask. Right now, the oxygen is primarily marketed to the elderly in high-altitude regions. But the idea is to take it mainstream: anytime you feel like a breath of pure air, you can snuff a hit.

When Esak listens to her describe it, his face tightens in full-throttle excitement. The ironies—of breath-obsessed yogis leading the commodification of the commons, of packaging thin air—never occur to him or are quickly dismissed. Instead he is entranced. "Fantastic." He turns to the group. "What a lesson in the abundance around us."

That night as we wall-walk, Esak convinces her to bring out her samples. As we bend, we huff oxygen. Passing the little canisters from person to person, he is giddy as kid.

Later, when he finds out I have a friend who is a movie producer, he immediately floats the idea of a Backbending Club reality TV show: *Last Yogi Standing*. Cameras in the Backbending nest. Women in yoga shorts walking around, chewing carrot sticks. Each night there would be a mini-competition; the loser gets kicked off their mat. At first I think he is joking. But the level of detail and thrice-repeated suggestion that I get my friend to come down for a visit indicate otherwise.

When we backbend, Esak sometimes videoconferences with his wife, Chaukei. She is a legitimate yoga champion in her own right. Beautiful and enthusiastic, just like Rajashree, Bikram's wife. Chaukei used to come

---

[10] Although Nikes not so much: his two biggest contracts are for companies selling pond algae and sea algae supplements respectively.

to Backbendings in person, but now stays at home to take care of their one-year-old boy, Osiris. In her absence, Esak sets up his laptop in the center of the room, and Chaukei appears on a little panel, coming in and out of view as she bends along with us at home.

When he is not in the center of a group, when he is not leading a seminar, coaching a Backbending, or scheming out an idea, Esak's intensity can vanish. Then we have the yogi as prankster, daredevil, and show-off. This Esak gets mischievous grins. He is fixated on *Star Wars* mythology and routinely refers to Backbending as Jedi training for the mind. He is the Esak who saw the movie *Inception* five times and who, after leading a seminar in Las Vegas, convinces a friend to videotape him in a delicate one-legged balancing posture on a tiny so-slim-it's-not-really-a-median slice in the center of a highway. Cars whizz by. Esak goes into the posture with a dark mask of concentration. After holding it in unbearable stillness, he emerges with a gigantic grin, yelling at the camera: "That's hatha yoga . . . pure concentration . . . spun-steel tiger meat!" A cop arrives on the scene to issue a ticket, and Esak's grin only grows wider.

So it's not that I want to *be* Esak. Not exactly. He has a diffident energy surrounding him. His intensity keeps him apart, despite his best attempts to connect. He lives without the small joy of candy and occasionally says Nietzschean things about individuals controlling the world around them that strike me as dangerously confident or hopelessly detached from true poverty and helplessness. We stare at him a lot when we practice, and he has to bear the weight of those stares. But I do recognize his energy. I do understand that on a fundamental level, his body hums in a different way from mine. And so I want to know what he knows, learn what he's learned.

My first real lesson comes late one night during the second week. We are backbending to Michael Jackson again,[11] chests against the wall, heads

---

[11] Which is what we always listen to when we backbend, because Esak loves Michael, because Michael is the perfect blend of optimism and vulnerability for backbending, because Michael was pressed into service roughly at the same age as Bikram, and because like Bikram, Michael spent a lifetime refining himself for others, and you can hear exactly that sad but incredible experience in

between the legs. On the fifteenth bend, Esak notices that I am opening my feet slightly into a V during my backbend, a tiny action that allows me to open my hips and take pressure off my spine. He takes a towel and wraps it under my feet to hold them straight. It is our first one-on-one interaction of the entire two weeks, and I don't know whether to be embarrassed or flattered.

When I persist in my poor form, inadvertently yanking the towel askew, he lets me know the answer is neither.

He calls me out in front of everyone. "Stop. We talked about this. Never come out of a backbend like that again. Make a commitment to yourself. Never do it again. From this moment forward."

Change your mind.

And so that is what I do.

A Sprite Intermezzo

In many ways, Esak is the definitional opposite of my aforementioned favorite yoga teacher. Courtney Mace is social grace. She is slapstick funny. She is kind and emotionally intelligent in the way that only professional therapists and kindergarteners tend to be in real life. When the bathroom window broke at my studio, she posted a sign that said,

Do not open window.
Broken.
(That means no pooping ahahahahaaha!!)

She does not believe in fifty backbends ever. She believes in doing two or three, but making them really deep and really count. She does not believe

---

his voice if you listen past the one thousand times you've heard each song before on the radio or in passing cars or at wedding receptions, which is of course the only way you can listen to a song while at the liminal point of consciousness that is backbending.

in raw spinach either, erring instead toward New Orleans shrimp po'boys. Instead of taking our water away during class, she often talks about fantasizing about having a Sprite while she is teaching. She talks about these Sprites in a way that makes it completely unclear if she is playfully taunting us or just indulging in one really deep personal fantasy. When she leads the advanced class, she makes us sing "Row, Row, Row Your Boat" in a round to serve as the count during several postures. I have seen Courtney sad; I have seen her bitchy; she is not bionic, nor made of chlorophyll; she is 100 percent completely human, in the way that I want to be human: someone who seems comfortable with that status and isn't hell-bent on transcending it.

She does share two things with Esak. She has a freakish body. Courtney has the height and bouncy blond hair of a shampoo model, but a girth that feels like it could fit into a shampoo bottle. She is skin stretched over muscles. Her legs look like braided nautical ropes. Her stomach is hard, plated, and slightly concave in a way that makes me think of a steel drum.

Her other similarity to Esak is that she was also an international yoga champion. She can do every posture to a startling level of beauty. Her pain tolerance is enormous. When she applies it, her willpower becomes almost a palpable force in the room. Watching her feels a little scary. It is almost as if the particles that make up her eyes firm together into a more solid substance. You keep expecting beams to shoot out of them.

For most of my practice, Courtney was just my favorite teacher. I loved her class, I loved how soft it was, how it held space but still made me push myself. I loved the fact that when a smart aleck asked why they did a certain posture in the middle of class, she responded by telling him that it was so he could finally blow himself. I loved that she seemed invested in her students. But mostly I loved that she never made us do anything she couldn't do herself.

There is nothing macho in Courtney's class, nothing excessive either on a physical side or a spiritual side: it just is a class.

I always knew she was strong, but I thought that was just what happened when you were a teacher who walked the walk and practiced what you taught. I knew she competed, but since she never talked about it, I didn't pay any attention. Then one day, shortly after she recommended I consider competing, Courtney took second place at the New York regional competition. Then four months later, she won the national competition. Then she came in first place in the international competition.

All of a sudden, my favorite yoga teacher was a yoga superwoman. Nothing about Courtney seemed to change, but everything changed around her. People who had been practicing with her for years started complaining her classes were too hard. That she was pushing them in ways they weren't ready for. Other people started showing up from out of town to take her class. In Advanced Class, I would sit out half the postures just to stare at hers. The studio started displaying her trophy at the front reception like we were a karate dojo, and soon after, she left town to go on an international tour.

Whatever depth I have in my backbends, I attribute to a sort of athletic extension of the concept of anchoring, developed in behavioral economics. In anchoring, our expectations for the price of goods are set by prices we hear prior, even if they are not at all rational or reasonable. Not knowing any better, Courtney was my concept of a pretty good yogi. For a fat stiff man, this was not rational or reasonable. Instead of pretty good, Courtney was amazing. Literally the best in the world. But I didn't know that, and thus my efforts to be a merely passable yogi were hopelessly skewed. Believe whatever you will about Esak and competition, but for me, Courtney will always be proof that comparing yourself to others is both an inevitable part of community and a positive one: instead of competition, I'd call it *learning from others*. Meaning we learn from others what is possible and then apply it to our own lives. In the best-case scenario, they, in turn, do same thing with your life. At the very least, it's the route to a pretty deep backbend.

Belonging

By the end of the week, Backbending has acquired its own rhythm. I wake every morning to someone's ankles. Usually the ankles belong to someone carrying on a conversation directly above me about the merits of alkalinalized water, or the perfect ratio of cucumbers to celery when making a green juice. Soon grogginess is replaced by pain. Then I spend my first conscious minutes awkwardly slathering various spicy balms and liniments along my spine.

When I actually make it off the floor, I inevitably discover that I am the last one to rise. By this point, the Backbenders have striated themselves by morning behavior. The most maniacal have long since silently disappeared to the studio to begin their work on postures. I am occasionally woken as their long bony legs stride over me on the way out the door. Then there is a more tortured group, Backbenders who clearly would like to be working out at the studio, but instead pace around the house, nursing injuries, wondering aloud in the guise of conversation what chiropractic adjustment they should be getting or which herbal supplement they should be swallowing. Then there are the Backbenders I can identify with: Fiona from Ireland, hair wet from a shower, nursing a cup of hot tea. Garland, a studio owner from Virginia, hunched at her computer checking emails. Brett, opening the wrapping on a contraband coconut-covered marshmallow product and eating it for breakfast. Finally there is Afton, the punk rock pixie, a group all her own. Afton is already proving to be one of my favorite humans ever for no other reason than she seems so normal. She executes her flawless postures, rips through Esak's additional work, and then disappears to hang out with non-yogic friends who have driven into town to visit her. All while I'm still scraping myself off the studio carpet. No alter ego ever hid their superpowers better.

I belong to none of these groups. But that's because I don't really belong. My morning routine consists of two parts: a bright yellow pee and a full-body panic. The two are related. First I panic because inevitably, no matter how much I drink, my pee looks like a liquid highlighter. This I take to mean I am dehydrated, so I follow my pee with a run to the kitchen to guzzle water. Only months later does a doctor explain that this supernatural yellow color is actually the result of the excessive quantities of vitamins I am consuming on a daily basis. If ever there was a metaphor for asinine American overindulgence, there I am, every day flushing away enough nutrients to abolish rickets in the third world. My second panic comes after

I have spilled water all over the front of my chest, and I realize our first class of the day is only minutes away and I haven't eaten yet.

And then it happens to me. After closing our routines early, maybe 10 P.M., I skip my chores. It is an unexpected decision, but suddenly and vehemently, I just don't feel like it. None of my postures are happening. My body crumples where it should remain firm and refuses to give where I ask it to bend. When I try to drink from my water bottle, it feels too heavy to lift, so I don't bother. While everyone else is working, I slip into the shower. I let the water drum against my brain. When I go to shampoo, it takes me several minutes to realize the extent to which things have gone wrong.

I put the shampoo in my left hand like normal, but then instead of raising my arm, I tuck my chin to my chest, trying to lower my head as much as possible. I use my right hand to push my left hand up by the elbow. It happens so unconsciously that I don't even realize the posture is weird until the back of my neck starts hurting from the tuck. I try straightening my head, but my left arm literally won't reach up to my hair on its own. It seems to have some upper limit. As an experiment, I stop using my right arm as support. My left arm just slides off the top of my head like a slop of rope. It is gone.

Rest reveals this is not just muscular exhaustion. Use of my left shoulder has simply disappeared.

The next two days are spent in wonderment and fear at this new development. It turns out that most of my range of motion is intact. Swinging side to side, pulling weight down, scratching my right ear, and zipping my fly all feel normal. But one particular motion—it almost feels like a channel my arm cannot pass through—is impossible. As if the muscles needed there have gone blank. Lifting my arm with the elbow directly beneath the forearm—the motion of shampoo applications and water bottle to lips—is simply unavailable to me. My arm begins the movement, gets to a certain point, and then quivers. Like it has been frozen midair by a magician.

It is a highly specific and completely painless paralysis.

Taking class with this absence is baffling. Despite the limited physical mobility, every action is even more exhausting than before. Instead of a rest for the muscles, the lack of movement drains me. And the harder I focus, the more exhausting it becomes. It is frustration I am unable to put into words until I find a description by neuroscientist Richard Restak of a recovering stroke victim:

> *Each small gain in ability to move the limb brought with it a sense of heaviness and resistance, as if the arm were being held down by heavy weights. The harder he tried to move, the greater fatigue and the greater effort required. This inner sense of exerting a mental force against a feeling of inner resistance was later described . . . "as a kind of mental force, a power of will. . . . As if there was a resistance which could be overcome . . . some kind of mental energy."*

Esak notices it in class the next day before I can tell him. I am sure this has less to do with his exceptional perception, more to do with the fact that my postures look deranged. When we talk afterwards, he is firm. First, I must stop doing wall-walks if I want my arm to return. I nod and silently note that he poses this as a question. Second, he tells me this is totally and completely normal. It means I am doing things right. He tells me it happened to him early in his training and his shoulder came back completely within a month. I nod again, silent at the prospect of a month without my shoulder.

Over the next few days, I become obsessed with regaining the range of motion, staring at myself helpless in the mirror as I make stunted gestures. I also become obsessed with whether other Backbenders believe me. The work we are doing is so hard and so exhausting that my shoulder seems like a convenient excuse. Like a psychological manifestation designed to save my body from this torture. But instead of wariness, the other Backbenders embrace my condition. David is especially warm. The same thing happened to him in a previous Backbending to both shoulders simultaneously. He tells me I'm holding up well and that he was terrified. And for the first time I start to belong.

What is amazing is that at no time do I ever get really get angry. Not with Esak, not with myself. I have this extremely worrisome, strokelike phenomenon that has debilitated my ability to function and that has a very clear and indisputable cause (i.e., doing wall-walks correctly). And instead of anger or doubt, I feel pretty calm about the whole situation. I have this weird sensation that my body is simply adjusting. That this is just part of the process. The only time I actually get scared is when I conduct a thought experiment: If this doesn't make me quit—what type of injury would?

When we line up to take Beginners Class—the basic series of twenty-six postures that makes up the Bikram regime—I end up next to Esak so much that it's a joke among the people in my car. I know why too, I'm always rushing in late, and nobody else wants to step into the spot. Everyone wants to take it easy during class, save their energy for the nightly routines. But nobody wants to let Esak down. That, of course, makes me perfect for my role. Compared to everyone else here, I already know I'm going to let him down.

During class, I notice Esak squirm a lot. I notice him grimace and pop out of postures a few seconds early. At first I think my presence annoys him. That he wants to bend next to someone who can inspire him. Then I think that he is lowering himself to my presence: the master teacher incrementally altering his instruction for each student. And while I'm not ruling out either possibility, I think there is another reason. The basic series of Bikram Yoga is just really, really hard. Even if you are the best in the world. That is what it is. Hardness as definition. Meaning, if it's not hard, you're not doing it right.

One of the few days I'm not lined up directly next to Esak, he is teaching the Beginners class. It's a 10 A.M. on a weekend. Members of the general public—non-Backbenders—are taking class with us, and the room is packed.

The density of bodies and Esak's intensity make the class feel hotter than normal. A big linebacker-sized fellow toward the back of the room is gasping. I can hear him huffing. Then stomping. Then there is silence as he goes down in a crumple. Esak keeps teaching the class without even a pause of acknowledgment. Eventually the linebacker gets up and stumbles toward the door to leave class for the locker room.

Esak stops him before he can make it. Instead he has the man kneel right by the lip of the firmly shut door. So close to relief. "You are free to leave right now," he tells the man, whose blocklike head is in his hands, and who is audibly wheezing again. "But you have a choice. Sometimes your yoga is in the postures. Today, your yoga is recognizing you have a choice."

Then after instructing us to come out of a posture, with a voice aimed directly at my heart, "Everyone else—stop listening! Stop thinking! Don't imagine his class is easier than yours. Don't flatter yourself with your effort. Right now, this is the person working hardest in this class. He is getting every benefit he can.

"What you need to ask yourself," Esak continues, "is whether you are getting the same benefits he is. Just because you're still standing doesn't mean you're still doing the yoga like he is. If you aren't putting the same effort into it, you're doing nothing. No benefits. You might as well walk out of the room, because if you limp through this series, you're flattering yourself if you think you're doing yoga."

It's a funny thing that way. Someone standing and looking very impressive in the mirror and someone sitting hunched over doing almost nothing. Same yoga.

Much later, I would meet a yoga teacher—Alison Tavares from Arizona—who would make this dynamic even clearer. We are sitting poolside in San Diego; it is seventy degrees with a slight breeze, impossibly far from the stink and oppression of the yoga room. Alison tells me about teaching a class with three men she loved. One, the first student she ever taught, was a triathlete in his late twenties, the type that might shave his chest to cut down his swim time. To his left was her father, in his late seventies, a few months in recovery from cardiac bypass surgery. His chest had been shaved at the spot where his doctors had sawed through his breastbone and implanted a defibrillator. And last in the row was her husband, an ex-marine, now paraplegic, out of his wheelchair on the floor balanced on the remainder of his legs. All three in the same posture. All three side by side. Watching them, she realized this radical, almost Vitruvian quality of the yoga. It was metric, adapting to the individual. Each of the men in front of her was a dedicated student; each spoke enthusiastically to her about the benefits they received from the yoga. But to an outsider, each appeared at an impossibly different place, and in the case of her paraplegic husband, potentially not even doing the same posture. What they shared was a commonality of exertion, and a commonality of form to which they poured this effort.

After class, I find the man in the locker room. He's sitting on the floor with his back against a corner. His face is red, and it's unclear if he's been crying. Everyone else is walking around him.

So it's the greatest relief to have Esak next to me, struggling. Legs trembling, occasionally coming out of a posture early to sneak a break. It's a relief because for the first time, I don't feel like such a clod. Because in the beginner series we're all leveled, all equal. But it's also a relief, because I know he's legit. Only a fraud could make it through flawlessly every time.

And then it's over.

On the last day of Backbending, Esak teaches class. There is a small moment in the beginning of every class where students are given a tiny break. The official Bikram dialogue calls it a warm-up, a moment where you walk your hips "several times, right and left and right and left." At Backbending, Esak has forbidden us to take the warm-up. The idea being that we are training to be champions, and champions don't need warm-ups— they go right into postures. In the last class, when we get to that part, he says for whatever reason, "Go ahead, walk your legs out. . . . Ah yes, a little treat." Despite being in class, I laugh out loud at the joke, and then, almost like I'm choking on the sensation, I suddenly start crying. It's inexplicable and actually the first time I have ever cried in the yoga room. These aren't tears of sadness exactly, more self-recognition: It is such a small, simple movement and it feels so good on my aching body.

Hours later, even after we have packed our things away, David's house retains a battered feel. The hardwood floors are visible again, but there are still small overlooked remnants hiding in plain sight. Reminders: a stray lime on a shelf, a forgotten pair of yoga shorts on a doorknob, a couch that may forever stink like Bengay. Everyone is circling around, giving hugs, promising to keep in touch, making rash commitments to come to the next Backbending, wherever it will be.

As thanks, a group of students presents Esak and David with custom-made T-shirts that read JEDI FIGHT CLUB—CHANGE YOUR MIND. Esak gets positively bouncy with enthusiasm. He sits on David's staircase, wearing the shirt, hugging people good-bye, accepting donations as they leave.

When it is my turn, I slip Esak as large a check as I can reasonably write and quietly tell him I wish I could triple it. The sentiment is real. I hug him good-bye with my gimpy shoulder, then quickly leave for the car. My body is wires at this point. I walk in stutters. I have learned a lot in the last two weeks, perhaps more about my body than in the preceding two years, but as soon as I pull out of the driveway, I decide to stop all backbends until I see a doctor.

The next day, driving back to New York, I find myself doing wall-walks against the aluminum siding of a rest-stop gas station. There is a moment, just prior to unbuckling the seat belt, where I wonder what I'm doing. But by the time I'm actually at the wall, I just shrug my shoulders, roll my eyes at the sky, and arch back to meet the pain like it's a moral obligation. When I'm done, my shirt is off and I'm smiling like a fool. Guess it turns out I'm a junkie too.

PART II

The Living Curriculum

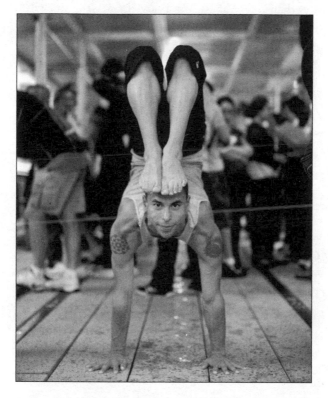

Joseph Encinia in handstand scorpion pose

Heartbreak opens for even breaking is opening . . . My spirit takes journey, my spirit takes flight, and I am not running. I am choosing. I am broken. I am broken open. Breaking is freeing. Broken is freedom. I am not broken; I am free.

—DEE REES THROUGH THE CHARACTER OF ALIKE

Emmy

Emmy is Bikram's oldest student, and theirs is a special relationship. Emmy is the only person left who can criticize Bikram in public. She is the only one who can scorn him. Who can reference the fact that his physical skills are in decay. That his ego has turned him into a cartoon. She can joke at him and not just with him. They love each other; they insult each other; they fight with each other. But above all, they need each other. Bikram is remarkable. And Emmy is remarkable in ways that complement Bikram without encroaching.

At eighty-three, she is almost regal in bearing: spine solid as a crowbar when she walks, white hair perpetually pinned up, single pearls on her ears. In her long, tight dresses, at the many formal events that dot the Bikram landscape, she introduces you to the concept of octogenarian sexy.

When Emmy teaches, she never rises to the podium, never sits on Bikram's throne. Instead she circulates the room, talking softly into her headset microphone as her voice broadcasts out through the mounted speakers on the wall. The effect, especially in the megarooms of hundreds, is ghostly.

Unlike Bikram, who is a focal point when he teaches, demanding even more attention than the mirrors, Emmy is everywhere and nowhere. She wanders up and down the aisles of bending practitioners, giving highly specific modifications, and it is impossible to know whether she is far or near until suddenly you feel a firm, bony finger pushing at your pelvis, and the voice from the speakers is telling the room to "push the hip forward. Really, now. It is just impossible to balance if you don't push it forward."

Where Bikram believed American students would never be ready for anything more than basic postures, Emmy wrestled the Advanced Series out him. She still teaches the class weekly at the International Headquarters. Occasionally she will demonstrate. Her postures are beautiful, her instructions clipped. "Stop fidgeting! There is no fidgeting in yoga. You look like a cat clawing around before it takes a shit." There is no class quite like Emmy's in the Bikram universe; she has mastered all the guru's knowledge and yet made it entirely her own.

She has the type of self-comfort that makes aging look attractive. In the middle of a talk about sex and reproduction to a room of three or four hundred young women, Emmy will suddenly spin off topic. "Oh, that reminds me, ladies. Kegels. These are very important. . . . You can live your whole life and not know about Kegels." And suddenly, this lovely old grandmother will be lying on her back onstage, staring at the ceiling, dictating into the microphone: "I'm tightening my anus, now tightening my vagina, now tightening my anus," and explaining to a room filled with women a quarter of her age the importance of vaginal grip for really high-quality sex.

"I take only the things that fit into my life as a modern Western woman," she explains. "The yoga is tremendously powerful. But I believe in bliss in this world. I believe in using it to strengthen the self. I drink wine, which is, after all, only fermented grapes. I will enjoy a coffee. I do not think more is better. I do not believe in holding a headstand for hours." She tells Esak she thinks doing repetitive deep backbends after the age of thirty-five is probably dangerous. "There is nothing to be gained by extremism. And that includes devotion to the self. There is nothing helpful in victimology."

If she has an operational principle for her vision of yoga, that's it. A Latvian who fled the German invasion of World War II, Emmy lost her mother as a child. Lost, in the potentially more terrifying sense, as in her mother was still alive and Emmy actually lost her amidst the waves of occupying German then Russian troops. She was placed with a host family, arrived in the United States, and taught herself English while running the hosting desk at a YMCA in Chicago. She married. Her only son died of a massive sudden heart attack. She moved forward. Every year at teacher training, she leads the pain lecture. It is her area of expertise, although she never mentions her personal history. She does, however, make overt comparisons between the ability to distinguish and hold on to different bodily sensations and learning to manage your life. "Never hold on to the bad sensations. . . . I always put the things I have survived behind me or used them to make myself stronger. . . . Learning to recognize the differences in pain sensations is learning to recognize the difference between anything: musical notes, colors, emotions. It is essential, and if you are going to practice yoga, you must learn to recognize and distinguish. Do not allow yourself to be held hostage by anything you don't need. Let it go."

Emmy met Bikram when she was a fully formed adult in her forties, when he first came to America. She had practiced yoga before but was entranced by Bikram's authenticity: not only as an Indian yoga master but also as a human. "He tells people what they know about themselves. And he has the charisma to make them own up to it instead of hiding." The Bikram she met didn't swear. He didn't brag endlessly about himself. He never spoke about sex.[12]

"When I first met Bikram, he had opened his studio for about a week. This was in the basement of a bank. He taught four or five classes a day, and there was a room in back where he slept. . . . He was a real workhorse." Although he never bragged about himself at this time, he did talk. And talk

---

[12] When I ask another of Bikram's oldest students if Bikram ever mentioned sex back in the '70s, she is aghast. "Oh, no. All the women were mad for him too. We gossiped, of course. But he never was vulgar, never showed any interest, not even a glance. I would say he was completely asexual. . . . We wondered for a while if there was something going on between him and his Mexican friend, Tony Sanchez. They were so close, and we thought maybe if he was gay that would explain everything."

and talk and talk. "Bikram would tell us, 'Old yogi eat little, sleep little, talk little. Me, I *never* sleep, *never* eat, but make up for it in the talking!'" This Bikram was a storyteller and jokester. The classes he taught were difficult but passed quickly because he was constantly entertaining. In between postures, he'd name-drop the celebrities who'd stopped by earlier, he'd sing, tell stories his guru told him, or jump around the room, testing people's postures by using their outstretched legs as a bench or pressing down on their shoulders, anything to entertain, to get a quick laugh, to prevent his students from remembering how uncomfortable they were.

But soon, the best technique he learned for holding attention was pointing out flaws. And so before her eyes, Emmy watched Bikram evolve into a master insult comic. If you were the target, you doubled down on effort, stung awake by his honesty. If you were anyone else in class, you laughed along with the group. He had an almost superhuman ability to detect effort levels—Bikram used to say all the time he spent avoiding work with his guru made him an expert in laziness—but effort wasn't the only thing he picked on. A messy divorce, a flat chest, a set of stretch marks, an awkward haircut: Bikram would sense the weakness, identify the source, and pounce.

"But you see, he was like a terrier pup—all growls, no bite," another very early practitioner, Bonnie Jones Reynolds, tells me. "He could get away with saying things nobody else could—not your mother, not your best friend—because he was a pup. He would make you laugh. And we just adored him for it. . . . You'd have famous actresses who he had just insulted bringing him cookies." And as Emmy notes, people put up with it because he was usually right. "He really holds a mirror up to you. It can be uncomfortable to look at yourself. But he never flinches."

In Beverly Hills, where idle bits of flattery were practically built into the local grammar, Bikram stood out as fearless. "It was the thing to do," Bonnie remembers. "At least half the class was Hollywood stars. . . . Hot Lips from *M*A*S*H* got me to my first class, and once I was there, I hid the whole time behind Shirley MacLaine."

The Hollywood stars brought their own adjustments to his teaching; Bikram learned to put swollen egos in their place. As more and more money flooded into his studio and as the entertainers gave way to superstar athletes, and everyone demanded his time, Bikram gained certainty: he held himself apart, refusing all overture for private classes, his sense of self growing in a direct arms race with the egos of his fabulous newcomers.

"We'd have the Lakers coming to Beginning Class, and they were so tall, they'd have to bend down at an angle during all the standing postures," another senior teacher from that era remembers. "But if they were five minutes late to class, Bikram would put them out. . . . This was while they were winning championships. Literally the most popular guys in town . . . Nobody else could do that."

But that was because Bikram could get them to laugh. The same teacher remembers, "Bikram would work with Kareem's father [this being Kareem Abdul-Jabar, captain of the Lakers at the time], and the old man loved him. He had the guy in stiches the whole time."

When he did get serious, when his voice dropped, it was to talk about yoga. He believed in it completely. That it was his gift. That it could actually change the world in the only way the world could ever be changed: by incrementally altering each person who practiced with him for the better.

His class was a laboratory for transformation. Bonnie remembers a man brought in on a stretcher and propped against the wall. "Basically for weeks, someone would bring him in and prop him up. The poor guy would make any little movement he could in order to try to do the postures," she laughs. "And that same guy, months later, was bouncing around like a kid."

This was a Bikram fresh with the miracle—still glowing from his twelve-hour training sessions with Ghosh, from his work as a healer sitting with elderly clients, hand behind their head, coaching them to breathe. He would walk around the room, giving hands-on modifications. He would jump into postures at every opportunity to demonstrate. His body was impossibly powerful and bright, and he showed it off constantly—"Best advertising," he'd say of his decision to teach class in a tiny Speedo. "This is what I do; this is what I sell." It was a Bikram who, after class, would retire to the backroom of his studio to practice the advanced postures he never shared with students. A Bikram convinced that spreading the yoga was his mission and that it was the most important thing he could do for the world.

"The absolute maddest I ever saw him, and actually this was a bit frightening at the time," Jimmy Barkan, Bikram's head of instruction for the late '80s and early '90s, says, "was when someone who was a regular student *skipped* class without telling him. I remember a woman who went away for two weeks without practicing, and Bikram was furious. He physically threw her out of class. 'Where have you been?! Where have you been?!' And he pushed her out by the neck. . . . But for the rest of us, it was a lesson in dedication. That was how much he cared. The yoga, having integrity to the yoga, it was everything to him."

This Bikram was a one-man operation, manning his studio day in and day out. Bonnie remembers, "He was absolutely intent on giving those twenty-six postures to the world. There was this true loving intent. I mean, you simply couldn't sit there like that—from eight A.M. to seven P.M.— unless you were dedicated."

And it didn't stop when class was over. "I remember going out to dinner one night in Miami, a big dinner party," Barkan tells me, "and one lady's father was there with arthritis. He was probably seventy-five years old, in real pain. And Bikram left with him, took him back up to his hotel room, and spent an hour and a half with him at nine P.M. at night in the middle of the dinner party. . . . You see, he felt like he had to, like it was his service. He couldn't not heal if someone nearby needed it."

"He thought everybody could benefit," Bonnie says. "He'd say it to us a million times: 'Never too late, never too old, never too sick to start all over again.' It was a quote his guru said to him. I don't think he envisioned the empire it would become. He didn't plan it. He just wanted to give it to as many people as he could."

The push to democratize the yoga, with the pull of maintaining its integrity, became Bikram's biggest difficulty. To Bikram, who had suffered through incense burns and preadolescent tears as he strove to meet his guru's demands, yoga was as fragile as it was powerful. The difference between a correct asana and silly stretch was one of minuscule degrees of intention. The power of Ghosh's yoga came from its exactitude—in the focusing on specific alignments, on subordinating the spontaneous mind to an abstract form, of the unity between physical attributes and mental focus that was created if that exactitude was achieved.

It demanded that practitioners push themselves beyond what they thought was possible. But that, in turn, demanded that the physical alignments of the postures be carefully regulated. Pushing the wrong way—especially over time— causes injury. To demand intensity, the alignments of the postures had to fall within motions that would be difficult but not harmful to move into.

In a Lululemonized world, where yoga postures "should never hurt," this focus on alignment simply doesn't matter as much. Practitioners who are taught never to push themselves will only rarely push to the point of injury in even the most irregular alignment. Instead, each invents a subtly different but specific posture within the more generalized form. To Bikram, arriving after twenty-five years of dedication to his guru's standard, that yoga was apostasy. It was hollow. A scam yoga that coddled American egos by refusing to push them beyond their comfort zones but still promised them the spiritual benefits of that struggle. To Bikram, to do a posture without a standard, without a form, and without precision was "cheating, shopping with no money."

Thus the most difficult and uncomfortable of his alignments—such as locking the knee in standing postures and maintaining perfect stillness between postures—became the aspects he held to most ruthlessly. To adhere to their form became an essential aspect of his yoga.[13]

This left a contradiction: yoga for the masses, but yoga without modification. It was a contradiction that Bikram negotiated with two twin sayings: "Ninety-nine percent correct, one hundred percent wrong," and its complement, "Try one percent the right way, get one hundred percent of the benefits." The latter opened the benefits of the yoga up to the world, especially when applied to his twenty-six-posture sequence. Everything in the sequence was within the normal range of motion, nothing would cause

---

[13]Or as Bikram says: "I don't care whether you live or die in Locust posture, just get your legs up and keep your knees locked. . . , People say I am a great businessman. That is wrong. I know nothing of business. I know 'lock the knee.' I know 'two hips in one line.' I know exactly what my guru told me, and I teach exactly that. . . . When you die, I do not come to the funeral. I come afterwards, late at night. And I jump on the coffin box and say, 'Lock the knee, lock the knee, lock the motherfucking knee' because only then do you do yoga and only then you can you get to heaven."

injury by itself, and by pushing toward the posture to the best of their abilities—even 1 percent—a practitioner would achieve the therapeutic benefits. The former ensured a focus on perfection, demanding forever an attention to detail. A posture that was 99 percent in alignment was insufficient. Only with total dedication to form, an almost unattainable 100 percent perfection of posture, where concentration knitted the mind to the body—with higher functioning baked to submission by heat—could a practitioner experience flickers of that elusive union.

This 99 percent wrong/1 percent right mentality created the classic Bikram dynamic. During class, internally, there is a perfectionism, a demand for an almost hostile conformity that works like metallurgy on the human form. Outside the hot room, externally, or from the teacher's perspective, the yoga is compassionate, open, and tolerant. Every improvement is praised because every improvement is hard won. Bikram himself plays both roles, toggling in and out from the demanding voice inside your head to the encouraging coach on the outside: the strict disciplinarian and the loving healer.

"Sometimes," Barkan tells me, "I think the worst thing that happened was he decided to hold his teacher trainings away from his regular classes. He used to teach everyone in one room right at Headquarters. His trainees lined up in the back, regular students off the street up toward the front. Then the students he was training would really see how caring he was during class. How compassionate he could be to someone elderly or obese or injured. Now his trainings are so large, he can't do that. Everything is in isolation, in a hotel, in a tent, and the teacher trainees don't see that side of him. . . . What they see is how hard he is on his teachers. Which he always has been—there is a hazing process, that's part of his training from his guru—you force your teachers to do extreme amounts of yoga and push their limits. But teacher training isn't what a general class is supposed to look like. . . . And so the message many teachers take away is—Bikram, tough, kill, hurt. They get all of the punishment, but see none of his love."

Emmy speaks to something similar when she talks about her own training. "Back in the beginning, there was no teacher training. There were just very accomplished practitioners who got pressed into service," Emmy says. "Bikram would just disappear—sometimes he'd just run off to India, and he would ask you to teach in his absence. That is how I learned. . . . There were days when Bikram would call early in the morning and say, 'Emmy, my voice, it hurts,' and you would have to step up, because people looked at you as a healer.

"He didn't believe that you could make a real yoga teacher in less than five years," Emmy says. "He was impossibly protective. That was how he learned."

But, of course, being protective was its own liability. Success was rising all around him, and there were no other teachers to help him manage the demand. "He was already losing his voice in 1974," Bonnie remembers, "teaching five or six classes a day. You could hear the toll it was taking."

Five years later, with business exploding, and still almost no teachers to sub in for him, Bikram watched the success take his own practice. "We would ask him about it," Jimmy Barkan says, "but he would always say, 'No, no, no, no. Interest in the bank. I practice yoga thirty years. Now run a little on interest.' But every once in a while, especially at the beginning, he would still take class with us. Emmy would coax him in. . . . He'd show-boat around; he loved it."

St. Luktananda

It is axiomatic in the yogic world that, instead of searching, a guru appears when the student is ready. This is called the living curriculum: a student learns what they need when they need it, because the universe provides it. Although obviously full of mystical overtones, there isn't anything necessarily extrasensory about the living curriculum. To some extent, it is a little like when you learn a new word and then suddenly see it all over the place. Or the way that general knowledge can crest to the point that several different scientists or philosophers can make simultaneous breakthroughs on different sides of the globe. It is a sign that there are an infinite number of connections to be made in our world, and that we weave narrative threads through those we are capable of comprehending. At its worst, the

living curriculum probably fuels groupthink, tribalism, and other intro-
verted self-satisfied approaches to understanding the world. But in the case
of our spiritual teachers, it's far more benevolent: As our brains begin to connect ideas internally, we become primed to recognize when other people
start expounding on those connections. They in turn open doorways to
new connections, and slowly, as we are able, the living curriculum allows us
to grow.

And so I found Luke. Or Luke found me. Or however it works.

An intense sage in tattoos, Luke has the body of Iggy Pop with the
well-jowled facial hair of Wolverine. Personality-wise, he is the ultimate
dharma bum: part poet-surfer, part beer-soaked goof, part deeply self-aware
mentor. All eager, all giving, and most important for me, someone with
enough self-knowledge and clarity to know when to shrug his shoulders
and laugh.

To give myself credit, I recognized his qualifications almost immediately. Unlike so many in the healthier-than-thou set who end up worming
their way into the yogic world, Luke is a fully realized survivor of his own
stupidities. Near-lethal carbon monoxide poisoning. Slogging through day
labor while drug-sick. Broken legs from leaping off bar tops. Stoned nego-
tiations with completely unstoned Eastern European gangsters. Hustling
art to tourists. And in general, a "lifetime of parties and bands and ware-
houses, wrecked cars, lost jobs, and black market abortions" that leave you
either hung by your own petard or hoisted slightly closer to a nonbullshit
perspective.

He has the compassion and instinctive giving that come from really
having suffered. Listening to Luke, I can't help but think of the Czeslaw
Milosz quotation: "In a room where people unanimously maintain a conspiracy of silence, one word of truth sounds like a pistol shot." And while I
wouldn't exactly call the endless chatter of self-betterment and self-promotion
in the yogic world a conspiracy of silence, Luke's story still manages to cut
through it and leave a wake.

The story begins with Luke drifting westward toward the end. After a
drug-addled tour of Eastern Europe, life savings exhausted, compulsively

using heroin and cocaine, he settled with a girlfriend in Houston. "It was the most American part of America we could imagine," Luke says. "We wanted sun, English, beer, and strong, close-to-the-border-of-Mexico, old-fashioned hard drugs."

Luke found work as a day laborer. Houston was in the endless middle of its housing boom, and unskilled jobs were everywhere. He navigated the city by foot, trotting each morning to a pickup location, where he would wait for the day's contractors to fill in their crews. He was white and hungry-looking, so he almost always got picked. This led to an eight-month string of persistence work: scraping the paint off prerenovated shanty houses, carrying stacks of lumber from truck to site, cleaning up debris after skill workers finished their skilled work. His girlfriend got a job as a bartender at a topless bar, which Luke was never permitted to visit and which he decidedly does not want to remember. "No part of me wants to suspect what really went down on those nights out. . . . We were trapped in a real mess of a life."

The couple never had the funds or the motivation to move into a place of their own, so they slept on the same couch in a junk house for months. They woke to dry mouths and a darkness cut only by the slender light cracking through the house's well-drawn curtains. Clothes and dishes littered the floor. There was never ever any money. Except for dope. Days looped. To the extent the routine was interrupted, it was just barely and totally predictably with the small overdoses Luke and his girlfriend experienced regularly—all handled with amateur self-assurance, cold showers or hard slaps, bodies propped on their sides and pants unbuttoned so ice could be shoved down between the legs—and by the solemn serious resolutions to get clean that followed those nights. It was a lifestyle with a narrow but definite focus, a mechanized junk-oriented stability.

The primary catalyst for breaking this stability was a generous dealer. The couple had a daily ritual. There was a slender three-hour overlap between the time Luke returned from work and before his girlfriend went off to work the bar. Each day after getting paid, Luke headed to a prearranged 7-Eleven, where he took five dollars from his sixty-five-dollar daily take to purchase a hot dog and a large blue Gatorade. Then he took the entire remainder of his wages and sat on the curb, eating his hot dog and waiting for his heroin dealer. His girlfriend was responsible for procuring their cocaine.

When they met at home, they would sneak to their roommate's room to borrow her bed while she was at work. The CD player would get started, the dope would get mixed, and like magic, from anticipation alone, the dope-sickness withdrawal symptoms would begin to disappear. Finally they would tap in: "watching the rose bloom of blood gurgle into the syringe, then waiting—riding the wave of excitement for a few moments more—until we plunged the drugs home."

On one particular night, a generous dealer upgraded their dope and pushed what would have been a small overdose into one just slightly larger and scarier. Luke remembers waking after passing out for just a few seconds, needle still in his arm. His girlfriend was next to him not moving, not breathing. Like many times before, he pulled off "a bit of poorly rendered CPR and dragged her to the shower." She came back to her body and headed back into the bedroom. To reward himself for his bravery, his efficacy under fire, Luke decided to give himself another quick shot to the arm.

At which point he "fell out for a moment."

Upon waking splattered on the bathroom floor, alone, scared shitless, and pulling himself up to the sink for a splash of water, "right in the mirror, right in front of me, was me looking back. But it was not me how I always saw myself in the mirror. Instead there was a younger me."

Luke stared at this clear vision of a younger self. And the morning afterwards, both he and his girlfriend decided to check into a state methadone program. "Which proved absolutely useless. . . . Lots of red tape, forms to be filled out, endless waiting, and a grossly inadequate dosage that left you craving for more and which were administered in the presence of some of the most well-equipped dealers in Houston, who were also 'recovering' and waiting in the lobby with you."

This program led to another program, which was significantly more successful, if only because it was experimental and deregulated and the administrators supplied such adequate doses that further attempts to get high were pointless. The couple would pick up their weekly maintenance dose and leave the offices buzzing. According to Luke, the operating premise of the program seemed to be "get them so high that if they try to get more high, they can't feel it." And it worked.

Totally energized and euphoric, the two began pouring themselves into sobriety projects. "It was time to fill the void. But after all the silverware is clean, the pens and paints are labeled and sorted, the late broadcast TV is over . . . what to do then?" His girlfriend headed to yoga. He began working at Whole Foods with a manager who also doubled as a tai chi coach. Together they began a transformation process that ended somewhere pre-transformation when he lost his job at Whole Foods after a three-month trial period. His tai chi coach was one of the managers who opted to let him go. So, in Luke's immortal words, "Fuck him, fuck Whole Foods, and fuck tai chi."

Without a job, his girlfriend dragged him to a Bikram class. His first class was a "macho dickhead disaster," where he lined up directly in front of the teacher and pushed himself as hard as possible from minute one, and where the only existential realization came shockingly early, after only the third posture, when suddenly he awoke to the understanding that "I AM GOING TO VOMIT." This led to him fleeing not only the hot room but the entire complex, out to the cool of the parking lot, where he sat on his haunches by the hub caps of an impossibly nice "top-of-the-line, silver Jaguar S-Type car" and puked his brains out. He did not return. He felt betrayed, ambushed by the class and his girlfriend, by the teacher, by a weak body: instead of energy, he felt flooded with resentment.

"Shame might be a predecessor to humility. But shame as a process is ugly, and this instance was no different," he told me of this time period. "It took a while for me to go back, but somehow my girlfriend persisted through my bitchiness and managed to convince me to step into the hot room one more time."

The second class left him for dead as well. But he made a connection that would change his life. Even though Luke himself was still unsure, the studio owner, Mike Winter, seemed to understand how badly Luke needed the yoga. He offered Luke an opportunity to enroll in his "Janitorial College of India." Luke would come six days a week and clean the yoga room, and in exchange, he could take classes if wished. Luke accepted.

It is an understatement to say he didn't fit in around the studio. Luke is a long man, over six feet tall, with buzzed hair and piercings. His pink body is all lean angles, all pointy intensity. In yoga gear, with shirt off, he is a messy pastiche of tattoos, which wraps around his chest and arms like the tatters of a costume. He does not channel "safe" or "soothing"; he mostly channels "hug your grocery bag tighter, old women." But nobody intruded on his practice. His teachers gave him space and encouraged him to come. The middle-aged moms he practiced alongside gave him the type of prolonged plain smiles that meant they had no idea what he was going through but wanted to let him know they were trying to be supportive.

His obvious pain was addressed in the same way all pain in the yoga studio was addressed: It was personal, unique, and factual. Nobody could help you through it, and it was not to be avoided. Pain was simply part of the routine. Concealing, glossing over, or denying it was as pointless as indulging it or letting it become definitional. And if you trusted in this routine, surrendered to it, the pain would become more bearable.

"Yoga practice becomes a mode of self-inquiry, self-healing, and self-actualization," Luke says. Bikram asks you to stand and stare at yourself during your most agonizing, day after day after day. The practice is excruciating, and instead of running from the trauma, you revisit it. "I study myself in asana. I examine my way of being, who I am choosing to be. . . . Where I am being absolutely authentic and beautiful, and where am I being less than honest and selling myself short."

After six months, things started to change. Luke softened. One by one, like ignored former acquaintances, his addictions dropped off: first heroin, then cocaine, then the dextroamphetamines. He watched this happen in the same way he watched himself in posture. He and his girlfriend broke up. He grieved. He founded a stable job. He started assembling the pieces of his life, so he could at least begin contemplating putting them back together. He kept practicing: attending class daily, burning himself to the ground.

His last addiction was methadone. Although proposed as a government-sanctioned alternative to heroin because of the more moderate high, in one of those bureaucratic ironies that uses good intentions as pavement, physical withdrawal from methadone is actually much more brutal than heroin withdrawal. Symptoms ranging from vomiting and tremors to full-body aching and intense sleepless hallucinations can last for weeks longer than a heroin detox of a similar dose. Luke compares it to "the sickest you have ever been, the worst flu, the worst, most throbbing headache, the sweatiest, sickest fever . . . multiplied by one thousand."[14] Luke was doing 80 milligrams of methadone a day. Cold turkey withdrawal at that level can and has killed people. There is a respected medical position that, given these side effects, reducing from methadone isn't actually necessary. That it is a perfectly acceptable outcome for addicts to simply maintain an indefinite weekly dosage, just like any other prescription drug.

For those, like Luke, who choose to get clean, reduction occurs at 5 milligrams per week, moving slowly through an agony that lasts months.

Luke went through the process on the Bikram floor. First gradually as the program suggested, but as his confidence increased, in a great enthusiastic push. When he got to his final 20 milligrams, just the point where the clinical literature recommends tapering reductions even more slowly (down to 1 milligram per week) because the withdrawal symptoms grow the worst, he gulped the rest of his prescription, enjoyed the last great high of his old life, and braced for fall. That night he crawled into bed and fell asleep weeping.

By the time he hit the studio the next morning, on what would turn into his final day of detox, the methadone withdrawal undid him. From the second posture, he went down to his knees, losing vision. He spent the entire remainder of class on the floor, "shivering, boiling, dripping,

---

[14] "Closed eyes brought an anxious void, open eyes brought paranoid illusions and hallucinations, none of which were so drastic as to be obvious, making them all the worse. There were always people's voices and they were always talking just out of range but on a subject matter that certainly regarded me. The corners of my vision revealed family members and neighbors, faces blank or filled with nasty scorn. Everything tasted horrible. And I was filled with a constant sense of shame and fear."

wheezing." He realized the class was over when he heard feet stepping gently around him and the cool air creep in from the opening and closing of the door. Luke continued to lie facedown. About an hour later, he heard the door open again, followed by feet shuffling, the pump of the spray bottle, and the sound of the squeegee on glass. The studio owner, Mike Winter, had begun to clean the mirrors, doing Luke's work for him. Luke tried to get up but fell back, listening while Mike silently and methodically completed his sole contribution to the studio. Then he heard the supply closet open again and the footsteps head for the door. He was convinced he had utterly failed.

Instead Mike reverted to the simple and factual. "Drink water, please. See you tomorrow, son," before shutting the door. Luke lay back on his mat for another hour. It was the only time anyone at the studio had modified a posture or an act for him. "When I was at the end, Mike gave me what I needed, just enough to pull myself up. Anything more or less, and it wouldn't have worked the same." When he finally mustered the strength to head back home, he slept the rest of the day, through the night, and so far into the next morning that he missed class.

But he showed up to clean the mirrors after it was over.

Eventually Luke became completely hard-drug free. He went on to attend teacher training, buy a studio in New York, and manage it successfully. His living curriculum kept unfolding.

Or as he says in an interview with the online magazine *Heyoka:* "Realization is an infinite process, it is a path not a destination." The mirrors help guide you, the postures help guide you, and, if you get out of the way and let it, the yoga will open you to it: "Trust me, I was there at the brink and I came all the way back again."

The problem with Luke is that he existed only online in that single interview for *Heyoka.* It was as if the living curriculum had played a joke on me. The interview was profound and simple. It told his basic story, it explained how he had used the tool of yoga to view himself, and it, in fact, introduced me to the concept of the living curriculum. But it also left me with tremendous questions I felt needed answering. Who was this punk rock yogi who saw the practice so clearly? Why wasn't he off giving seminars? Posing for *Yoga Journal*? Or at least maintaining a Facebook account? The more I searched for clues about Luke, the less certain I was that I hadn't just actually imagined him. On the Internet, there were a billion potential Lukes but no trace of one whose life was saved by Bikram. At a certain point, I found a deceased blog that seemed a tantalizing lead, but it contained only poetry. And it was (god bless) a poetry devoid of reference to yoga in general and Bikram in particular. So there was no way to be certain. Pieces would fall at me every once in a while. When a friend prepared to go off to teacher training, she directed me to a blog that contained a single sentence about "an amazing man named Luke who taught class and reduced us all to tears." But that was it. I went in search of the Chelsea studio the *Heyoka* article mentioned he owned. But when I visited and asked the teacher behind the desk about Luke, he looked confused and explained the studio had changed ownership several times. For two years, the only evidence of Luke remained this ghostly interview on a ghostly webzine.

Then one day, I was doing what I typically do when I decide to write, which was not to write and instead play Scrabble-like games on Facebook, when I stumbled on a status update of yoga friend: "Just took amazing tape recorded class by Lucas M."

I clicked her profile, and at the very top of her friend list there was profile picture of blue fuzz with the label Lucas under it. I clicked on the blue fuzz. There appeared a man in sunglasses, board shorts, and a cardigan. He was holding an oversized beer stein. Beneath the picture, he had decided to comment on himself and wrote:

Yo yo yo, Hey wuddup, bitches?!
My name is DJ Luke and I clean the dishes
Make 'em shiny like childhood wishes,
Swimming though yer dreams like magical fishes . . .

I emailed immediately, asking if he was, by chance, a yoga instructor once featured in *Heyoka* magazine. Within ten minutes, Luke had replied.

The living curriculum was alive.

Oddly, however, the first place my interaction with Luke sent me—through the simple mention of how far his life had come, how radically people could change—was to essentially the opposite type of yogi: Joseph Encinia.

Joe and Sol

"My mom's still in touch with a couple of my doctors," Joseph Encinia tells me. "She sends them links to the YouTube videos of my postures. They're happy for me, inspired and all, but at the same time totally baffled." He laughs.

"They're like: 'What! Him! That kid! What happened?'"

It strikes me as he talks: Joseph is beautiful. He is stretching out in the near splits, torso rising straight up from the floor. His body isn't muscular like an action hero, it isn't fatless and magnificently articulated like some backbenders. Instead it has fluidity; when he moves, his muscles ripple like pond water at the point of disturbance.

It's a body that Joseph clearly takes pride in. He pulls the shirt over his head; his mood changes. He absentmindedly begins stretching his body in disorienting ways, the sides of his smile widen by a few millimeters.

A lot of the joy comes from simply knowing he can.

"When I was a teenager, doctors told me that at twenty-five, I would still be living with my family," Joseph says, "that my parents would be my caretakers. I remember being told that by thirty, I would need a walker."

The doctors had good reason for their pessimism: At eight, Joseph was diagnosed with pediatric rheumatoid arthritis. The sterile white synovium that capped his bones was being eaten alive. In rheumatoid arthritis, an unknown trigger causes the immune system to attack itself; his white blood cells were literally digesting the cells in the tissue surrounding his joints. And as each of these cell exploded, they unleashed a chemical cascade into the joint cavity, causing swelling and raw inflammation. To move meant to hurt.

So instead he mostly slept and ate. "I wasn't allowed to play. No gym class, no sports, no horsing around. Everyone told me I would hurt myself more." He pauses. "And the last thing I wanted was to hurt myself more. My body was already broken. I had knees that would swell up like grapefruits."

This form of arthritis is supposed to be a modern curse, a disease of the elderly, common only to the extent that medical advances have made it common to reach old age. For Joseph, it was his boyhood. He was channeled from bed rest to doctor's offices to hospital waiting rooms. There was a major surgery on his knee. There were warnings not to play outside. There were lots of lollipops for being a good patient. Instead of comic books, his memories of the time are filled with the superhero-like brand names of all the painkillers he took. Vioxx, Celebrex, Ultram.

Taking the pills was better than the pain, but they just reinforced his feeling of being hopelessly sick. Even now he can't differentiate between their side effects and his depression.

By thirteen, Joseph was a pill-swallowing machine. His register of daily painkillers, antiinflammatories, and antacids (for a stomach ulcer he had developed) grew every time he saw the doctor. "Something was always being added," he says, "something adjusted."

But it didn't last:

"I was at home during summer vacation. Of course, that's what summer vacation meant to me at the time, being home while everyone else was out playing. . . . And I just felt really sick. All day my head was hurting, my breathing uneven, I got dizzy. So my mom took me to my pediatrician. We waited. He thought it was a combination of a summer flu and a cold. He just ordered more bed rest.

"Later that night, I woke up, and I was having even more problems breathing. This was different. I was taking deep breaths, but each breath was killing me. I remember my mom putting me in the car. I remember us starting to drive. Then I blacked out. . . . I woke up the next day in the ICU, attached to every machine in the unit."

Joseph had just had a heart attack at the age of thirteen.

For the last forty-eight hours, his coronary arteries had been in spasm, a condition known as variant angina. The narrowing in the coronary vessels blocks blood flow to the heart muscle cells, starving them. As these cells shut down, circulation throughout the body slows.

Although Joseph had exhibited textbook symptoms of the disease, it wasn't until he was hooked up to life support that doctors at the Children's Medical Center in Dallas realized what had happened. Variant angina isn't supposed to happen to teenagers. It is a condition for elderly smokers, men with histories of high blood pressure, high cholesterol, and alcohol abuse.

It's easy to imagine this being the final straw in Joseph's chances at life as a normal kid. If his family was protective before, it's hard to imagine angina relaxing the situation. But instead of driving him deeper into his medico-Dickensian childhood, the heart attack marked a small turning point.

"First of all, I got a lot of attention all of sudden. Nobody was quite sure why this happened." The hospital assigned him two cardiologists: one pediatric, one adult. As Joseph stayed recovering, attached to his beeping machines, a debate over his condition was happening just out of earshot. "The pediatric cardiologist, looking at my medical records, my weight, and my diet, essentially saw this as a forgone conclusion. The other cardiologist said, 'Wait a second. This kid is on way too much medication. We're suffocating him. We're medicating this heart attack.'" The result was that Joseph emerged from the hospital with decreased dosages from some of his more heavy-duty painkillers.

Off the medication, Joseph was clearer. But he kept gaining weight. And both cardiologists agreed that with his arthritis compounded by a cardiac condition, sports were out of the question. "I spent high school eating. I was depressed. I was lonely. This was especially true, because my brother was this all-around all-star: good with sports, good with girls. And I was none of that."

In the grand tradition of alienated, anti-athletic students, he poured himself into his studies, especially the sciences. "Being in a hospital my whole life, I had all these fascinations. I wanted to understand all my conditions. I wanted to understand what it meant to be healthy. It was really a chance for me to open up and come into my own."

His junior and senior year, Joseph got the opportunity to spend every other day working at the hospital as an intern. First with a nutritionist and then with an occupational therapist.

"As I got more confidence, I just woke up. And when I woke up, I was fed up. Fed up with social status. Fed up with my brother. Fed up with no girls. So I started testing the boundaries I was always told I shouldn't break. I was still taking painkillers, but I realized I had to take control."

This boundary crossing culminated when a girl he met out at a concert dragged him to a Bikram Yoga class. "I knew nothing about yoga. I grew up in a Roman Catholic household that was very interested in academics, very invested in Western medicine. But I mean, if she invited me, of course I was going to go."

He died his first class. "Like I really thought I was going to die," he says. A claim that is far more believable, given his previous brushes with cardiac arrest. "It destroyed me."

But two hours later, he felt amazing.

He went back a second day and upgraded to a monthly pass. The studio owners noticed him coming every day and they offered him work-study: clean the studio on Wednesday and get free yoga for the week. From there it really took off. "For the first time in my life, I felt my body improving. I felt myself becoming an athlete."

Joseph began a daily practice and watched his body transform. He lost fifty pounds in the first six months, lost his depression for good, and most important, stopped being afraid. "I was always told, especially with the heart attack, I couldn't do certain things. I was always told I had to limit myself."

Around the one-year mark, his arthritis went into remission. It wasn't that he was pain free, exactly. It was that for the first time in his life, he could deal with his pain. "Doctors taught me to cover my pain. Bikram has taught me to accept it," Joseph says. His knee might still swell up if he overstretches it during an advanced class, but his instinct isn't to reach for a pill bottle.

"I started the yoga six years ago, and for the last five years, I've taken no painkillers. Which is a huge step for me. To be honest, my parents actually weren't very happy about that at first. They thought I was behaving recklessly. But," he laughs, "they've come around."

The reason they've come around, and the reason he can laugh, is because looking at Joseph today, there is no evidence that a transformation has even occurred. He shines. He glows. He's excited. I try to picture a tired, pudgy boy with cotton balls stuffed in his brain, but I can't quite do it.

So I ask him, "Do you have any connections with that past? Is the kid still in you?"

Joseph is upside down, having just glided up into a handstand. He stays there for a second and then pours himself back onto two feet. "He's still there. I just wish I could go back and tell him things. You know, you don't have to be the way you were brought up to be. Your life doesn't have to be that way."

A few weeks after talking to Joseph, I start having these visions.

The first time it happened, I was in a Wawa convenience store. There was an extremely fat woman behind the counter. Her body was swollen tight against her clothes. When she turned, it looked like her ass might contain lions—it bulged in torment. Her face bulged too, almost disorienting to look at. The same universal human features we all share were blown up and distorted.

But when I got up to the front to pay, got face-to-face with her, the disorientation went away. Suddenly—and weirdly, and unsettling in its clarity—when I looked at her, I saw a skinny twelve-year-old girl. Her fat remained, but it had lost its dimensions of human skin. It became something of a gelatin: molded on but not attached to another face below. We exchanged our pro forma pleasantries, she swiveled to get my change, but what minutes before had seemed like a physical property suddenly looked as artificial as a puffy winter coat. Her fat was a costume. When she turned back, I saw both her jawlines at the same time, overlapping each other: one swollen, one slight.

I'm not given to spontaneous visions, or even staring into other people's eyes for prolonged periods of time, so this whole interaction unnerved me. I literally had to push off the counter to check the length of my gaze.

I collected my change and shuffled out.

But then it happened again. And again. To paraphrase *The Sixth Sense,* I saw skinny people. Not everywhere, not even often, but every once in a while when I wasn't expecting it. I would look at someone, catch their eyeball, their eye socket, and suddenly feel like I could see a face within their face. A younger face.

Crack-up. It was weird.

Anyway, before it sounds like I started throwing my visual stimuli in with the dietary police and other health fascists, I want to be clear that, one, these were visions, and thus a sign that I was going a little crazy. And two, they didn't happen with people just because they were monstrously obese. There was no organizing principle. It just happened.

Either way, I am sure it would have been all a minor fascination, a phase forgotten, until it happened with my friend Sol.

Not only does Solomon King Prophete undeniably have one of the all-time greatest names, I'm going to go out on a corny limb and say he has one of the all-time greatest hearts as well. Sol is a Dominican-Mexican mensch. Community seems simple when you're with him. He likes people. People like him. There is not a store within walking distance of his home where the shop owner doesn't greet him by name. There's not a neighbor in his building who hasn't stopped by his second-floor apartment for a conversation on their way up the stairs.

I met Sol in college. We lived down the hall from each other freshman year. Sol grew up in a housing project just off 125th Street in Harlem. I came from suburban Maryland. This is probably the only way our lives would have intersected, but luckily for me, they did. Sol tutored me for my first G-chem exam. I played video games in his room. We got high together and threw cake from the rooftops of buildings. We got drunk together, and I puked out his window. Fifteen years later, I was in his wedding party when he married the cute blonde who lived across from him on our freshman floor, Ashley.

Sol's fundamental goodness operates on many competing levels. As a husband, he does the dishes and keeps the kitchen immaculate. As a Super Bowl host, he gets up out of his chair to give you the best view of the game. He is a seriously good son. His father passed away when he was young, and Sol rose to the occasion. He does his entire family's taxes. He cares for his sister's mental health. At one point, while I was busy getting fantastically drunk and sleeping through my classes, Sol dropped out of college to pay for his mother's bills. He got a forty-hour-a-week job with benefits and funneled money toward her rent. Later he dropped back in and graduated. But even then, I realized Sol was a man, in ways I wouldn't have to face for years.

But when it comes to describing Sol's fundamental goodness, one particular story stands out from the rest.

Back before their marriage, when Sol was dating Ashley, she bought a pug puppy. Pugs, for people who don't know, look nothing like dogs (more like weird furry larvae) but are fantastically cute anyway. Ashley loved this pug, named him Mu-shu, and he became something of a sensation in our friend group; I immediately thought I'd be hilarious and feed him Kahlúa, resulting in a memorably hard slap from Ashley.

Anyway, Ashley was devoted to this pug, Sol was devoted to Ashley, and one weekend Ashley asked Sol to pug-sit while she went into the office. Sol dutifully responded. He walked Mu-shu to the local dog park, chatted like a mensch with some strangers on a bench, and then watched appalled as a pit bull, off his leash, walked up to Mu-shu and bit half his face off. Everyone at the dog park started screaming.

Sol shook off his initial shock and grabbed the pit bull by its jaws. Blood was leaking out, but the grip was too tight. So Sol dropped the snout and began kicking. As he kicked, the owner of the pit bull ran up and tried to push Sol away from her beloved pet. But Sol kept at it. Finally with Sol kicking, the owner pushing, and the whole park screaming, the pit bull just kind of gave up and coughed. Mu-shu rolled out. Sol scooped him and ran. Then he ran back to pick up Mu-shu's left eyeball, which had popped out of its socket and scooped that up too.

At this point, regardless of how you think he handled the situation so far, Sol assumes superhero proportions in my eyes. At the edge of the park, cradling Mu-shu's limp body under one arm, he stepped directly in front of oncoming traffic, his other arm straight out.

A woman slammed on her brakes, and Sol climbed in her passenger seat. He showed her Mu-shu's body and said, "Lady, I need you to take me to my vet."

They bonded on the way, and celebrated later on the phone when, against all odds, Mu-shu pulled through. The detached eyeball was implanted successfully. The vet, impressed with Sol's heroics, charged the young couple only one hundred dollars for the whole four-hour operation and follow-up visits. And eight years later, Mu-shu is still going strong, both his bulging pug-eyes intact, perpetually scanning the world for food.

Anyway, as a long digression about a pug demonstrates, it's hard for me to say enough good things about the man. I'm sure you have someone like this in your life. The point is, Sol is that guy in mine.

The other point, in relation to this book, is that Sol had also been getting really fat. Not by the Wawa standard; Sol wasn't buying multiple tickets on airplanes or anything. But he was heading that way. Quickly.

In many ways, this is a totally unfair observation, a backhanded maneuver from a historical ally. For years, I had been one of the more unhealthy influences in his life. If Sol wanted to order an extra beer, I got us a shot too. If we went to the movies, I smuggled in the jumbo bag of peanut butter cups. We once, on a whim, on a bored Sunday whim, had an eating contest where we each ate (in order): fifty buffalo wings, two ice cream sandwiches, a beef patty, about a quarter of Ashley's fabulous 7 Up cake, and, AND an entire tray of Entenmann's Raspberry Strudel.[15] I know that is exactly what we ate, because we cared about it. We took pride in it.

But even back then, I always balanced my eating with exercise in a way Sol never did. I would wolf down two plates of hash browns and eggs during a 4 A.M. trip to the diner. But then I would hit the gym the next day. Punishing myself for the indulgence, minimizing the damage to my waistline.

Sol never did any of that. Instead of the gym, Sol would hit a fat Dominican cigar. Instead of minimizing damage, Sol would zone out to late-night CNN. Lately, in fact, Sol was barely walking. Their pugs, fantastically round themselves, would get walks around the block. Sol would return breathing heavy from the trudge up his single flight of stairs.

---

[15] Despite orchestrating things to end in a tie, and despite the fact that Sol subsequently puked about half of his portion up, I've always felt Sol won that contest because his wings were CHEESE WINGS, an absolutely revolting and short-lived concept that involved buffalo wings being smothered in easy cheese.

Anyway, all this came to a head in my head, one evening over dinner. Ashley is from Memphis, and cooking is her stress relief of choice. Her food is phenomenal but never ever healthy. Ashley vocally believes in a culinary principle that requires the use of butter and bacon in every dish, including most desserts.

This particular dinner was at the height of my yoga honeymoon. Ashley knew I was trying to eat healthy, and so instead of her usual potpie, meat loaf, or ham-soaked collard greens, she made a salad. Naturally the salad was heavily mulched with shredded bacon. But I appreciated the effort.

Years ago, in college, Sol had shown me his high school identification card. On it there was a picture of an absurdly skinny Mexican kid staring back. Even back then, Sol was pretty heavy, and the picture looked nothing like him.

But sitting across from him at dinner, munching on that bacon-infused salad, that's who I saw. The skinny kid. Not the whole time, but in flashes, especially as Sol chewed. I hadn't seen the ID card for years, but my vision was so vivid, I had no problem placing it instantly.

I didn't know what to do with this vision. So I sat on it. I figured I'd wait and see if it was there the next time I saw him.

It wasn't, but that's because the next time I saw him, he was in the hospital.

Only a few days after our bacon-salad dinner, I get a call from Sol. Ashley has gone to walk the dogs, and I was about to walk into the subway on my way to work. But then there was Sol on my phone.

"Hey, man." He sounded faint. "I'm really sorry to ask you this. But do you still have that van?"

I hadn't had a van in years.

"I was thinking if you do—" He stopped talking for a long five seconds. "—if you do, it would be great if you could come pick me up. . . . I need to go to the hospital. It's really bad."

This is not a phone call you ever want to get from your friend. Not only was Sol not making sense, his voice was so quiet I could barely understand what he was saying. So I did the only sensible thing a friend can do in that situation.

"Sol, what the fuck are you doing calling me? Hang up and call 911 right now! Can you do that? Do you need me to do that for you?"

It turned out he had an extreme gall bladder infection and was delirious from pain. It had exploded on him all at once while Ashley was out walking the dogs. He went to the hospital for emergency surgery, and the next time I saw him he was under heavy sedation: a massive mound of gray flesh with a sheet draped over him, breathing quietly. Sitting there, with cheeks sagging and eyes shut, he had that essentially ageless helpless quality hospitals cast over newborn babies who look exactly like grandparents, and grandparents who suddenly revert to infancy. Only Sol was twenty-eight and sick, so it was very hard to look at him for too long.

The gall bladder is involved in processing fat. It stores bile from the liver, which is the body's primary means of breaking down fat during digestion. And while it is impossible to know what caused his particular infection, the fact that he was morbidly obese and consumed absolutely stunning amounts of fats, at the very least, could not have helped things.

A week later, when he was back home, deposited on his comfy chair in front of the television, basically intact, albeit slightly paler and with a grotesque little drip bag plugging through his skin to collect fluids his body could no longer process, I took him aside. It was something I was thinking a lot about.

"Would you ever be interested in coming to yoga with me? Might help get you back on your feet."

Sol sat there thinking. I felt like I had just proposed to him.

"You know," I continued. "I'm working on this book, and I'm hearing a lot of amazing things."

He shook his head and said, "Me, yoga? You gotta be kidding me." And then to my eternal surprise, "Why not?"

There were a few problems with this: One, Sol was lazy. Two, Sol hated pain. Three, Sol worked a lot.

Four, one or two yoga classes wouldn't do anything for Sol. He was in deep.

But it was worth a shot. Any sustained form of exercise would be good for Sol at this point. And we had one really big asset on our side: Sol practically lived on top of a Bikram studio. It was literally a thirty-second commute door to hot room.

With that in mind, we created a schedule for sixty days of yoga over approximately two months. It would start after his recovery was complete, after the little bag of drippings had been removed and the incision healed up. Each week, Sol would do six days in a row and then have a rest day. He wouldn't change anything else about his life. He would eat the same, drink the same. Just add ninety minutes of bending first thing in the morning.

The reason we decided to keep diet and beer the same was not some misguided attempt to make this a scientifically controlled experiment. That would be folly. Sol was one big man, not a cohort. We left diet the same because the one thing I did not want was for Sol to attempt to radically transform his life in one heroic shot.

When a dedicated fatty goes on a health kick, odd things happen: Headbands come out. Short walks turn into impromptu jogs. Vitamins get popped. Whole bottles of soda find their way down the drain. At first, in all these little things there is a mini–snowball effect. The fatty starts feeling good! Health breeds health, he hums to himself, having figured it all out. And suddenly abstaining from little poisons like a doughnut in the morning or three Skittles proffered by a coworker seems like the easiest thing in the world. In fact, during a health kick, something like a doughnut starts to feel crazy. As in, why on earth would anyone every want something like a doughnut? Are we all mad?

But then almost invisibly it all starts creeping backwards. First there is complacency based on the modest success. Then complacency gets replaced by frustration. Hormones out of whack from years of poor eating are screaming biologically misguided messages to eat. Eventually the fatty fudges, perhaps literally, perhaps just a bit. But if the fudge is big enough and progress lost sad enough, hopelessness takes over. Suddenly little poisons like doughnuts are basically the only things that make sense. At least they taste good! At least they stop the feeling that I'm starving myself! And finally, the fatty ends up fatter than ever and more demoralized.

I knew all about this from personal experience, and this was exactly what I didn't want to happen. I knew the yoga was powerful stuff and I knew if he actually went through with it, there would be a ripple effect on his lifestyle. But I did not want Sol to think about that. I didn't want him wasting precious willpower abstaining from a burger or worrying about a beer. If he really got hooked, that stuff would work itself out regardless.

As motivation, I decided to take class alongside him. The trip to his studio from my apartment was about an hour. That meant if Sol skipped class, he was essentially standing me up and would hopefully feel tons of guilt. Which was perfect, as far as I was concerned.

The project built from there. We stayed up late, discussing hydration strategies. I explained the cycle of pain he was likely to face. I told him in advance which parts of his body would hurt like a muscle ache and which parts of his body would hurt like he had done something so bad, he should see a doctor. I asked Esak for advice, and his one-sentence response became our mantra: "Take it easy once there, but get there every day." We decided to spread out in class, so we could both pretend the other wasn't there. We made vows never to leave the room, no matter how much it hurt. Then we got the rest of our friends involved.

The key to the effort was sustainability. The more people who knew, the more people invested, the less Sol would be tempted to cheat. I created a spreadsheet, and friends of ours volunteered to come and bend for a week with Sol and me. They were our pit crew, an unexpected face in the locker room, ready to give support to help turn this life around. As word got out, the weeks filled up. We had friends coming in from out of town, we had friends volunteer who swore up and down that yoga was for sissies. There was great momentum. Everyone was excited.

Everyone, that is, except Ashley. She knew her husband. And she knew all about Hector's stroke and why exactly I was writing the book. The night before the sixty days were about to kick off, she called me around midnight.

"Look, this is great. And I am behind it one hundred percent if it's going to help Sol. But I want you to be careful." There was genuine fear in her voice. "First, I want you to promise to stay nearby after class. He can barely make it up the stairs without resting. I don't want Sol coming out of class so exhausted he slips and hits his head on the curb or passes out with nobody around. Second, I want you to know I'm going to pull the plug on this if it gets too extreme. Do not kill my husband with your fucking yoga."

PART III

Not Dead Yet!

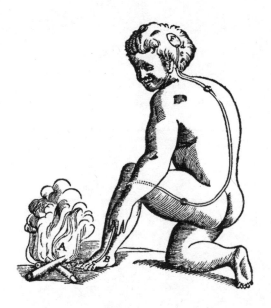

Descartes's Pain Pathway

If we take man as he really is, we make him worse. But if we overestimate
him . . . If we seem to be idealist and overrate him, and look him at
high . . . You know what happens? We promote him to what he really can
be. So we have to be idealists in a way, because only then do we wind up as
true realists.

—VIKTOR FRANKL

Mary

I will forever think of Mary Jarvis as a blessed human for this: ripping
apart her nori-wrapped vegan burrito and smuggling the contents onto
my plate. "Shhhhhh, don't say anything, just take," she says, and hands me
a clump of the burrito's raw squash and fermented cabbage innards. "If I
don't like, I'm passing to you." I shovel her offerings into my face as quickly
as they come, careful not to let anyone see. Mary, I think, is being secretive
because she is being polite to our hosts. I, on the other hand, am merely
worried other people might find out there is more food available and ask
me to share.

I have briefly joined another two-week Backbending session, eager for
the opportunity to meet up with Mary, and after only one day, I am delirious
for calories. Somehow Esak has convinced the owners of a local raw restaurant to cook us a group dinner "as service," and out of the kindness of their
raw little hearts, they have obliged him. Like most things during Backbending, I don't know exactly how or why this is happening. It both makes sense
(raw, vegan, altruism) and is totally inexplicable (service to self-indulging

yogis? in the form of food that is essentially noncaloric?) But either way, after ten hours of yoga, we arrive en masse at their adorable sunflower-covered café to sit down for our first meal of the day. Sweaty. Aching. Bewildered. And, in typical Backbender fashion, bursting at the eyeballs with energy.

The energy radiating out of their bodies is almost oppressive. I feel like a grumpy grown-up being assaulted by a six-year-old with a camera. All around me, human flashbulbs are popping. As soon as we get settled—introductions and thank-yous made—the restaurant fills with the chattering, laughing gossip of a high school cafeteria. It's hard to reconcile the giggling with the fact that just an hour ago, the same group of humans worked themselves to a point of absolutely depletion. Sweating and crying and struggling to keep their knees from crashing into the carpet.

I, unfortunately, am still depleted. And as each course comes out, tiny, delicate, and looking far more ornamental than culinary, I start freaking out. We get kale leaves folded like gluten-free origami, then a half cup of cashew soup, then a single cigar-sized roll labeled "burrito" by the waitress. While everyone else is praising the nuances of flavor and freshness, I am gauging whether or not I can fit the entire meal in my mouth at the same time. This is my first raw experience, and while I am finding the meal delicious, I have no idea if that has anything to do with the food. Spam's delicious if you've been hiking all day.

And so Mary Jarvis will forever be sacred to me. While I am self-digesting and desperate, while everyone else around me is rejoicing at their prissy bounty, Mary is taking her big fingers and ripping apart her highly nuanced food to give me the morsels she doesn't care for.

Mary is one of Bikram's most senior teachers. She attended his first official training program, received his wisdom back when he was dispensing it one on one. On top of that, depending on whom you ask, she is also: a bona fide saint, a healer, a scientist of compassion, a slut, and/or "a really pushy bitch." Those last two were Mary, by the way, appreciating Mary.

Young Mary was a lioness: blond, strong, and lean. She started taking yoga classes with Bikram beginning in 1984, before his formal training program. "There was no brand back then. There was no hot yoga," she says.

"Now, it's so weird—people talk about Bikram like it's different, like it's a brand like Kleenex or Xerox. Back then, it was just yoga.

"Everyone was family. We just hung out and practiced. Nobody really knew anything—it was just fun and you felt better. And then every once in a while, Bikram would come by with this enormous surge of energy, and he would sit and talk yoga for eight hours. . . . He had this incredible message to deliver and couldn't rest until he had passed it on. Believe it or not, he talks less now. At this point, he doesn't have to convince anyone."

During that period, she remembers "one, maaaaybe two compliments" buried in between far more insults, admonishments, challenges, and lectures on her deficiencies. "If you want to understand one thing about Bikram, understand this: He is the standard bearer," she says. "He will always be out there holding higher expectations for you than you hold yourself." That was how she learned her postures, and that is how she decided to teach.

As a result, Mary knows the physical aspect of the yoga with an intimacy very few senior teachers can match. If you want to perfect your practice as it exists, there are many teachers who can correct your technique. If you want to push your practice further, become the type of yogi you never thought you could become, then Mary is the person to see. She has been there, and she has trained others.

Which is why eight years ago, when Esak began to train for the competition, he sought Mary out.

"Esak asked Bikram what he should do to prepare for the competition," Mary tells me. "Bikram thought about it and said, 'Mary. You want to be champion, go see Mary.'"

Which was a huge disappointment to Esak. He didn't know Mary, he didn't live near Mary, and he didn't love the idea of being coached by an older woman. But he dutifully followed Bikram's advice and showed up at Mary's studio, hoping to convince her to let him apprentice with her.

"He was so cocky back then," Mary says. "All the girls adored him. Everyone was telling him how good he was. I just remember thinking, 'Jesus'— and he had Jesus-length hair back then, by the way—'who does this guy think he is?'"

Meanwhile, Esak remembers wowing her. "I was in class, going into Standing Bow, just really feeling great, kicking into it. And I knew she was watching. And sure enough, she opened her mouth and—"

Mary cuts him off. "—I said, 'Esak, that is the worst Standing Bow I have seen.' And it was! He was totally crooked, but you know, everyone had been telling him how great he was."

Esak stuck around and listened. "He did everything I asked. Never complained once. And he worked hard. I knew he was in pain."

"Oh, yeah," Esak says, smiling. "I thought I did permanent damage to my back. It hurt so bad. I remember walking just dumbfounded that I could have let myself do this to my body."

If young Mary was a lioness, old Mary is more of a fairy godmother.

Her home studio, Global Yoga in San Francisco, is a shrine to her twin principles as coach: exacting technique and motivation. The walls are covered like a crazed yoga scrapbook with images of flawless postures, news clippings of incredible human achievement, and weird homemade banners with slogans like 202 CLASSES IN 101 YOGA DAYS! The postures and pictures are often labeled like *Monday Night Football,* with arrows and circles, indicating vectors of force and areas of muscular contraction.

Compared to many of the newer studios, Global Yoga is unique. It sweats to the heat of its own furnace, as it were. There is a bathroom in the hot room. The studio might have a shower, but I couldn't find it. There are no lockers in the locker room. And Mary doesn't sell water. Which, for a hot yoga studio, is like a movie theater not selling popcorn.

I imagine the decision probably does similar things to her revenue stream. When I ask Mary about it, her answer is quick.

"Don't need it. Not in class. It'll sit in your stomach like a pastrami sandwich. Have a green juice instead. . . . And drink it later, when you're not practicing something that requires stillness."

Mary sits behind the desk at her school, elbow deep in the worn-out index cards she keeps student information on. It's a precomputer holdover, hopelessly more complicated than necessary, the type of system that in Mary's hands ends up both creating debates over whether a student's package has run out of classes and then instantly resolving those debates by her offering a free class.

"Just come today," she says. "We'll figure it out next time. . . . Love you."

Mary's use of the L-word falls just short of the pathological. Students are greeted with it when they walk in and then universally a second time when they stagger past her desk on the way out. Old students whose names she has long forgotten get it when they stop by to say hi, strangers on the street get it if Mary notices them doing something nice to someone else. Often the exchange is initiated by the student: "I love you, Mary." If you get missed, it's only because there was a more substantial conversation taking place. This is the exact polar opposite of the corporate *buh-byes* and service thank-yous we've become culturally inoculated against; each "I love you" from Mary sounds unique and sincere; it is no doubt a practiced art. Mary pauses and smiles, and you can feel the statement build in her smile. Standing next to her, as a mere mortal who has trouble signing emails to his parents with the word *love,* it is also bewildering.

There is a point in every Mary Jarvis seminar, after everyone is good and tuckered out from the yoga, sitting on their mats, sipping on coconut waters and other restorative concoctions, when Mary brings out the pictures. These are pictures of practitioners in their prime, practitioners she coached personally, in postures everyone admires but can't quite imagine themselves embodying. She takes each picture out of a folder carefully, admiring it as she tapes it against the mirror. When she is finished, she pauses for a minute to take them all in.

"No matter what, I always start by thanking Bikram." She pulls out a final picture and puts it up in the lower corner.

This is a picture of a young Indian man in a baseball cap and sparkling black and red T-shirt. He is staring away, looking carefree in the way a boy running out of the house to meet up with his friends is carefree.

Mary paws the picture. "So thank you, Bikram. Thank you for coming to America, thank you for bringing this yoga. Without Bikram, there would be none of this."

Then she looks away for a moment. "Some people confuse this by thinking you need to always be near him. They think that surrounding him makes them important yogis."

She looks back at us and laughs. "I like to have Bikram near, but not too near."

Where does Mary's faith come from?

It's simple. If young Mary was a lioness, in 1994 that lioness got T-boned by a driver running a red light and almost died. She remembers the moment as unusually quiet. She was stopped at a red light. When the light turned green, she drove forward. And then was lifted. The cab beside her just disappeared from her peripheral vision. Her last concrete memory was thinking, *That's so weird—where'd the cab go?*

She landed in chronic pain. Her spine was badly damaged, her vertebral discs herniated. She couldn't lift her arms above her head. Her surgeon warned her against physical exercise and prescribed a battery of painkillers. Mary, trying to avoid an invasive surgery, dutifully followed his recommendation and stayed in bed.

The result of the medication and the decreased ability to move was depression. At the time, Mary owned a chocolate factory just outside of San Francisco. "I had a storage closet that I turned into a cave; it had a cot, a futon. . . . The pain was so great, the fatigue was so great, I just hibernated. . . . I would wake up in the darkness of that little room, and everyone else would be gone for the day. They would close up the whole shop for me. Other times, I would walk out blinking, and it was almost a joke because everyone else would have to tell me the time of day."

The problem was it wasn't a joke. If Mary hadn't owned the factory, she would have been fired. Miserable, she scheduled another appointment with her doctor to go over options.

After reviewing Mary's current state, her doctor was adamant. Mary needed surgery. Her doctor explained her spine would continue to deteriorate if left alone. In two years, she might be in a wheelchair. But when Mary asked for details about the surgery, the doctor couldn't give her any answers.

She asked, "Am I going to be pain free?"

The doctor said he was not sure.

She asked, "Will I be able to move the way I did before?"

He said he did not know.

She asked, "Will I be able to stop taking the painkillers?"

He explained he couldn't guarantee it.

And then the doctor stopped the line of questions. He put up a hand. "Look, your back will never be the same." He explained she had been in a life-altering accident and that failure to accept life-altering consequences was denial. When Mary brought up the idea of using the yoga as rehab, he dismissed it. When she persisted, her doctor shuffled around his desktop and handed her a business card for a psychotherapist and suggested she visit. It wasn't the smoothest response in the history of doctor–patient relationships, and suddenly they were in a fight. Mary swore at him. The doctor swore at her. She stormed out of his office.

Alone on the elevator, she began crying. "I kept thinking in my head, 'Mary, what have you done?'" She says, "I was in tremendous pain, and here I went and pissed off one of the few people who could actually help me."

And then, *bing,* the doors opened, and Mary just knew. "I heard my voice tell me, 'Okay, Mary, you're going back to yoga. If it worked so well when you were healthy, why would it desert you now?'"

She had a ten-year knowledge of the yoga at this point. Before the accident, she was a full-fledged Bikram devotee; she haunted her local studio, expected to be the best in every class she took, and sold the yoga's ability to heal to everyone she met. But now she would have to live it. Up to that point, her practice had been entirely based on choice. Now it was based mostly on desperation.

But she did it.

The next day, Mary hobbled into her studio in a neck and back brace and began pouring herself into her practice, taking the beginner class seven days a week. Her postures didn't look anything like the other people in the room. "It wasn't pretty at first," she says. "I would do what I could do." Which at first was basically nothing. It was mental. "Plenty of days early on, I was just locking eyes in the mirror and thinking through the posture." Other days, she could muster maybe a tiny Half Moon, bending barely visibly, feeling enormous waves of pain through her spine. When class was over, she would lie on the floor as the agony crept back in.

"Most of the teachers who were around at this point really didn't understand what I was going through. They thought I was really hurt, not yoga hurt. They would get that nurturing voice you use when talking to dying kids or cute animals: 'Mary, I'm worried about you, Mary, how are you? Are you sure you can do this?'"

But it was working for her. She felt something. "The only time I was pain free that first year was when I was in a yoga class. It was a sign I was on the right track." And so she doubled up on the classes, going twice a day. She also went, as she calls it, "full hermit." Mary explains, "I stopped talking to other teachers. I stopped talking to people who wanted me to doubt." Dealing with the anxiety she was producing in others was almost as difficult as the pain. "Asking me if I am okay fifteen times a day isn't supporting me. Asking me if I'm in pain isn't supporting me. Trust me, I knew I was in pain."

And pain wasn't actually the worst part. The worst part was the nothing. "After the car accident, there would be days when my leg would be paralyzed. I couldn't use it, I couldn't feel it. My left leg would just sit there limp like a tail. Especially when I just woke up."

On those days, she would drag herself around to the side of the bed and hold on to the mattress and lower herself back into a backbend posture called Camel. I can picture Mary there, knees tucked almost as if in prayer, but instead of leaning forward with head tucked, she is slowly lowering herself backwards, arms stretched out in her holy backbend.

"I would hold that posture, desperately grabbing on to the mattress sometimes five minutes."

And from that early-morning bending, she became convinced that backbending was at the core of her healing. "I would be against my bed, hold it and hold it, first there would be a tingle, then the leg would get fuzzy, then there would be a weird stabbing."

In two years, she was doing the full series again. Her postures had returned, even if the pain was still present when she wasn't in them. And her faith returned larger than ever: "Everyone can do this yoga. That's what makes it so awesome. The beginner postures are all so simple, unless you're dead, you can do them."

Pain

I've heard a lot of conflicting things about pain in the yoga world. First there is my almost unconscious YMCA-yoga cultural bias, dreamlike and pervasive, which tells me yoga should above all be relaxing, that all pain is bad, that I should "take it easy, baby." At this point, I can't remember if I ever actually heard this vocalized, or if I just absorbed it during various latte-soaked conversations. Or maybe it's just good old-fashioned nonsadistic common sense. Either way, the notion that "if you hurt in a posture, you are doing it wrong" feels very yoga in the sense of the word that gets confused with yogurt.

Then there are my young beloved Bikram teachers who repeatedly echo their guru in class, conflating pain with authenticity, calmly explaining that a posture "should hurt like hell." These are the wide-eyed and gung-ho. Teachers, often derailed from a primary career by their sudden passion, standing in the back of class, arms conducting up and down as they urge us to push deeper and deeper into the burning sensation. Here pain is validation, a blaring trumpet in my thigh announcing I have hit my edge.

Then there are the older, potentially wiser Bikram teachers, embodied by Emmy. "Most pain is your mind labeling a sensation it never had before," Emmy says. "You need to learn to relabel the agony of stretching into the luxury of release." When I ask about other types of pain, the result of something other than stretching, she looks at me like I am a dolt. "Of course you don't go and hurt yourself. It's a fundamental job of the yogi to learn how to distinguish between different types of pain. The bad ones, you must avoid."

Then there is Esak telling me all pain is a phantom. All pain is in my head. Then there are the advanced practitioners walking around with constant backaches and smiles. Then there is Mary, Esak's coach and mentor, who tells me it is impossible to feel pain in a yoga class if I'm doing it right. Which would make me wonder if I've gone full circle back to the YMCA, except Mary is the person guiding those advanced practitioners into their backaches.

Last there is me in class. Who pretty much listens to everything my teachers tell me, except when I decide it crosses an invisible line, in which case I back off and feel like a wimp.[16]

All of which begs the question, what is pain? Why do we care about it?

This is actually a surprisingly hard question to ask. Mostly because it seems so obvious, it's hard to muster up the necessary faux-naivety to tackle. But also because once we start to look at our expectations closely, we see pretty quickly that they don't line up to our experience at all.

The English word *pain* comes to us from Poena, a dominatrix goddess responsible for vengeance and atonement. Perpetually depicted by the Ancient Greeks in modern-day dungeon gear (maiden's skirt, lace-up boots, and "coils of jangling chains"), Poena brought the pain. Literally. To be visited by Poena was to pay a price for something you deserved. It turns out etymologically *pay* and *pain* are more than just sound-alikes. To the Ancient Greeks, pain was revenge the person deserved. It was their receipt. This is a sense that my vertebrae highly commend during Backbending.

In many ways, because we are better acquainted with ego than with compassion, we have just barely outgrown that notion of pain. When we look at people in pain, especially ourselves, we have to fight to get to empathy. It may not be pretty to acknowledge, and it certainly is not universal or unrelenting, but lots of times our gut reaction to pain is an expectation that the recipient is somehow weak or deserving.

The extent we have outgrown this notion is limited to the extent that in our own lives and own skins, we've connected Poena to Trauma.

Trauma is of course why, when we're not in pain, most of can say something like: Pain is helpful. Pain warns and teaches, steering us away from scalding liquids and against our macho-judgment toward our doctor's of-

---

[16] And then there is Bikram himself. Who says: "People come to me and think yoga is relax. They think little flower, little ting sound, some chanting, hanging crystal. . . . No! Not for you! Waste of time! Here I chop off your dick and play Ping-Pong with your balls. You know Ping-Pong? That is yoga!"

fice. Even in its more bratty forms involving knees against coffee tables, pain awakens us, pulls us into present focus. In the larger spiritual sense, this is why the great religious seeker and children's book author C. S. Lewis called it "God's megaphone." Pain has a unique ability to pull lives otherwise too busy to stop, out of their banality, toward their great cosmic humility.

As such, unlike any of our other sensations, pain operates both inside and outside of us. It is separate but apart, of us but against us.

This dualism is pain's most essential quality to a yogi: It exists without integration. In this way, pain is unique as a sensation, sharing far more with our more unsettling appetites: sex, hunger, and sleep. It is modular, functioning parallel to our sense of self. Like a weather system in the environment we inhabit, like an ill-fitting pair of shoes, pain is definitional to our experience—demanding adjustment, but never integrated.

Listen to neurosurgeon Frank Vertosick Jr. talk about pain. A dyed-in-the-wool materialist, so phobic of anything resembling the mystical slash nontraditional that he snarks about visiting chiropractors and acupuncturists only "under assumed names, of course," Vertosick suddenly joins the Age of Aquarius when discussing pain: "When I'm alone with a chronic pain patient, it feels as though three entities are in the room: the patient, the pain, and me. So palpable is the pain, even to an outsider, that it becomes another living creature to deal with, not a disease to be treated but a conscious demon to be exorcised."

With the right pain, we all become junkies striding down the corridor, observers of our actions, just removed enough not to stop them.

Writing in 1664, Descartes encapsulated what, for many of us, still feels like an accurate explanation of physical pain: the Pain Pathway. In Descartes's theory, an injury is received at the tissue, then "passes along a delicate internal thread" until it reaches the brain, whereby the mind produces the sensation of pain. Think tin-can telephone. Like Newton with his apple, this theory was the result of an insight Descartes had outside the laboratory, while walking in a trick sculpture garden. He stepped on a tile in the floor and suddenly water squirted out of a statue into his eye. He stepped again and it came to him again: cause, hydraulic pathway, effect. Or in the human body: we get injured—cut, burnt, or bruised—a message is pumped along our nerves to our brain. Then we squirt out a curse word like the water from the statue. In his later writings, Descartes likened the sequence of events to pulling a rope to ring a church bell. The harder you pull, the louder the bell clangs.

Given how closely this explanation reconciles with our common sense, it is difficult to express how radical these ideas were in their time. Up until Descartes, descriptions of the senses, including pain, were left to the philosophers and poets. Scientists and doctors were still uncovering details of the physical anatomy, and not yet ready to tackle phenomena that couldn't be labeled or measured. This gap between poetic theory and scientific practice was not fun if you were a patient. In Italy, for instance, in order to silence "the pain energies," it was common practice to prepare a patient for surgery by placing a wooden bowl over his head and hammering on it until the patient passed out.

Descartes's insight changed that. If pain was essentially physical, it could be connected to anatomy and studied. For the next three and a half centuries, the scientific community was dominated by experiments doing just that. Researchers classified pains based on the subject's description of the experience (sensory—*sharp, stinging;* affective—*draining, annoying*), based on the quality of the insult (thermal, mechanical, chemical), the duration (acute, chronic), and region of the body (head, shoulders, knees, and toes). They then steadily connected these classifications to objective structures within the body.

By the twentieth century, specific pain receptors called nociceptors were found. Just as taste buds are specialized to detect a distinct flavor, these receptors fired only in the presence of a distinct type of pain. When activated, they sent electrical energy up the nerve to the brain. Using tiny probes, researchers found that firing a single nociceptor, like a tiny tug on the rope, wouldn't generate much of a response in the brain. But when hundreds of receptors were fired at once, as in the smashing of a toe, the bell in the brain would start to ring.

Three and a half centuries later, this basic Cartesian description still dominates how we treat pain. From mothers on the playground to doctors in the ER, if someone runs up to us in pain, we immediately and reflexively search for a source. If we notice a twinge in our thigh when stretching, we scan back in our memories, searching for a moment we might have pulled something. A feeling of pain always results in a search for the injury pulling the bell.

But pain is tricky. And although the dominant Cartesian description may be helpful, it is decidedly inaccurate. This became apparent even in the early days of pain research to those who were watching. Researchers noted a "volunteer effect" in their pain labs, whereby first-time volunteers who were asked to undergo a procedure (like a precise shock to their fingers) reported experiencing a higher level of pain than the subjects who had volunteered many times before. Similarly, in experiments where subjects were lucky enough to self-administer pain, they ended up demonstrating a far higher pain tolerance than those where the patient sat passively watching as someone else ratcheted up their dose.

But these observational asides didn't make much of an imprint. After all, the actual results of the experiments all still supported the Cartesian hypothesis. It wasn't until scientists stepped out of the laboratory and began studying what the pain response looked like in practice that the metaphorical rope began to fray and its bell began to crack.

Consider, for example, the fifty-two-year-old machine shop foreman cited by Ronald Melzack and Partick David Wall in their study of pain in a Canadian emergency room. A piece of heavy machinery had collapsed in his shop and landed on his boot, severing the entire front half of his foot. The wound was gruesome; his toes were gone, the remainder of his foot mangled. A Cartesian would expect every nociceptor in the neighborhood to be ringing its corresponding bell at top volume. Yet, when asked by the attending physician whether he would like anesthesia, the foreman demurred, stating he was in no pain. In the words of Wall, the foreman with his mashed foot "was coherent, sad, and thoughtful." Instead of moaning or complaining, he would softly murmur regrets like "What a fool they will think I am to let this happen" and "There goes my holiday." The only time pain did come up was when the foreman complained about a small pain in his *uninjured leg,* which he hoped would go away with a light massage.[17]

What makes the foreman interesting is that his reaction, while certainly unexpected, is not some freakish exception. In fact, Melzack and Wall were conducting research in that ER precisely because of a previous observation indicating that the foreman's reactions might actually have been normal.

This was the experience of Dr. Henry Beecher during World War II. Dr. Beecher was manning a care unit one station removed from the front lines. The men he received had devastating injuries—bones shattered by gunshot, limbs torn free from explosions—and with their survival in question, Dr. Beecher's first instinct was humanitarian: to ask these soldiers if they were suffering pain and determine whether they required anesthesia. During the frenzy of triage, he was surprised by how many men calmly rejected his offer. But when he looked back over his notes, he became astonished. Almost 70 percent of the severely traumatized soldiers had rejected his offer of anesthesia, describing themselves as feeling only slight pain at the sight of their massive wounds.

Weirder, Beecher remembered many of these soldiers wincing, yelping, and cringing when he approached them to insert intravenous needles to supply fluids.

The image of a solider with his leg blown off wincing as he was approached with a tiny needle stayed with Beecher after he returned to civilian life. And together with Melzack and Wall, he ushered in a new theory that changed the course of pain research.

The new theory, known as the gate control theory, proposed pain, as it travels up the rope to the bell, hits a checkpoint (or gate), which acts a bit like a Ma Bell operator in the spinal cord. At this checkpoint, the pain signal is evaluated. Depending on the circumstances, it is allowed to progress upward intact, dialed up (as in an extremely powerful reaction to an unexpected paper cut), dialed down (as in our stoic wartime heroes), or stopped completely. Even more fascinating, when researchers began looking for the

---

[17] It did!

physiological mechanisms behind the gate control theory, it turned out there was a host of signals traveling *down* to the checkpoint from the brain. Meaning the decision to allow a pain to progress upward is active: as if the brain can tell the Ma Bell operator which calls to let through. Factors such as emotions, memories, beliefs, mental suggestions are all channeled to the checkpoint, mediating our experience of pain. Finally and most important— actually overthrowing the gate control theory itself—researchers discovered there are pains that exist *only* in the brain. Phantoms. Bells that ring without a rope being pulled. Neural routines that misfire.

In this new era, instead of a straightforward transmission—from injury to rope to bell—pain exists on a continuum. On one extreme, there are classic Cartesian pains tied directly to an injury; on the other end, there is the entirely psychogenic pain that lives in the brain, disconnected from any physical injury. And in the vast blurry middle where we spend most of our lives, we have pains mediated by factors in both directions: connected to the flesh but controlled by the brain.

In this context, the pain-aware yoga of Backbending no longer seems an unreasonable method of retraining the mind. Might the repetitive deep spinal bends provide an opportunity to explore pain perception? Might the overwhelming—but voluntary—pain rewire otherwise damaged neural pathways?

It's not as crazy as you might think.

One of the extremely helpful qualities of neural networks is that they get stronger the more often they are activated. This efficiency through repetition is one of the reasons a black belt in karate or a concert pianist has such blinding speed where the rest of us experience routine clumsiness: Their motor neurons have practiced the same sequence so many times, the paths have become etched into their brains. Or as the neurological ditty goes: "Neurons that fire together, wire together."

The same understanding means that the longer the pain pathways relay messages, the more efficient those pathways become. In chronic pain patients, this means greater pain is transmitted quicker and deeper into the spinal cord the longer the pathways are activated.

It also explains why hanging out in a deep backbend, focusing on exploring and observing those pain pathways, might weaken those connections. In a backbend, the pain is initially intense, but you learn to actively move that focus elsewhere. You start down one pain pathway, but then divert those neurons elsewhere. You pull the rope, watch it travel to the checkpoint, and then practice reconnecting it elsewhere. You take ownership over Ma Bell: from stabbing burn to deep breathing.

Five years after Mary's desperate self-experiments at home, in 1999, the Physicians Neck & Back Clinic in Minnesota began thinking along similar lines. The clinic conducted a study in which sixty patients whose doctors had recommended back surgery delayed the surgery to first participate in a ten-week program focused on strengthening the key muscles that support the spine. Of the forty-six members who completed the study, only three decided to continue with the surgery; the rest were able to significantly reduce their pain. Within the world of rehab, the results were exceptional.

But that was because the Physicians Neck & Back Clinic in Minnesota was pioneering a new type of rehab. When I talk to Dr. Brian Nelson, founder and medical director of the Physicians Neck & Back Clinic, he speaks of four ways the clinic bucked the conventional wisdom in back pain. Each resonated with a lesson I'd learned from the yoga.

First, they avoided surgery. "We found that 85 percent of the time, we couldn't determine the exact cause of pain," Dr. Nelson tells me. "Yes, a CT scan will show areas of abnormality in patients. And lots of doctors will interpret those abnormalities as the cause of the pain. But when you look at the CT scans of patients without injury, people who have no back pain, they will often show identical types of abnormalities." And because the clinic couldn't link the pain to a discrete injury, they believed surgery should be a last resort rather than a default option.

Second, they believed in a different kind of rehab. "We believe in an intensive rehab. You need to overload the muscle, work it to failure," Dr. Nelson explains. "At failure, there are neural muscular channels that get activated, the muscle adapts. The patient will experience soreness and may believe that is damage . . . but it also promotes healing." This was a big departure from the prevailing wisdom of the time, which essentially taught patients in pain to take it easy.

Third, to complement the intensity, they believed in precision. "Chronic back pain typically involves the weakening in very specific muscle groups. These can be very difficult to isolate because many other muscle groups protect them." To target these muscles, very carefully prescribed strengthening exercises were needed. At the Physicians Neck & Back Clinic, these are done using precisely adjusted Nautilus machines rather than precise alignments prescribed by an expert teacher/guru, but both the principle and the muscles involved are strikingly similar. "It turns out that by avoiding those muscles—which often can be quite painful to exercise—the muscles atrophy. You get patients who are extremely good at compensating, but are in actuality making their recovery more difficult," Dr. Nelson says.

Finally, they accepted that to complete these exercises, patients would experience pain, even deep pain. "One hundred years from now, they are going to laugh at how we understand pain," Dr. Nelson tells me. "Pain actually changes the pain. The perception, the experience of pain, alters the way the brain reacts to the pain. Patients need to be retrained so that hurt does not equal harm." In many cases, even if a patient's back pain originally sprang from a physical cause, the pain signals became lodged in the higher recess of the central nervous system. The Cartesian bell was ringing out of control regardless of rope. In these cases, spinal surgeries devoted to burning nerves or fusing discs were futile. To dislodge the pain, nerve fibers need to be "reeducated." "We've found that trying to live without back pain is exactly the wrong idea. Patients need to see that this pain—precisely delivered to the correct muscles—is a good thing. It changes the way they perceive all pain," Dr. Nelson tells me. "You can see this effect on an fMRI, by the way. You can see the parts of the brain light up handling the pain, and you can see that explaining the significance of pain shifts the parts of the brain lighting up."

Listening to Dr. Nelson discuss the chemistry of a vertebral disc produces another lightbulb. "The disc," he explains, "is living tissue, but it has almost no blood supply." This lack of blood flow means that getting nutrients and healing agents into it, especially when damaged, can be very difficult for the body. Instead the body relies on relatively huge blood flow to the vertebral body located directly above and below the disc. Nutrients circulating in the vertebral body diffuse through to the disc itself. When the muscles of the back atrophy, the discs compress down, reducing diffusion even further, making it even more difficult for nutrients to penetrate and for the damaged disc to repair itself.

And what enhances diffusion? The backbend! "Backward bending creates a huge pressure differential," Dr. Nelson tells me, "which has a corresponding huge positive effect on diffusion. It gives nutrients a chance to slip in there." Not surprisingly, the deeper the backbend, the larger the pressure differential. I find it impossible not to think of Mary gingerly placing herself into a backbend off the corner of her bed, her body sensing that it was doing something necessary. "In fact," Dr. Nelson tells me, "backward bending and forward bending are probably the only ways we know of to increase diffusion to the disc."

And the Rest Is Reefer Madness

Descartes's interest in the pathways of the body was actually only a side project in a larger obsession. Descartes was intent on solving the problem of dualism. Dualism in Western philosophy asks us to reconcile the idea that man occupies both a spiritual and a physical place on the planet. By tracing the physical pathways of pain, Descartes hoped to find the intersection point where they mediated with the soul. In this way, Descartes was on a very similar quest to that of our sages from the Vedas. Yoga is after all concerned with the yoking between man's primary dualities: the immediate physical reality of his senses and the expansive immortal reality of the universe.

And although dualism has never been terribly successful in locating a plausible gateway for the soul in the physical body,[18] thinking about pain provides another, slightly more materialistic way to think about this union. Yoga

---

[18]Descartes ended with somewhat comical precision, pinpointing the location of the soul in the pineal gland.

can be seen as an attempt to unify the rope and bell. To create a consciousness that is not divided with one part located in the raw material world of our surroundings and one part located in the messy interior world of our brains.

Instead of pain being some exceptional outlier, the more modern neuroscience probes the workings of the brain, the more it appears all perception operates within the anti–Cartesian principles of pain and the gate control theory: *Our reality is created by the brain as much as it is perceived by the brain.* Vision, our bedrock sense, can be lost to people with perfectly functional eyes, or deconstructed so that patients lose isolated aspects: Men and women who are suddenly without the ability to sense motion, recognize a particular shape, or see texture. Perception of our body parts can be altered, famously in disorders like phantom limb syndrome, where amputees continue to feel sensation from appendages that no longer exist, or more wildly in disorders like Apotemnophilia where people with perfectly functioning limbs suddenly disown them, fail to recognize them as their own, or become filled with an intense desire for amputation. Our most private intense sensations like orgasm can be stimulated without pleasure during seizures, or on the flipside, generated without any physical stimulation, by thought alone. Even belief itself—spirituality—can be elicited in atheists by stimulating specific areas of the left prefrontal cortex. The more we learn, the more it appears our experience of the world is built out of fragments cobbled together like a tile mosaic, our consciousness only an interpretation, minimally corresponding to the stimulus external to our brains.

The result is disquieting. Neuroscientist V. S. Ramachandran talks about the essential dilemma this dichotomy produces in his patients. "Science tells us we are merely beasts, but we don't feel like that. We feel like angels trapped inside the bodies of beasts, forever craving transcendence." Yoga offers an essentially secular materialistic pathway to stitching together this divide. By acknowledging and indulging in the sensations that line the edge, it gives us an opportunity to practice regulating the more bestial aspects of ourselves while also recognizing those areas beyond our control. It is a physiological serenity prayer.

Jill Bolte Taylor took a decidedly less pleasurable route to this same realization. At thirty-seven, she experienced a massive stroke effectively wiping out most of the characteristics we ascribe to self, including the ability to read, write, walk, talk, process emotions, or recall memories. In her book *Stroke of Insight,* she details the opportunity her recovery gave her:

> *The number one question that I am most frequently asked is, "How long did it take you to recover?" My standard response, and I don't mean to be trite, is, "Recover what?" If we define recovery as regaining access to old programs, then I am only partially recovered. I have been very fussy this time around about which emotional programs I am interested in retaining and which ones I have no interest in giving voice to again (impatience, criticism, unkindness). What a wonderful gift this stroke has been in permitting me to pick and choose who and how I want to be in the world. Before the stroke, I believed I was a product of this brain and that I had minimal say about how I felt or what I thought. Since the hemorrhage, my eyes have been opened to how much choice I actually have about what goes on between my ears.*

Losing access to the physical qualities hardwired inside her brain empowered her to differentiate and choose between them. This "learning to choose," as Esak calls all yoga, gives us an opportunity to resolve Ramachandran's dilemma: not as angels or as beasts alone, but as unified humans: where instead of feeling trapped by our animal spirits, we pay respect to their hoof stomping, but also understand the power we wield over them.

Back in the Real World

"Actually, I wouldn't be surprised if someday lots of athletes use heat as a training tool," Santiago Lorenzo explains, "just as athletes use altitude training or hypoxic tents now, heat acclimatization could provide a very real edge in the future. A powerful nonchemical way of boosting performance."

It turns out while I was Backbending with Esak and Mary, the Human Physiology Department of the University of Oregon published the first scientific paper demonstrating that the benefits of heat acclimation carry over to a cool environment. Santiago Lorenzo, the lead scientist in the study, is explaining to me the implications. He is excited. Unlike Susan Yeargin, with her background on the sidelines tending to heat stroke victims, Santiago is a former Olympic track and field athlete. He is used to pushing limits, comfortable with punishing workouts.

"We found seven percent increases in performance. Seven percent is a gigantic gain in competitive cycling."

The study examined the performance of twelve trained cyclists after ten days of heat acclimation. The cyclists were tested in both hot and cold environments while their vital signs were measured by a complex rigging that looks something like the cross between a bicycle-powered airplane and an asthma inhaler on steroids. It turns out that compared to matched controls, the cyclists who exercised in heat improved almost every area of their performance in both hot and cold environments. They could go faster, harder, for longer. Just as important, these improvements were mirrored by corresponding changes to the cyclists' physiology: increased blood plasma, increased maximal cardiac output, and increased power output at lactate threshold.

"In many ways, heat acclimatization is more practical than altitude training," Santiago tells me. "And, at least in our study, produced more robust results."

When I tell him about the yoga, it is the first time I don't feel bashful. Indeed, he immediately gets it. "Yes, of course. I certainly don't know anything about yoga, but I can absolutely see it increasing the athletic benefits."

When I ask if the cardiac benefits are real, he is equally adamant. "Of course. You are stressing the cardiovascular system. It doesn't matter if you are using a marathon, a stationary bike, or a yoga pose to get those results."

He also immediately jumps to therapeutic implications. "It's conceivable that this type of training could be used to give cardiovascular benefits to patients who can't otherwise get them. Like patients with paralysis or other injuries that prevent them from exercising. It could give them a way of getting benefits when their bodies otherwise won't allow it.

"Of course," Santiago adds, "you have to be careful extracting too much from one study. Everything we did was in the safety of a lab. To get benefit from heat acclimatization, you need to get your core temperature up. Which obviously carries inherent risk and requires caution."

He's of course right. It's a modest study, in a highly controlled environment, certainly nothing that speaks to mental clarity or improvements to memory. But it's no longer the unstudied area it was when I talked to Susan Yeargin. And hearing Santiago's excitement instantly seals my decision. The researchers at the University of Oregon think they have discovered a radical new therapy for bringing cardiac benefits to the injured, but—just like the pain-conscious rehab pioneered by the Physicians Neck & Back Clinic—it's something Bikram has been doing for the last forty years. Rather than wait for medical science to confirm or deny each aspect of the yoga, I decide it's time to go to the source and see for myself. And so, throwing my common sense—and credit card statements—to the wind, I take a nine-week leave of absence from work and pony up the eleven thousand dollars to register for Bikram Yoga Teacher Training. It's time to bend with the master.

PART IV

Like Kool-Aid for Water

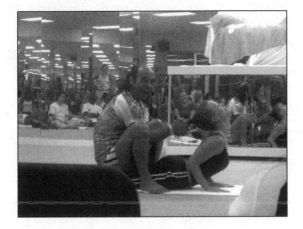

Bikram Choudhury adjusting postures

"We talked of everything," he said, quite transported at the recollection. "I forgot there was such a thing as sleep. The night did not seem to last an hour. Everything! Everything! . . . Of love, too!" "Ah, he talked to you of love?" I said much amused. "It isn't what you think," he cried almost passionately. "It was in general. He made me see things—things."

—JOSEPH CONRAD, *HEART OF DARKNESS*

The Outer Circle

The Fall 2010 Bikram Teacher Training is held on a peculiar belt of aging 1950s resort-hotels circling the I-5 superhighway in San Diego, known collectively as Hotel Circle. I say peculiar but mean wretched. The Hotel Circle concept seems to be the result of some quarantine movement in urban design. We will isolate you from all that is nice about our city, and you will pay extra for the experience because you will be at the mercy of your hotel for all your needs. It is a concept where everyone wins except the guest. Hotel Circle is not even particularly close to the airport. It was just deposited like some giant pile of contractor's excrement along an otherwise unoccupied section of the interstate. The resorts themselves sit recessed from the access road like great concrete castles, all ringed by monstrous unfilled parking lots. There are no shops or restaurants along Hotel Circle Road. There is no nightlife. The ten-minute walk between each hotel says it all. It is a walk marked less by decay than desolation: a space for exactly nobody, built into each hotel's design like a DMZ.

Within this wasteland, we stay at the Town and Country Resort and Convention Center.

Unlike some of the resorts on Hotel Circle, the Town and Country is very definitely a hotel in a senescent state: a few decades past its prime, a little less than one decade ahead of offering an hourly rate. You can still see vestiges of what must have been a proud past—at one point, a family thought it spoke highly enough of them to remark that it was family-run. It is massive in ambition. A tangle of underweeded wending gardens, bungalows, drab conference rooms, shitty chandeliers, and overbleached swimming pools. At this point in its devolution, size is its only draw. If you are trying to host a large group on a bargain basis, overinvite for a wedding/bar mitzvah, the T&C is your place. The staff is unfailingly polite and earnest and looks just similar enough that it makes me wonder how large the original T&C family was and whether or not there was a founder's instinct toward brood. There is an eccentric's whimsy, something of a shuttered carnival: bellhops and room service boys pedal around on bicycle-powered carts, trolley cars zip around carrying luggage with drivers who never miss an opportunity to stick a head out to wave hello. But the eccentricity is mostly obscured by a feeling of drab decay, where every curtain is slightly sun-bleached, every carpet only 80 percent clean, and paint flecks collect in the crevices of every wall.

As time goes on, we will come to know the Town and Country very well. We will know where stray gardeners go to get high. We will know which portraits are repeated in every third room and which ice machines clog when pushed too hard. We will uncover the pattern of the rotating specials at each of the five themed restaurants and coordinate our visits to take advantage. We will learn the life cycle of the hotel's magnetic keys and make friends with the bicycling boys who come to unlock our doors after they demagnetize. There will be mini-wars with the bitchy groundskeepers who complain about yoga mats hanging from the balconies and awkward birthday parties for old Mexican maids who almost assuredly loathe us and our college-dorm attempts at cookery. Nine weeks is way too long to spend at any one hotel. And the T&C is not any one hotel; it is a hotel going through a prolonged, likely terminal, "rough patch." But like an old madam, worn to the point of authenticity, completely self-assured for what she is, the Town and Country actually seems to gain some dignity over our stay. I leave with a grudging respect, somewhat influenced by the fact that upon checking out, I find its aged system for tracking room service charges has awarded me a couple hundred bucks in free meals.

Flexible travel dates and a cheap fare bring me to San Diego a day early, but after investigating the T&C and evaluating its merits, I decide to stay at an adjacent hotel along the circle. So on Day One, I find myself trudging along the otherwise empty Hotel Circle sidewalk to my home for the next nine weeks. When I get to the periphery of the Town and Country, I notice a guy with a huge rolling suitcase and two bursting bags trudging along similarly. One of his bags is full of bottled water; the other contains a juicer. Bingo. When he struggles to lift the suitcase over the curb, I break into a sprint to help him. I want to make friends.

It turns out his name is Daniel, he is from London, he has been here three days, staying, like me, at a hotel on the other side of the circle. We walk slowly across the giant Town and Country parking lot, discussing the unknowns of the next nine weeks. I am enormously relieved to find Daniel sane. One of the first things he tells me is "I don't know why I like this yoga. I can't barely explain why I am here. All I know is it makes me feel great when I do it on a regular day and makes me feel like shit when I do it hungover, which means I don't drink nearly so much anymore. Which is something I really needed to do."

The closer we get to registration, the more potential yogis I see. The men: all thin, gauntly muscular faces, stick arms, thick legs. The women: squeezed into tight jeans or in sundresses, weird webbed tattoos peeking out along shoulders or down arms. Everyone: dragging enormous suitcases, faces a little unsure about the plunge we are about to take, standing surprisingly silent, occasionally making awkward conversation.

Then we are given room keys. Amazingly, and thanks entirely to my impulsive last-minute registration, I am given a double room all to myself. I was the very last person to register for training, and there is no one to pair me off with.

First Principles

Soon after, all 380 of us are gathered together for orientation. Immediately we are told Bikram will not be attending. Immediately, it becomes mind-drubbingly dull. The room, with its plastic chairs, spare decorations, and pull-down PowerPoint screen seems to be channeling a Holiday Inn conference center. Instead of Bikram in the flesh, we have a stage with three cheaply framed portraits wreathed in flowers: one of a young Bikram straddling a skinned tiger; one of his guru, Bishnu Ghosh; and one of his guru's guru, Paramahansa Yogananda.

Our orientation consists of a parade of speakers wearing headset microphones, all slightly bored with the information they are imparting, all pacing before us. We learn the schedule for the next nine weeks, as simple and all-encompassing as basic training: a morning yoga class, an afternoon lecture, an evening yoga class, and then a night lecture. In the cracks, we are responsible for finding food, sleeping, and memorizing the official Bikram Yoga "dialogue"—a forty-five-page transcript of a single Bikram class we have to be able to recite in order to graduate. We learn that under no circumstances are we to leave the hot tent during class. We learn that all Teacher Training staff are unpaid, serving their nine weeks as service to Bikram. We are told repeatedly that the single best thing we can do to enjoy Teacher Training is to hold no expectations.

This extends in particular to Bikram himself. A senior teacher tells us that Bikram, the man, will be unlike anything we have ever seen. He explains that Bikram is "a fully realized human, a true master." A second senior teacher follows that encapsulation by explaining that we can't actually see Bikram at all. "What you see is not Bikram," she says. "It is a mirror." This prompts a third teacher to reverse the whole dynamic, explaining that Bikram will be able to see right through us. "When you stand in front of him, he will read your whole life in an instant. He will see your future and understand your past." This teacher concludes the whole Bikram expectations–visibility discussion by requesting we restrain our curiosities and never approach the guru outside of lecture. "There are three hundred eighty of you and only one of him," he says. "Bikram will try to give, but you will just overwhelm him."

Finally—after a cringe-inducing pep talk where the head of sales at the Town and Country explains to us that we're inspirational—Rajashree, Bikram's wife, gets on the microphone. Just before she takes the stage, several mannequins are placed onstage beside her. These are wearing Bikram-branded yoga shorts and spandex bras. Rajashree's speech includes lots of sensible advice ("This is not the time to experiment with a new diet, not the time to detox") interspersed with Hallmark platitudes ("Here is a tough time, the best time, the time of your life!"). She is an impeccably pleasant-looking woman, unmistakably in middle age, but the type of woman who at first glance you mistake for having arrived there smooth and uncracked by life, and only at later glances, who you recognize is perhaps well cracked, but then caulked up sufficiently tight. Watching her speak, I decide she reminds me very much of another remarkable woman married to a powerful man, Hillary Clinton. It's not just the feeling of a muzzle over her obvious intelligence, but the way it feels like she is submitting to a role—a whole way of presenting herself to the world—that left on her own, she would never seek out, a role that she is also game to make the best of because she understands, however unnatural it comes, she is still better at it than most.

When Rajashree is done speaking, I watch with some horror as she pushes her two teenage children in front of the microphone to say a few words to us. The sense that they are getting groomed for some eventual yoga takeover / succession of the guru throne is undercut by their painfully shy reluctance. I feel an instant almost clairvoyant twinge as to what the Choudhury dining room table is like. As the daughter talks, I notice the son almost visibly shrinking, a cross between a middle school dance recital and one of those old *Mad* magazine cartoons of a human caught under a giant magnifying glass. Relative to every other speaker, it makes me like all three of them a lot. Perhaps because in a room full of posturing, and announcements of fully realized mirrored invisibility, this is finally an interaction I can relate with.

Eventually, Rajashree retakes the microphone and points to the mannequins. "You will be losing weight and gaining weight and so of course need to be buying very stylish clothes," she instructs us. "We will have lots of changing outfits with the best styles and you will have to buy." Then she points to a young male aide-de-camp and explains he will be manning a Bikram-brand shop doing business out of a hotel room. This aide-de-camp, Rajashree informs us, will give "a really honest opinion. Because us girls need honest opinion from boys." At this she laughs a laugh so stilted and awkward and so oddly long that it must be authentic. The audience responds with actual hoots of enthusiasm.

A few more senior teachers rise to re-inforce the no-expectations rule. Finally, we are given a chance to ask questions. A single girl raises her hand. The room goes quiet.

"What if we are going to vomit? Can we leave the yoga room if we are going to vomit? Is that a problem?"

A senior teacher nods seriously. "Excellent question. This will probably happen for a lot of you at some point. Go quickly, come back quickly."

Rajashree chimes in: "Let it happen. Let the process move through your body. Let it attack your mind. . . . You will experience big changes over the next weeks. I am sure in a few days, you will think you have made a terrible mistake."

The next day, sitting packed in the same chairs, I realize I'm way ahead of schedule.

Where yesterday was boredom, today the room is practically exploding with anxiety. The tremulousness in the feet beside me is actually threatening. We are waiting for Bikram. In flesh. Looking down my row, knees are jostling up and down like a player piano. It is an electric contagious antici-pation; I am sure if I had iron filings to sprinkle around the room, they would instantly arrange themselves in field lines.

Listening to the buzz gives me my first sense of how international the yoga is. There are representatives from thirty-three different counties float-ing around with especially large blocs from Australia, Japan, and Mexico. Despite the inability to communicate directly, everyone is smiles and eager eyes, connected to everyone else by a common, almost primal bond. We all get it. Whatever scary, tremulousness-inducing understanding *it* may be. Outside of Las Vegas and maybe the UN, you don't get this wild collection of cultures mushed together by an authentic common purpose.

An aide comes onstage. "Boss will be down in another five minutes." And then, almost before the aide can make it offstage, there he is. Bikram. Bounding into the room with a "Check, check! Check one, two, three, four . . ." coming from his headset microphone. Leaping onstage just as all sound is drowned out by cheers. And we are on our feet in San Diego.

The very first thing I hear when the crowd dies down is: "I want to make you rich!"

Bikram is standing beaming before us. He walks up and down the stage. He smiles, showing every single one of his teeth. "Welcome to . . ." All of a sudden he is blinking helplessly at his staff, a rock star lost on his perpetual tour. "Country, country, town, place, city . . ."

Someone in the audience shouts out, "Town and Country Resort, San Diego!"

Bikram: "All I know is my shower is shitty!"

The room explodes in laughter. Like a bomb of laughter. Like we are projectile vomiting laughter to dislodge a feeling we would otherwise be choking on.

Bikram grows brighter from the laughter. Suddenly he is asking, "Is it hot in here?" and we watch Bikram take his jacket off. "Should I take off more, ladies?" Which he instantly does, revealing a moderately fit brown belly and producing shrieks from the 70 percent female audience (as well as an actual palm-to-forehead from the senior teacher who just yesterday told us Bikram was a mirror).

The rest of the introductory speech is frankly a blur. We learn Bikram's last breakfast was in May of 1964. We learn that just prior to that meal, Bikram taught Pope Paul in India for a month. We learn that although it is not his habit, he slept maybe two hours last night. And that twenty minutes before this very introductory speech, Bikram was in his room fixing the brim of his favorite hat. A factoid that, both in content and delivery, I find very endearing. Bikram drops the hat-brim knowledge on us offhand, as an example of how clever he is for maximizing the time he saves by not sleeping. We learn that his weight almost never fluctuates and that, based on a dog-year-like calculation of Bikram-hours slept relative to normal-person-hours slept minus formative years when Bikram slept like a normal person, that his true age is 220 years old.

All of this is delivered with Bikram bounding around onstage, hopping on his orange throne to crouch for a moment, hopping off, eyes glowing, cackling with laughter. When he is not bounding, he is recovering from bounding, reaching back, hand on hips like a stiff old man. In between the bounding and bracing and sharing factoids about his life, he is flirting with us: picking out people—men and women, the young and the middle-aged—from the audience to tease, to flatter, to shower with special attention.

Bikram concludes his introduction with a series of fist-pumping decla-rations. "Teacher training! Your body! My brain!"

There is one last roar of applause at this, one more time people get on their feet. Bikram stands beaming in the center of the stage. Then we sit. As he walks offstage, headset microphone still on, the audience rapidly fad-ing into a postcoital buzz of side conversation, we hear Bikram one last time: "I did okay?" Then, softer to himself, "Thanks again, everybody." Then, "I think I did okay," before the microphone is finally switched off, and lips still moving, Bikram walks out into the afternoon alone.

You Put Your Hand on Shit Just a Little Bit, It Still Smells like Shit

I return from Bikram's lecture and begin arranging my room for the next nine weeks. Blessed as I am with a single room, I spread out. A little library of books on the dresser, a second library of protein powders on my night-stand, little piles of folded clothes on the bed.

Then I hear a key card fumbling at the door. Then, through the paper-thin walls of the Town and Country, in an accent I will soon recognize as Latvian: "Please excuse me, my English is no good. But I have question for you. Is this how you run hotel? In my country, I think we call this a robbery."

Enter Janis.

Janis is the very last cadet to arrive at teacher training. He arrives without registration. He arrives without a room. He arrives unable to balance on one leg and unaware of what most of the postures are. And most important, he arrives not caring about any of that nonsense.

Janis is here primarily because he made a two thousand-euro bet with a friend that he could lose eight kilos in nine weeks. He tells me he has taken only five or six Bikram classes in his life before now. His son, an elite high school hockey player in Sweden, recommended Bikram to him as the toughest off-season workout he had ever experienced. After taking a class, Janis recognized immediately that it also helped with an old injury of his own.[19] He also tells me he thinks he might open a yoga studio. This urge he cannot explain. He just has a feeling. A woman in Latvia who takes sauna with him has a property that would make a good yoga studio. He trusts her. He wants to open a good business that helps people. He says "good business that helps people" in the way of someone who has maybe opened a few bad businesses that ended up hurting people. The thought had been growing in his brain ever since he took class with his son. Then he finds out there is a training that starts in five days. Then his friend makes him the bet.

So naturally he is here.

We shake hands. I offer him a few nori crisps, which Janis finds delicious. His surprise at enjoying seaweed is palpable. He seizes the entire box and brings it up to his smiling face. As Janis scans over the ingredients list, I tell him that I'm a little tired from my flight and about to go to bed. It's something like 9 P.M. In reality, I'm just disappointed that my paradise of a single room has been violated. But I lie down in bed and close my eyes.

And Janis does what any new roommate would do in this situation.

---

[19] The one area where Janis is equipped to compete with the other trainees: his injury story. In addition to tearing the ACL on his left knee, he shattered his lower leg into four distinct pieces, leaving him with a metal rod running the length of his calf to bind it together while it heals. Doctors told him he would never walk normally again, and indeed, if you know what to stare at, there is a slight limp to his gait.

He sits down on my mattress, high up by the pillows, and starts to show me pictures of his American friends on Facebook. Then he goes over his son's hockey career. Then he announces he is staying only one night and getting a single room for himself.

This is Janis.

I love him. We bond. He never gets the single room. He is a thickly built Latvian: squat body, big weight lifter arms, and a pudgy roll of fat around his waist: essentially the opposite of the lean Bikram-body walking everywhere else. In personality, he is essentially the opposite as well. As might be expected from his impulsive decision to come to TT, Janis does not believe in the yoga. He thinks it's a good workout—but he does not think it is the best. He thinks it helps with his injured leg—but he is not completely sure. Mostly he thinks this will be an adventure. He is thirty-six and retired. He was a lawyer. When the USSR dissolved and Latvia reverted into existence, he discovered and exploited a loophole that allowed him to buy back land that had been appropriated by the communist government. This made him a tremendous amount of money. Then he retired. He loves to push himself. He boxed as a youth and tells me at one point he is always looking for a challenge that matches up to the pre-fight fear. Bikram Yoga fits the bill, and it doesn't hurt that this particular challenge involves being marooned at a hotel with lots of nimble, extraordinarily well-waxed women. It turns out that this type of impulsive inclination toward the extreme marks all his endeavors. He flies helicopters ("Forty hours of training. Almost solo!"); he is taking stunt-driving classes in L.A. ("You learn drift. So *easy*! Maybe we go on Sunday? I pay."); he raced in the Gumball 3000, a multicontinental overland car race. He plays high-stakes poker and won an ATP Poker Tournament. He Jet Skis. He walks around perpetually dripping with electronic accessories and cables, iPad, iPhone, laptop, portable hard drive, several cameras. He is seemingly unconcerned with money, occasionally pulling out big clumps of cash—say five hundred bucks in twenties—from his pockets and depositing them on the nightstand. At first I think this is the product of a foreigner's confusion about currency, a Monopoly money disassociation. But quickly it turns out Janis is merely filthy rich.

The next day he greets me coming out of the shower, explaining: "I think I buy us a scooter. We use for groceries, help get around. Then at end, maybe I can give to you?"

When I shrug and tell him it might be difficult to take the scooter back to New York, he thinks.

"Okay, maybe I give to a friend of mine in L.A.!"

We don't get a scooter. But Janis does promptly rent a car. A cherry red convertible. He puts the keys on my nightstand for safekeeping. "This is good car. Our good car."

Later, especially when Janis discovers that San Diego has a few underground poker clubs, his money habits grow to farce. The drawers of our nightstands will fill with loose cash. I will borrow the car and open the glove compartment looking for the parking validation ticket to find literally thousands of dollars in crumpled hundred-dollar bills shoved in. On more than one occasion, I fish actual spendable large-domination bills out of our trash can.[20] It is educational. It is my first time spending serious time around someone who has an entirely different relationship to money than I do. It is paper to Janis. If it grew on trees, he might afford it more respect. There is something vaguely yogic about it all: just as the old high school trope has communism and fascism looping around into each other, Janis's relationship to money is essentially nonmaterialistic. It doesn't cloud or define his character. He is still needy, petty, generous, and supremely patient. He uses the cherry red convertible to cart people to and from the grocery store like a soccer mom. He buys flowers for the mothers who are away from their families on their birthdays. He picks up the tab for people who are struggling. He asks an endless parade of women if they are interested in coming back to our room to massage him.

But on day one, I don't know any of this. I know he has arrived in San Diego having taken five yoga classes at a training full of people who have been practicing for years. I know he is sweet and loud and excitable. But, with my back still bruised from Backbending, I decide I am more than a

---

[20] When we have guests over to our room, I often find them staring at a single stray hundred-dollar bill Janis has spilled about, engaged in some personal morality struggle. Should they quietly slip it into their pocket? Should they alert Janis? Side benefit: we get exquisite maid service.

little worried about Janis when it comes to classes. It's clear he doesn't know what he's in for.

Training begins the same way it continues for the entire nine weeks. Every morning I wake Janis. And every morning he is first to be dressed and out of the room. While I load up my water bottles, Janis runs out to the elevators and holds the perpetually closing doors for me, yelling "Come on come on come on! Elevator is waiting for you!" I run over and announce that we are late. We ride down in silence and when the doors of the elevator crack open, we smile and say "late, late" to each other, me speaking in the adopted Latvian accent I use to communicate with Janis, and then, together, we force our creaking bones into a slow jog toward the hot tent.

As we pass the other sleepy stragglers, Janis's energy grows, and he's yelling, "Come on! Come on! We late!" sometimes slowing our pace so other people can jog with us, sometimes smacking them with his rolled yoga mat as we pass by. We arrive at the tent just in time for class. We bend. We stagger out. And then I avoid him for my own sanity.

No matter how crippled he looks, no matter how grueling the class, every class ends the same for Janis if I am around. "What you think? Me? *Easy!*"

After class we disappear to separately memorize our dialogue, and we rarely see each other again before the second class.

At night, we sit in lecture listening to Bikram. Afterwards, if the lecture ends early, Janis runs off to go play high-stakes poker. Then he returns with the big wads of cash that he dumps all over our room before crawling under the covers for sleep. Then I wake him up and we do exactly the same thing again and again.

Here Is a Steeple

In San Diego, to accommodate the 380 students, we practice in a giant tent erected in one of the many Town and Country parking lots. It is the chapel of our megachurch.

The tent itself is huge and white, stretched sheets of plastic held erect by massive belts and bands, themselves secured to I-beam-sized tent poles. There are two double-door entrances, each with tiny alcoves for shoes and personal possessions, although after experiencing the crush of 380 bodies bolting for the door after a hot class just once, everyone learns not to bring anything except flip-flops into the alcoves.

When you walk in, especially when the tent is empty, the space is un-expectedly vast and extraterrestrial. Black Astroturf carpeting.[21] Giant plastic tubing running rafterlike across the ceiling. Vast flapping sheets of plastic. And although from the outside, the tent rises at least three stories, inside, a thin plastic ceiling truncates the space, stretching oppressively low over our heads. It is insulation to trap the heat, and it ripples like a low liv-ing sky when the heaters begin to blow.

The front of the room is lined with paneled mirrors, cheaply affixed to plywood frames. The mirrors will steadily warp over the weeks, giving out an increasingly nauseating reflection. A few will fall off completely. The re-sult would be more unsettling, but the truth is that in a room of 380 people, almost nobody can actually see themselves in the mirrors anyway. Rising in the very center, above the paneled mirrors, is the teaching podium. It juts into the front row. And in the very center of the teaching podium, visible from all sides, Bikram's throne.

The throne is befitting only Bikram: lord over this room of plastic and mirrors, prom king of the apocalypse, our very own babbling Lear. The base is a thick black leather sofa chair that looks stolen from a suburban basement. The upholstery long cracked from the humidity and temperature changes, it is accordingly, always draped in several bright orange beach towels. A small table on the right holds a small bowl of hard candy, which Bikram likes to suck on during class to soothe his throat, and a tall glass of water,

---

[21] Made of some highly synthetic material obviously designed to be impervious to bacterial growth despite the epic sweat being deposited on it daily, the carpet is somewhat itchy to look at. Definitely the type of substance that in civilian life I would avoid touching with bare skin out of fear of devel-oping a rash.

which will grow almost erotic at our most desperate points. But the real magic of the throne is above: two ribbed plastic ventilation tubes hang down. They connect to a personal air conditioner, pumping cold air down on Bikram's head as he teaches.

As the tent gets warm in preparation for yoga practice, everyone stands on spots marked by plastic tape. We are packed tight: mat to mat, row to row. To do the postures correctly, you will invade another's space and you will be dripped on. During the later hazier weeks when everyone is operating closer to a point of failure, and bonding under adversity reaches physical proportions, there is lots of touching for support, hand squeezes, toes being tweaked, and water passed from those with excess to those in need.[22] The density on the line is enhanced by several irregularly placed

---

[22]Like everything at TT, water consumption escalates from terrifying into farce and back to terrifying. I start training taking class in proper Esak–Mary Jarvis format, without any water. But classes are indeed hotter than normal, and we are repeatedly told that water is important and we will experience cumulative dehydration without it. So I quickly begin lugging a single bottle. On Rajashree's advice, I add salt, lemon, and honey, making a cheap, unprocessed Gatorade. This is the Eden period of my water consumption. Later, inspired by classmates who are lugging huge four-quart thermoses into class, I graduate to two water bottles. A few weeks later, I break down and buy a thermos of my own. The exhaustion of training builds on itself and the mental strength needed to refrain from guzzling water is one of the first things to go. By the final weeks (sorry, Mary!), I am lugging a four-quart thermos plus original water bottle into each class. Sucking down the entire 4.5 quarts over the ninety minutes. My body at this point is totally fucking confused and betrayed by my behavior: the decision to indulge in plus or minus three hours of extreme heat while also swilling gigantic amounts of water results in cells that are expert at storing any residual hydration. At my maximum, I have fourteen-pound swings in weight loss from a single class. Twice a day. Between classes, when my body goes into storage mode, my fingers start swelling so much, it becomes difficult to make a fist until I've sweated through the first twenty minutes of a class. Still, despite this obviously crazy relationship to water, I am too terrified of dehydration and mentally blahzo to reduce water consumption until I return home. I am not nearly the worst either. Many in my training will cart entire ice chests into class. They become water and ice fairies, offering a handful of melting cubes to anyone nearby and in agony. The first time this happened, I was stunned. It was like cheating. I was totally self-absorbed in my practice. A woman next to me tapped me on the shoulder during the floor series. She dropped a few ice cubes on my chest. They felt like gifts from an icy goddess. I watched her dig back into her cooler and take another handful to give to the person on her other side. Finally, she attended to herself, snapping open her bikini bottoms and shoving a handful of ice in. It being the seventh week of training, this behavior didn't strike me as odd at all. In the "water consumption as metaphor" department, I meet a visiting teacher and studio owner who explains he has trouble opening his eyes if he skips class for two consecutive days: his lids swell shut.

gaps, where no one lays a mat. These are the spots directly underneath the heating vents, where the hot air beats against the skin so harshly, it feels like it may actually cause a burn. Inhaling here, you feel the distinct sensation of nose hairs smoldering. By week four, they become my favorite spots of all: not for the space, nor due to my obvious growing masochism, but because I discover, if you can suffer through the beginning blast, later in class, the mere existence of any airflow against the skin feels downright luxurious.

All lights in the yoga tent lie behind the plastic sheet of the ceiling, giving the interior a soft muted glow.

Sometime, by the middle of class, when the tent has completely warmed and the sweat from the 380 bodies has risen into a dense moist blanket of humidity, when the rushing white noise of the furnaces matches the rushing blood at the ears, there is a moment where all 380 people lie flat on their backs in the tent and tuck their knees into their chests. It is pavanamuktasana, it comes every class, and all 380 of us lie there fetally, following commands that boom down from the speakers above, each a curled dot in the massive room, winding back to an earlier state, another time when we surrendered to the loud incoherent babbling of outside noises while cloaked in heat—but instead of evoking the warm comfort of the womb, lying there, looking up at the oppressively white plastic ceiling, body straining in discomfort, ribbed plastic tubing shooting around the field of vision, sweat running from the corners of the eyes, you feel all the horror of a preemie baby screaming in his bubble.

It is horrible and choking and dystopic and exactly how Bikram wants it.

After all, if you can create peace in the hot tent—if you can locate the grace in your inner preemie baby—you can probably create it anywhere. Or as Biks would say: "I push I push I push I push and then, when you are right up to the edge, half foot on, half foot off, I give you a great big kick and you fly off. . . . But instead of falling, you float. You levitate. You are yogi now."

Things I Learn about Bikram Within the First Three Days of Teacher Training that Will Make the Rest of This Section Make Sense

That Bikram is a man without a vocabulary for moderation. That when he says, "Every yoga in the United States is fake yoga," realize he is also the same man who in the next breath says, "You know the most repulsive creation ever made in the West? That thing called blue cheese dressing." For Bikram, no idea of his is not the greatest, no acquaintance is not "my very best friend," every punch could kill someone, every rich man is a multi-multibillionaire, and any random thought that might come out of his mouth could be "the most brilliant sentence ever created in the English language."

That he will make you believe that charisma is a physical quality of the universe. That it can actually radiate off someone.

That you are not immune to his charms. That's how real charisma works. You may decide you don't like him or that you find him cartoonish and silly, or you may decide you love him and want to run away to join his circus—it doesn't matter. When you are around him and actually experience him, unless you are jaded to the point of a clinical pathology, you will be surprised. Impressed by his variability, aware of his attention to the present moment, his ability to pick up and react to the people around him. He will, in short, undermine your expectations whatever they are and make you curious about what exactly will happen next and then convince you that this quality of curiosity and unpredictability is authenticity.

And that it was none other than Bhagwan Shri Rajneesh, the proudly deviant, ultimately monstrous force of twentieth-century charismatic wisdom, who famously decreed that "authenticity is morality" just prior to diving right off the high board of sanity into the deep end of withdrawn madness, eschewing his life as a yoga guru to become a Valium- and whippet-addicted, ubermaterialistic, sexually abusive fiend slash international bio-terrorist who was exiled from twenty-one countries. And that although nobody except Rajneesh who thinks about the implications of the statement "authenticity is morality" can rationally accept it, it does subconsciously align with our most self-righteous notions of self and is very helpful in understanding why Bikram can appear warped, egotistical, and charming at the same time.

In other words: he's got it figured out for himself (even if that means the rest of us are fucked).

That he does not tolerate the color green in his presence. That he will occasionally recognize that this is illogical and no matter what, never try to defend it, but will, depending on mood, fly into caustic rage if you momentarily forget and accidentally wear green in his presence or bring a green object into a room he is occupying.

That by the end of the third day of Teacher Training, he has announced he "invented the disco ball," "was responsible for launching Michael Jackson's career," "brought Bruce Lee to America," "is number one in the world in hits since the computer started," "cured Janet Reno's Parkinson's," and was "best friends with Elvis."[23]

That he dresses only in complete outfits, never the discrete suburban options I grew up with, whereby pants, shirts, and socks were pulled from separate drawers.

That his sartorial style might best be described as a concerted effort to make disco balls cloth.

That beyond disco ball as cloth, Bikram limits himself to the colors of orange, red, and black. That, without irony, he wears shirts with tigers and flames. That he loves fedoras, pocket hankerchiefs, and wing-tipped shoes.

That, again on the clothing, he never wears anything restrictive enough to prevent immediate removal should an opportunity present itself for him to strip down to brown flesh either to show off the preternaturally preserved condition of his body or to literally give the shirt off his back to a deserving, demanding, or mildly confused man who happens to be standing in a room full of people Bikram wants to impress.

---

[23]In order: nope, nope, nope, nope, tragically nope, and actually, if it was late fat desperate Elvis, and you count spending a lot of time together on the phone as best friends, maybe.

That I have personally stood behind him when he thought he was off-mic and heard him muttering to himself over and over that he is "Bikram, a gangster like Cagney, like De Niro, like James Caan, like my most favorite Mr. James Caan, Sonny Sonny Sonny Sonny Boy" while rubbing his hands and cackling to himself. That I have no qualms about revealing these essentially personal mutterings, because I have heard Bikram mutter an identical rant of gangster comparisons to an audience of hundreds while on the microphone. And that this merger of public and private mutterings is just one example of a gigantic merger that occurs when you elevate into the truly weird sphere of being a full-time guru, where private and public selves by necessity must be blurred into one because that nonduality is precisely the product you are selling.

That when it comes to yoga, he is foremost a servant. That he is compulsive in his desire to help people achieve benefits from his postures. That this is perhaps the greatest reason for his success.

That he truly believes yoga will change the world, and his love of money and glitter and gangsters aside he will do anything to further this goal.

That he is a man who has been so successful at this goal that he once got in an argument with the adjacent passenger in his first-class seat of his Delta Airlines flight back to Los Angeles over his own identity. An argument where the adjacent first-class passenger insisted politely that there must be some language problem because it was impossible for his seatmate to be Mr. Bikram of Bikram Yoga, because there was no single Mr. Bikram, thereby encapsulating a belief widely held by those not in the know that Bikram Yoga is one of the ancient systems, a lineage passed down by the generations, a lineage where it is assumed that the *Bikram* in Bikram Yoga is either the name of a long-dead sage or, more likely, is some yuppie-appropriated Sanskrit word of the type now thrown on jeans or soaps or ergonomically branded office furniture. That the argument in the first-class bay escalated—as the man continued dribbling inaccurate details about the yoga into the conversation, details that he knew for a positive fact because his niece was deeply involved in this ancient Bikram yoga—and was settled only because by chance the Delta inflight magazine was doing a story on the sensation of Bikram Yoga, which featured an imposing picture of the real and nonancient Bikram in exactly the same fedora he happened to be wearing at the moment.[24]

That although that is what Bikram relayed to us and it seems probable, as there have been many stories about Bikram written in many in-flight magazines, I have no idea whether it is true. That Bikram routinely mixes stories that are definitely true ("I kick Robert Flack and Shirley MacLaine out of class for being late!") with stories that could very well be true ("Ronald Reagan called me for advice about his daughter," Patti Davis, who was a serious student of Bikram's and who went on to marry one of his most senior teachers) with stories that are almost certainly not true ("I get Bruce Lee his role in *Enter the Dragon!*") with stories that are false and told tongue in cheek for laughs ("Best client, Statue of Liberty. Hundred years she stands without bending the knee. Tough cookie.")

That he is the greatest example of sage-as-child I have ever come across.

That as sage-as-child, he skews toward the awkwardly horny, early-teenage child, who has just discovered masturbation and exaggeration but who is still really, really excited about video games, instead of the perhaps more wholesome wide-eyed and innocent child who fingerpaints and runs around in grass whom people tend to imagine when imagining their sages as children.

That he certainly has those wide-eyed and innocent moments too.

And that really, when you think about it, there isn't that big a difference between those two versions of sage-as-child, since the salient quality isn't exposure to sexuality or running through grass but the degree of wonder and curiosity and energy that occurs when an ego that hasn't been bashed aside yet by the wearies of maturity, the responsibilities of caring for one-self, and the learned boredom of sophistication is left to explore a universe it believes it is at the very beating center of.

---

[24] In another loss of identity moment related by someone who was there, Bikram is driving late night in Vegas in his Bentley and pulls into a gas station where his car is quickly surrounded by hookers. The gas station attendants vocally refuse to serve him and threaten to call the cops because based on dress and car and mannerisms they are convinced Bikram is a pimp and very much don't want him to think that he can use their gas station as a place of business.

That his understanding of America and what it means to be American has largely been formed by the Beverly Hills elite of the 1970s and '80s and their corresponding mannerisms in Hollywood movies. That because of this, he shares the same weird cultural warping you see in Japanese rock stars and/or Scandanavian jazz and/or hip-hop's adoption of Italian mafioso mannerisms, in that he's grasped a small, essential, and extreme part and used that part as a lens to frame the whole.

That the result of this sociological synecdoche is a Bikram who believes Las Vegas is the apex of American culture, thinks that name-dropping is a valid rhetorical strategy, and has trouble believing that his students are motivated by carrots beyond money and self-aggrandizement.

That he really believes it when he says he loves himself so much because it allows him to love you.

Both because he really, really loves himself and because he really, really loves you. As long as you stay as you a concept and don't morph too much into you an individual with needs that may conflict with his own.

That his love for you as either concept or individual will never, ever, under any circumstances allow you to outshine him.

That he was by his own admission a virgin until the age of twenty-eight, whereby he experienced his first orgasm when several women brought him to climax against his will. That who knows what that particular series of events does to someone's neural pleasure center, but that developmentally and behaviorally at least it resulted in him promptly going on an early-thirties sexual binge whereby he explored this new sensation to its utmost with many of Hollywood's leading ladies and many of his most devoted acolytes.

That he is the type of man who thinks that announcing in public that he has had "seventy-two hours of marathon sex, where my partner has forty-nine orgasms, I count" makes him appear more, rather than less, virile.

That he is incredibly, achingly lonely. That he can't stand to be by himself. That he misses India. That his need to be surrounded by people begins with senior teachers but quickly extends to essentially unknown newbie practitioners should senior teachers desire to go to sleep or otherwise have some personal space. That he will tell us not once, but hundreds of times from his throne, that he believes "loneliness is the number one punishment in human life" and/or that he can endure any amount of physical pain, "but put me in a room by myself, and I will kill myself."

That one of his most senior teachers describes his teaching method as "he takes a pin and finds the softest part of you, and he will prick you again and again at that point, never actually penetrating, never hurting you, until that part of you is the hardest place on your body."

That already in just a few days, one of his most junior teachers can see that although his instinct for finding the softest spot on people is unerring, almost genius level, he occasionally and very definitely misapplies the whole pricking part—and has ended up hurting people very badly.

That even among people who feel hurt, cheated, or injured—the people who seek me out as writer with grudges and curses and to expound on the reasons he is dangerous—even these people will typically have a moment when they think about him and their eyes grow big with memories and say, "but it's true, you know, the guy broke my heart, and I love him anyway. I can't help it."

That he never drinks alcohol. Abhors cigarettes. That there is something very touching about the way he is saddened when people close to him use those substances.

That by all indications, he does not practice the yoga class he is famous for creating. But that he clearly does exercise in other formats, including, bizarrely, doing thousands and thousands of stomach crunches in the sauna.

That he possesses an absolutely transcendent singing voice. That Quincy Jones wanted to record him, at a time when Quincy was at the height of his creative powers, in the mid-1980s, having just put out *Thriller* with Michael Jackson. That Quincy found himself crying when Bikram sang to him at the end of their classes together.

That Bikram can be both kind and terribly cruel in the same moment to the same person. That this push–pull is his métier and essential truth. That it operates on fragile, needy people like a drug.

That he is in no way anything but a human. And a particularly small human at that. That he is a man who through great personal effort has whittled away his humanity into a small, sharp point. That as with many great men, this has left him both mesmerizingly effective and totally and completely imbalanced. That it could be perceived as irony that yoga would be the skill that led to this imbalance, but that implies a misunderstanding both about the type of yoga Bikram is teaching and exactly what it takes to teach and spread yoga to millions and millions of people.

And with That as Background and Foreground, I Dive Wholeheartedly into Teacher Training

This is how lectures at Teacher Training begin. After a long, restless wait, after announcements about endless mundanities like laundry or postal delivery that are necessary but taxing to listen to, after his throne has been properly assembled and outfitted with fluffy blankets and his tea has been brewed, Bikram strides in. He will enter bundled up, hunched inward like he is perpetually cold, with a cap pulled down tight over his head, then he will look around left and right a few times, then strip down to reveal leopard-print gold lamé–lined short-shorts. Which he will show off with an excited ass-waggle or two to his now screaming trainees before bouncing up into his cozy throne to swaddle himself in an avalanche of orange blankets[25] and begin the night's lecture.

Instead of a specific topic, Bikram will come with a single idiom he wants to expound upon. This idiom typically comes directly from his dialogue ("What does it mean 'pulling is the object of stretching'?") or has a Rudyard Kipling *Just So Stories* quality to it ("Let me tell you something incredible but true: the heart hate the lungs") or a mathematical precision ("99 percent right is 100 percent wrong") or really requires no explanation at all ("Best food is no food"[26]). Bikram does this because as he puts it, he

---

[25] A construction cone orange that he will later earnestly describe as "saffron, the color of all yogis, a symbol of giving up material possessions and dedicating your life to teaching."

[26] Which is the idiom that inspired my favorite exchange of all training, which I feel encapsulates the essence of what it feels like to sit in a lecture with a rambling yoga guru and 380 people in various stages of mental and physical decay. Bikram: "Tell me what is the best food in the world?"

can "tell you with idiom in ten seconds what it would take another teacher ten minutes to explain. So simple." Of course, in real life, it is not so simple. Instead Bikram relates the night's idiom in ten seconds and then spends an hour and a half unpacking it, and explaining how it relates to sex, yoga, pleasing women, and/or the lives of various wealthy and influential friends of his. However, just as surely as a slot machine pays off with the variable reinforcement that keeps the suckers suckling, regardless of the inanity of the lecture, during his hour and a half babble per idiom, Bikram will make at least one offhand comment that registers as pure gold. It will gleam as it trips out his mouth, bobbing to the surface in an otherwise muddy stream.

Tonight's lecture is on the art of teaching. Bikram is explaining who our prospective clients will be. The idiom, to the extent there is an idiom guiding the lecture is one of Bikram's favorites: "Having doesn't mean a thing if you don't know how to use it." The lecture rambles from a discussion of the famous people Bikram has thrown out of class to the reason he hates San Francisco and Ashland, Oregon, and the "dirty hippie artists" who live in both places. Finally, talking about hippies, women with "armpits like a second pussy," there is a moment of coherence:

"The worst, dirtiest people in the world will come to your class. Physically, mentally trash, spiritual garbage, minus ten thousand mental attitude. You must be very nice to them. They pay very well. But expect a bunch of vegetables to come in wheelchair.

"Many will have tried to commit suicide even and were unlucky enough to fail. You will tell them: Don't worry, I will help you commit suicide very quickly—and kill you with this class!"

The audience laughs. Bikram grows serious.

"You laugh, but you don't know. . . . The saddest part of my life is that I know your lives. I know my power. I have used some of it—not all. But you—" He leaps out of his chair. "—your grandfather left you a

---

"Squash!" screams the man behind me. "No food!" Bikram booms back. "Best food in the world is no food!" "It's true," says the man behind me, nodding his head enthusiastically. "So many people die because they don't eat enough squash."

trillion-dollar investment, and you don't know how to get it, you don't know the life you could be living.

"God gave you everything, but you don't know how to use it. It makes me so sad." He sits back down, looking instantly older. "Why should I care? Because that is my karma yoga, that is my purpose. That is the promise I made to my guru.

"Yoga is the key. You already have the sports car. You already have Rolls-Royce. But you don't know how to turn it on. . . . The people who come to class, the vegetable garbage in wheelchair, it is unbelievable at first, but they have sports car too." He pauses. "But having sports car doesn't mean a thing. . . ." Here he stops as the audience roars back with the conclusion to his couplet:

"If you don't know how to use it," the room obediently and joyously chants.

"Yes! See, you learn something. God makes everyone a gold mine. That is your trillion-dollar investment. Your job is to dig it out and process it. To make it from dirt into gold. Have you seen gold directly from the mine? It looks like mud. You can't even tell it is gold, you need a geologist to tell you it's gold. That is the role of guru, sensei, master . . . to help you see the gold in yourself that you have been mistaking for dirt. Guru helps you process it, clean it, shine it.

"Then you take gold and make a necklace . . . and I promise you someone will buy!" He cackles.

At this there is a moment of silence; then he bursts into song. It is his theme song. A love song. We hear it almost every day, often in class at our weakest moments. With his soft voice, it is always unexpectedly beautiful, always mocking, always a little funny.

Don't look so sad,
Don't look so lonely
Long way from home
To kill yourself
That's what you pay for,
That's why I am here. . . .

Bikram lets the song trail off. He putters for a moment around the stage. Then we move to the next idiom.

Each night, this process is repeated with two or three idioms, the lecture extending into its third or fourth hour of babbling sermon, the room of four hundred people sitting in a state of sunken exhaustion, eyes blinking to wipe the growing fuzz from their lenses, legs beginning to knot up from iterant cramps, butt cheeks flexing to sustain blood flow, even individual hairs beginning to ache from fatigue.

Finally this is how lectures at teacher training end. Not with a whisper but a groan. Eventually, when Bikram has exhausted himself, just past the point when even butt-cheek flexing has grown unbearable to his audience, when he himself is no longer sure what his original point was, a fact he will often gleefully remark upon, he will announce with a blaze of enthusiasm that he is finished with the night's lecture.

And that he wants to show us a movie. A Bollywood movie!

Without exception, this will fill the room with huge groans and a few cheers. The cheers come from raving sycophants. The groans are filled with a loving grouchiness from the adults who realize they are stuck no matter what. The vast decaying majority remains silent, uninterrupted in their attempt to try to sleep with their eyes open. At our training, these movies never start earlier than midnight, often much later, and never finish until the room has been reduced to a refugee camp. Huddling trainees slumping on each other, wrapping themselves in bedding stolen from rooms, curling on the floor in the spaces that aren't visible to the rotating aides who circulate to ensure everyone stays awake. Although we never see an actual sunrise during my training, and despite a plethora of 3 A.M. bedtimes, I learn we get it easy. In the previous Palm Springs training, cadets suffered through week upon week of bedtimes that hurt my hair to even imagine: 5 A.M., 4 A.M., 5 A.M., 6 A.M., 5 A.M. All with the yoga bright and early in the morning to greet them, all to be repeated again and again day after day, week after week until they broke.[27]

---

[27] Every training has its own particular horror. In Acapulco, the yoga room was so poorly ventilated and the humidity so stifling that the back of the room was lined with "puke buckets" for students who needed to disgorge quickly and then get back to class. In Palm Springs, there was the punishing

Movies were not an original part of teacher training, but have always been an authentic part of Bikram the man. He loves them and sits upright in his chair, eyes glued on the screen, occasionally chortling at slapstick jokes, often demanding like a deaf grandfather that the volume be raised. Invariably, there is a woman standing beside him massaging his back, or a woman on her knees by his side massaging his calves and thighs. Or two women massaging both at the same time. He has watched movies late into the night for as long as anyone can remember. It is part of his insomniac drive. Back in the 1970s when he was training Emmy, it was Elvis films. During the 1980s he watched gangster movies. Now it's all Bollywood. Originally, however, they were a personal affair, just for Bikram and whichever senior teachers he invited back to his home or up to his hotel suite.

But then as the trainings grew from thirty to three hundred people, someone showed Bikram that the projector purchased for guest anatomy lectures could also be used to project DVDs. Suddenly Bikram could give more of himself to his cadets. As with everything at Teacher Training, the movies are not optional. (Unless Bikram is in an exceptionally good mood, at which point the entire room clears out in a stampede for bed, leaving him alone with a few die-hard movie fans and a few die-hard massage girls.)

The nonoptional late-night movies do serve one purpose besides Bikram's whim. They keep us awake and wear us down. The longer I am at TT, the more its operational principle becomes clear: cumulative exhaustion. No single day at Teacher Training is very difficult. Taking two classes a day is taxing, but by no means devastating. Similarly, the consecutive late nights are uncomfortable but nothing more awful than typical end-of-term frenzy at any university. The memorization takes effort, but it is liter-

---

late nights. In Hawaii, lectures and yoga classes were held in the same disgusting room, ensuring that cadets remained sweaty and sticky all day long. Ours in San Diego? Like I said, we get it easy. Probably the single most difficult aspect is the Hotel Circle isolation and associated lack of access to healthy food. Also, in combination with heavy rain and recklessly swilled Gatorade, there are truly epic amounts of ants in the hot tent.

ally the only intellectual requirement for nine weeks and therefore probably actually serves to ward off decay.

But although no single facet of Teacher Training is remarkable in itself, the routine builds on itself. Class after class with no rest, and muscle strain grows from minor to wretched. The lack of sleep eliminates opportunities for repair. The subtle electrolyte and mineral imbalances that come from sweating fourteen pounds of water a class accumulate and then swing wildly as people overcompensate with supplements. The stress of memorization and endless public speaking suddenly becomes uncomfortable. Someone catches a cold, and the moist incubator of the hot room accelerates it into a plague. Suddenly, a daily routine that shouldn't be too hard starts breaking people.

And boy do people break. Some just disappear: pack their bags and decide to forfeit their money for home. Others become aggressive. Others hypersexual. Others mournful. At least one man seems to be descending steadily toward a schizophrenic break right before our eyes. He started out cheerful, if perhaps a little overvoluable (memorably and oddly offering to write a poem with me after the first lecture), but by week four devolved into a muttering, withdrawn, increasingly paranoid ghost: perpetually pacing around with the hoodie of his sweatshirt tightly drawn, occasionally screaming out during posture clinic, signing in to lectures and then running off. Others are going through deep and regular emotional traumas. The bushes outside the tent after class always have at least a few people weeping into them.

Physically, the overtraining has other effects. To the horror of many women, despite doing epic amounts of yoga, weight-loss ceases: their stressed-out bodies hoarding nutrients and their heat-acclimated circulation retaining maximum water. In the reverse effect, many of the fittest men watch their muscles atrophy, the stress demanding too much energy to both repair and maintain their carved physiques. Without much time for meals, diet goes to shit. Protein shakes, supplement pills, shelf-stable products from Trader Joe's, and the basically fast, definitely overprocessed food of the Town and Country's theme restaurants dominate at the time when our bodies probably should be eating the healthiest, most balanced meals of our lives. A stressed-out system allows latent problems to rise to the surface. I hear about a rash of ovarian cysts among women. Sunny San Diego produces at least one case of pneumonia. Bacterial rashes flare up. Acne is everywhere. I get a single pimple on my ear one week and then a 'roidal outbreak across my back and chest so intense, it looks like I've been napalmed. Diarrhea, fever, puking, and perpetually runny noses are so common, they almost don't bear mention.

Emergency rehydration is delivered during almost every class.

But then the body adapts. It grows stronger. Suddenly by week seven, when all math and logic indicate that things should be at the very worst, you find yourself sprinting with joy.

That too is Teacher Training.

But ultimately, for me, all real joy from teacher training comes not from the yoga, but from the people. For nine weeks, the otherwise drab courtyards and poolsides of the Town and Country are transformed into a mixing ground for the amazing and bizarre. Burning Man has nothing on Bikram. I meet J.C., a yoga teacher who arrived weighing three hundred pounds and lost seventy pounds over the course of his nine weeks. I meet a man who sits in lecture, systematically eating a bag of popcorn with a spoon. I meet former heroin addicts, former meth addicts, former shopaholics, former alcoholics all using the yoga as replacement therapy. I meet, while folding laundry, a mother using the yoga to grieve the suicide of her son. I meet people with perfect bodies and such smooth, round muscles and tight bikini lines that they seem almost dissonant with the drab reality surrounding them. I meet people so skinny with such obvious eating disorders that staring at them evokes a similar if more queasy reaction. I meet a doctor from Utah, walking with crutches and wearing a wicked-looking knee brace, who tore every ligament in his knee wakeboarding, and whose own doctor told him that under no circumstances should his brace come off and under no circumstance should he kneel. Nonetheless, on his first day visiting training, he takes class with Bikram—who promptly, almost psychically, asks him to take off his brace and kneel to complete a posture. It is a command that the doctor obeys: slowly ripping off the Velcro then the larger clamps of his brace while the whole room applauds. His daughter, a trainee, the reason he is visiting in the first place, is beside him, terrified at his movements. I meet Jeff, a junkie turned plumber turned yoga studio owner, who has such forceful calm that he quiets a room of forty people in seconds by standing in front of them in a T-shirt. The ropy veins on his forearms somehow signaling that he is a man to be listened to. When a woman screams hysterically from the balcony of her hotel room as a man sprints across the parking lot, a yogi takes off in pursuit. And when a half mile later, he catches up with the panting burglar and wrestles the woman's computer away from him as the thief screams, "I have a gun!" the yogi simply bows to him and says, "but I have the laptop," before calmly walking back toward our hot tent. I meet yogis working through childhood abuse, financial ruin, and all manners of abrupt midlife changes. And although at some point I realize that—of course—a yoga based around self-transformation is going to attract a lot of people who needed to transform, what all these amazing crime-stopping, self-transforming yogis teach me again and again is the process of witnessing, discussing, and reveling in personal transformation never grows old.

The best part is how it catches you unaware. I meet Denis when we are running late to a lecture. Each lecture at Teacher Training includes a sign-in sheet to ensure attendance. Given the exhaustion levels floating around, there is a huge biological incentive to head back to your room and curl up in your bed (instead of, say, staying up until four in the morning, listening to Bikram talk about how he doesn't need to sleep). In order to thwart this temptation, trainees must sign in before each event. The penalty for failing to sign in—or for signing in even a minute late—is an additional class. Since, from the end of the first week onward, everyone is already exhausted, cramping, sore, and already taking two classes a day, nobody wants to be late and do an extra class. In fact, the entire idea of an extra class provokes a crisis in my brain.

Anyway, racing against that threat, Denis and I charge over to the tent. We make it, hastily scrawling our names at the sign-in table, and I look up to see Denis grinning. He tells me that was the first time he'd run since his accident. That it has been three years since he was told he was never going to walk again.

As we walk into lecture, he lets out a shriek. "I love this place! I love these people!"

On May 13, 2008, Denis decided not to wait for insurance before taking his new motorcycle out for a spin.

"I've always been a bicycle guy. But I got fascinated with the image of a motorcycle. The wind in my hair, being able to just pick up and go. So I bought one. . . . It's funny, I bought a cruiser because I thought I'd kill myself on a sports bike."

He hadn't even had the bike an hour. He was living in Vancouver and had taken delivery of the motorcycle at the marina where he worked repairing sailboats. This was the start of a new life. He had quit a corporate job as a sales and marketing director, and started woodworking. The money at his previous job was good, but it wasn't satisfying. He realized that without a family to support, this might be the only time he had to live his dream. The motorcycle was a key part of the dream.

"When it arrived, I just stared at it for a while. Then I called the insurance company, they gave me a price, and when we hung up, I thought, 'I just want to take it out for a quick ride.' There was a voice in my head that said this is not a good idea. But . . ." He spreads his hands. "I cruised around the parking lot. It was cold and windy. I remember the marina boats were rocking back and forth. Then I went against the feeling and left the parking lot." Just as he was leaving, it started to lightly rain.

"I busted out of town, and this is Canada so it didn't take long before I was at some beautiful scenery. I was taking it easy, maybe seventy—eighty kilometers per hour, but at a turn, I hit a little bump on the road. I lost control, I remember knowing that I was going to tip over, and as I was sliding, I looked up and realized a car was going to run directly over me."

Which it did. Front wheels crushing over first his tangled legs and then his chest before coming to rest directly above him. He was in and out consciousness the entire time, his only lasting memory the light creeping from the sides of chassis. He lost 60 percent of his blood before he reached the hospital. His right femur was broken in three places. His right hip dislocated, with the knee shattered at the tibial plateau.

"One thing I do have a memory of is my leg sticking out at this crazy angle. You have forty-three percent play in your tendons—mine was ripped, just dangling at eighty percent."

His left leg was in far worse condition, and when he arrived at the hospital, doctors wanted to amputate below the knee. Denis doesn't remember it, but his tibia had snapped completely and the calf stuck out to the side like an *L* just below the knee. His scapula was broken. Then due to a head injury, his frontal lobes started swelling, robbing him of most memories for the next five weeks.

When he stabilized, they hadn't amputated his leg yet. But his life as he knew it had been cut off. He entered into a convalescent's limbo, where he was wheeled from room to room, where his head was always exactly fifteen degrees above his heart unless he used buttons to raise it, where he marked time in terms of surgeries rather than weeks or months. "Hospital was home. The nurses, they cared for you. They were my best friends," he says. "God bless the Canadian health care system. They patched me up, connected all my broken parts together again."

But the lubricant that would eventually get those parts moving in a normal pattern was Bikram: "The yoga didn't save my life. That was the emergency response team, the surgeons, the nurses, and rehab specialists who waited with me as I learned my exercises and adjusted my medication. The yoga didn't give me the drive to recover. That came from some place inside me. A place my amazing friends who would visit and bring me joy could tap into . . . What the yoga did is allow me to use the life I had been given back. . . . And what's the point otherwise?

"It's exactly Bikram's favorite quote—'Having doesn't mean a thing, if you don't know how to use it.' What good are the blood transfusions, the hours on artificial respiration, if you live the rest of your life in pain? What good is having a body if you can't use it? . . . And so three and a half weeks after my fifth surgery, bandages still around my tibia, I hobbled into a Bikram class on crutches to start using my body."

Denis had practiced the yoga before the accident. He enjoyed it, the focus and meditation, reminding him of the clarity he achieved while woodworking. The heat and sweat appealed to his sense of rigor. But back then it was at most a curiosity. An eccentricity that made good conversations with girls.

"I had no reason to do it before. It was exercise. It was a thing to do. But now I poured myself in. I put one hundred percent belief into it. I knew I had to do it if I wanted my body back."

Every day his parents drove him to the bus station,[28] where he slowly boarded, rode, slowly exited to transfer to a second bus, and then in a maddening lonesome exertion, hobbled off the bus through a train station to catch the train that would deliver him to his yoga studio. Altogether, including time in the hot room, getting to and from a single yoga class was an eight-hour block of time. But one that he viewed as essential.

"The thing is, it's your body. It really comes down to the fact that it's yours. You need to believe. You need to see it and fix it. . . . At first the pain in class was unreal. There were sharp pains like I was doing something terrible to myself. I am still not good at describing it. But eventually I learned to be good at handling it. . . . If I saw someone else with these injuries today, I'd probably tell them take it easy. I'd say, please don't push yourself. But when it's you, and you are inside the pain, and you believe in the process, there is a helpful denial. The denial allows you to push. And if you push enough, in the right ways, in ways where you see progress, eventually things change."

One Hot Class

This was day one of week two. I positioned myself about three rows from Bikram, directly within his line of sight, directly underneath a heater. Bikram begins the class in an especially angry mood, picking on everyone

---

[28] "My father showed me what it means to love by taking care of me in a way only he knew how. He would bathe me. Push my commode chair to the bathroom and prepare me. Take me to appointments. He would do all this plus more and never complain. . . . We talk about what it means to love, care, and support in yoga so much. I was witnessing it firsthand, and it has made the accident the greatest gift of my life."

around me, but graciously saying nothing to me. "Ms. Boobs,[29] why are you so lazy? I hate lazy people. You disgust me. . . ." Then, "Senorita"—spinning toward a rather lovely if chubby Mexican woman—"suck in that fat stomach. The only reason you can do this posture is your fat ass and fat boobs balance you out." Then he spins back to Ms. Boobs. "Do your boobs speak English? What is wrong with you? How did you come to my training? You look like you never practiced a day in your life." Possibly in response to these failings, possibly because it is his whim, Bikram holds our warm-up postures far longer than normal. My legs get quivery doing poses I have done thousands of times. The heat continues to rise.

The first sign that things tonight are headed for weird occurs when a man to my left simply drops from the first balancing posture like someone

---

[29] It is impossible not to take a moment to dignify Ms. Boobs aka Ms. Vancouver, a woman who aside from hailing from Vancouver and having truly enormous pie-tin-sized bosoms, represents something hard to quantify but extremely important about Teacher Training: the difficulty of understanding where exactly on the four-axis scale of love, discipline, ridicule, and sexual weirdness Bikram's crosshairs fall at a given moment. Ms. Boobs was instantly singled out by Bikram for her sloppy postures and for being oddly resistant to any corrections—her nickname branded onto her by the end of the very first class. As someone who frequently practiced next to Ms. Boobs, I can attest that her deafness to correction was truly stunning; Bikram would tell her exactly how to move her body, and often she simply wouldn't change a thing. This frustrated Bikram to the point of rage and he would, in turn, demean her day in and day out, identifying her only as Ms. Boobs and saying really truly hurtful things to her about her intelligence, appearance, sexual hygiene, to say nothing of her abilities as a yogi, comments that she would bear with a nobility and facial expression that resembled a Hindu cow, but that in me at least continually produced a personal gut check, Asch conformity level of self-reflection, in that Bikram's comments were decidedly funny in situ but bullying and transparently mean-spirited in reflection. Yet, every day in a room with over 380 people, Ms. Boobs made the conscious decision to position herself directly in front of Bikram. She definitely felt some critical relationship with him. She made few friends. She wore tighter and more revealing clothing. Bikram, who would often show affection to people he insulted, especially outside of class, had nothing but disgust for Ms. Boobs and her determination to persist in the face of his anger. For instance, in the middle of one lecture, apropos of nothing but her existence, he stopped the lecture, turned to the room, and said, "When you get a person like her, you don't worry. Don't spend time. Take the money and go. They are expendable," before returning to the rambling topic at hand. He hurt her, she hurt him, and the level of bile he threw at her and the level of silence she threw back were raised to such uncomfortable levels that at the end of the training, during a routine announcement that brought up her name, everyone else gave her a spontaneous five-minute standing ovation in acknowledgment of the weird determined sad place her position taught us about the Bikram crosshairs. An applause that decidedly and cowardly occurred while Bikram was not in the room.

cut his legs off. He hits the floor hard. One moment he is standing; the next moment he is down. Out. Two aides rush in from the back of the room and carry him out of the tent by the armpits. The class moves forward without even acknowledging the exit. It is a normal-enough occurrence, although this is certainly early. By the sixth out of the twenty-six postures, the weirdness has grown exponentially, the heat continuing its manic ascent. Already I can feel my field of vision narrowing. I manage to hold each posture but begin crouching between sets. This is my second sign that I'm struggling a lot more than normal. At the time, I assume I'm taking stress off the legs. Later I will learn that what I am doing is shortening the distance between my heart and my brain, making it easier to pump blood. By the eighth posture, I am crouching for a whole new reason. Standing is unstable. The small stabilizer muscles that I have been relying on my whole life to keep me upright are failing. Unless I concentrate on the act of standing, I lurch around like a drunk, my legs stamping the ground like a restless horse. So I go down. From my crouched position, I notice almost two-thirds of the room is on their knees. This is amazing. We are barely a third of the way through class, and the majority of this class of teachers is unable to continue. Bikram notices this too and gives us several opportunities to drink water. He is showing mercy. The heat continues its ascent, and I begin to wonder if the heater is broken. To prolong our rest, Bikram asks a woman, who I conclude must be incredibly strong to be able to do anything at all, to demonstrate a posture while the rest of the room watches. I look up at her posture for just a second. She is beautiful. The girl in front of me seizes on the gap to walk out. Two other people within my field of vision get up and stagger out with her. The postures continue. Then we hit the halfway point and move to the floor.

Rather than being a blur, the whole second half of that class has been seared in my brain, all static images, as if the heat in the room heated up every discrete moment of time like a brand and then plunged them into my brain. I can remember details of Bikram's face—half concern, half determined—I remember him dancing crazed on the podium, hair in his top knot, like a devil, cheeks slightly sagging, gaining energy from our devastation. My water bottle, which had been filled with ice at the start of class, is now warm to the touch. The lemon juice, honey, and salt mixture tastes gummy. During the first few asanas on the floor, I keep telling myself to move carefully and let the yoga do the work. When I lie on my stomach, my bladder pushes. A woman's foot keeps turning bright yellow out of the corner of my eye. When I look at it directly, it becomes skin again. I need to pee and keep wondering if I have the muscular strength to hold it. Despite exhaustion, I am still terrified of Bikram correcting me. By the twentieth posture, the woman who had demonstrated the beautiful posture during the standing series lies motionless and then twitches. Bikram stops class a second time, and we all stare at her. This time, however, he demands that she get up. He is checking on her to make sure she doesn't need immediate medical attention. When she doesn't respond, a student practicing behind her dumbly walks over and prods her on the shoulder. She lifts her face sobbing, and Bikram is satisfied. She collapses back to her mat, twitching again in her sobs. My own postures are impossibly weak, legs barely lifting, body flopping. I realize from the way the smell won't go away that there is a very real chance that the lean tattooed women near me has shit her leotard. The rest periods between postures have become more unbearable than the postures themselves. My heart beats even faster. This is a sign I've switched over to anaerobic exercise. My heart is trying to recover from the oxygen deficit created during the posture by madly pumping oxygen at the opportunity of rest. Then amazingly my brain empties. I am here. Very here. I fill with a mantra of persistence: *This is your posture. This is your class.* At some point, I slip out and wonder why I am chanting in the second person and began repeating more forcefully, This is *my* class, in my brain. Although I begin pushing very deeply into the postures, my camel backbend produces none of the usual energy, no crackling of electricity, no pain: just swollen heat. I feel my lower body go numb during the final stretching. My whole leg is pins and needles. This is shunting. It means all blood has been diverted away from my limbs and into my brain and heart to keep me alive. The nerves in my extremities are correspondingly shutting down. I used my arms to push my legs around manually to get back into savasana. My whole body feels feverish, a distinctly different sensation from the regular heat, meaning my core temperature is creeping upward. I kept thinking of Backbenders talking about how they'd occasionally feel their entire field of vision black out. I remember reprimanding myself, thinking I probably would have experienced that if I hadn't crouched down so much. During spine twist, somehow, Bikram produces a little blond boy. He's maybe five or six years old in bathing trunks onstage. Bikram claps his hands, and the boy jumps into different postures. I think I am dreaming. Bikram places the boy in a perfect Bow posture and picks him up by the arms, twirling him around like a helicopter, screaming, "Look, look, look, at what I can do!" I keep stretching. The room is silent. Bikram is screaming about the boy. We move into the second side of spine twists, our very last posture, and I notice the boy's mother has come onstage to retrieve him. I almost can't believe I'm not hallucinating.

During final savasana, the class over, Bikram plays a song—about sadness, loneliness, and love—a monstrous, malicious decision. At Teacher Training, there is a rule: Out of respect, you do not get up to leave a class until the teacher has left, and teachers don't leave until the final savasana is finished. The song Bikram plays is eight minutes long. Every single cell in every single person's body in that room wants to run from the tent, and we are being held captive by a whining, oversynthesized Bollywood love song. My body feels hot and blurry. I can hear muffled sobbing on all sides of me. At a certain point, I realize I cannot lie still for even a second longer. I pull myself upright, and notice three-quarters of the room doing something similar. One man in the back of the room, whom I later recognize as a teacher and studio owner, is standing, pacing in circles around his mat, mumbling to himself. No smiles. No relief at being finished with class. I lie back down. The heat swells up again around my face. Eventually the song ends.

People stampede toward the doors. Bikram keeps yammering into the microphone about his sandals, but nobody seems to care that he's still in the room, and we aren't supposed to leave yet. People leave. Three-hundred-eighty bodies funnel through two small doorways, bumping into one another, falling. In the cool air of the shoe alcove, I look around at the faces of my classmates for the first time. They are sobbing, sober, red, drained.

It's the sweetest relief I can imagine. It means I wasn't alone. As I put on my flip-flops, a girl in a bikini top crumples at my feet. She says, "I'm sorry. I can't stand anymore." She lies motionless on top of five or six pairs of shoes. I grab my stuff and continue shuffling past her. Another girl sways and swoons, her knees buckling until she is deposited on the floor in prayer. We just step around her. All of us. A red cooler labeled FIRST AID lies empty on its side, everything resembling aid or rehydrating fluid raided.

Outside, there is a wreckage of bodies. People lie on the concrete. Splayed out. Leaning against the tent, shaking. A row of men sit on the curb, sobbing into their palms. I keep walking toward my room. I want to be away. Stalking steadily, picking up power from the cool air. My brain is returning. My thoughts begin rotating around recovery. Usually I make the mixture of grapefruit juice, seltzer, and ice that Lauren from Backbending taught me. But after this class, I am not hungry. I am hot. I want to plunge in a pool. Which, given the many sprawling pools of the Town and Country, is more than possible. But I am worried about rapidly cooling my heart. I once heard, or imagined a story about a marathon runner who cooled his heart too quickly after a race and went into cardiac arrest from the sudden contraction. As I walk, this terrifying idea replays in my brain like a song lyric I can't escape. I ask the women striding next to me if there is a heated pool. She tells me that yes that was the hottest class she had ever taken. I agree it was hot and ask her about the pool again. She tells me she agrees with me that it was the hottest class she had ever taken and then begins crying. Another woman breaks into the conversation and keeps saying she doesn't understand what happened. Repeating the phrase endlessly with an uplift like it is a question. I ask a third woman about the hot pool, and she looks at me like I am crazy. There is a pool, I am going, but it isn't heated, I hope, she says to me. I follow her. We plunge in. I try to move slowly so as not to overwhelm my heart and cause cardiac arrest. But that is impossible. It feels so fresh and amazing. It is worth risking a totally implausible death. The pool is filled with bobbing yogis. Nobody is speaking except to occasionally say, wow. A boy with curly blond hair starts giggling. I get out of the pool, suddenly glad to have avoided cardiac arrest. I walk to the elevators. Typically this is a huge bottleneck area. A giant clump of people serviced by two elevators. I almost always skip the line and walk. Today there is nobody. Both elevators are stationed on the first floor. No line, nobody. Bikram has killed us so completely that after thirty minutes, no one has made it back to their rooms yet. I press the button; the doors open. A group of crying women approaches, so I hold the door. One woman who is crying the hardest keeps saying to another crying woman that maybe she just needs to cry. I reach my arm to her bare shoulder and tell her to go to the pool. This is my only advice. I keep repeating, "The pool feels great," as she keeps crying and repeating to the other woman, "Maybe she just needs to cry." I get off the elevator on my floor and leave them. My skin begins to hum with heat again. This time a warm, almost lovely glow. It is a survival. As I walk to the ice machine to begin preparations for my grapefruit and selzer elixir—my body wrecked but dignified somehow—I keep thinking, Well at least I got my eleven-thousand-dollars' worth. And for just this class, it is true.

The Seventh Siddhi of a Master Yogi Is the Ability to Project Himself into the Body of Another

The core learning experience of Bikram Yoga Teacher Training has nothing to do with yoga. At least as it pertains to postures or history or philosophy or therapeutic modifications or spiritual ramifications. It has nothing to do with pain. Nothing to do with flexibility or persistence over adversity.

Instead, the single defining feature of Bikram's Teacher Training is memorization. Rote filthy memorization of the internal monotone, eyes-to-back-of-head variety, whereby student after student is expected to ingest words in and then spit them back up before an audience. Upon paying the approximately eleven thousand dollars to enroll, every proto-yogi is sent a copy of the official Bikram Yoga "dialogue." A forty-five-page soliloquy whose grammatically moronic but instructionally precise English is the copyrighted intellectual property of Bikram Choudhury. It is the distillation of a single Bikram Yoga class as taught by Bikram himself, and the goal of the entire Teacher Training enterprise is for every single graduate to go forth and recite the class exactly as copywritten.[30]

The single most common sight at the yoga training is the parades of potential teachers walking around with little booklets of the dialogue stuck in front of their noses, mumbling to themselves. The text becomes a constant companion: beside the plate at meals, on the thighs before a lecture, on a towel in the tent before class, and, of course, on the pillow, in bed before sleep. It is a bona fide rite of passage to discuss dreaming "in

---

[30]Bringing up a topic that I'd be remiss in not covering, since everyone except me seems to think it is fascinating: Bikram has a copyright on not only the words of the dialogue, but also on the actual sequence of yoga. He believes his beginning yoga class is his intellectual property and uses a battalion of lawyers to enforce his claims. When it first came out in 2002, this decision prompted epic controversy in the yogic world, especially because Bikram promptly began suing former teachers who were using his name. Yoga teachers everywhere began rending their spandex and shrieking in mantra that Bikram was trying to own yoga. Personally, I'm not bowed over with sympathy for these claims. In fact, for the most part, I find them disgustingly self-serving. The urge to copyright or trademark comes from the typical capitalist corporate mentality that we all have to bend over for once in a while. I'm not here to laud it, but I rarely hear the open-source yoga community rallying in opposition to the brand names on their sexed-up bikini bottoms. Bikram has never tried to copyright the individual postures. In fact, he has gone out of his way to point out these are universal and eternal movements, "gifts from the gods," physical expressions to the body-whole as music notes are to the vocal cords. Copyrighting the postures would indeed be perverse and folly. But when someone comes up with a unique arrangement of musical notes (or words or images or movements of the body as in a choreographed dance), we honor it. More important than the social ethics, however, barring some 1984-style Big Brother development, Bikram's copyright is never going to interfere with you as an individual practicing his yoga series in the privacy of your home. It is enforceable in a reasonable sense only with those studios who choose to teach it to large groups of people for money. So if your understanding of yoga precludes selling it to make money, then Bikram's copyright will not affect you; it affects only people who do as Bikram does. Further (now that I'm wound up) as someone who does not think Bikram's series is magic or holy or perfect, and who very much sees it as a human product, developed by Bikram and his guru within the limits of their time and place, I fail to see why these persecuted studios/teachers can't improvise from it to express either their individuality or to address some of the sequence's weaknesses. The fact of the matter is that Bikram's Beginning Yoga Class™ is a fantastic yoga class, a wonderful starting point for anyone looking to become more physically fit and spiritually whole, but it has some noticeable flaws. It doesn't strengthen the arms, chest, wrists or ankles terribly well. It doesn't feature internal bandhas or offer overt opportunities at meditation. It isn't an AIDS drug being withheld from the third world or a surgical procedure reserved only for the rich. It is an innovated yoga sequence, which in the spirit of Courtney Mace—style yoga competition, will hopefully inspire some of his best, most knowledgeable students to create enhanced innovations of their own—that is, once they grow a pair and get out from under their guru's shadow.

dialogue," an experience I never had, although I certainly often drifted off to sleep with the weird catchphrases uncoupling from context to echo in my head.

What's remarkable about the dialogue is how much of it is intended to remain as unexplained catchphrases. The hows and whys behind the instructions are not for trainees. Not yet. And perhaps, not ever. In Bikram's concept of a yoga teacher (or at least one trained less than five years), understanding is at best a tertiary concern. Which of course leads directly to the biggest truth of the dialogue: The goal of Bikram Yoga Teacher Training is not to make good yoga teachers. Nor is it to make teachers who are good at yoga. It is to train people called teachers to lead a good yoga class.

The distinction is crucial, to understanding both what happens within Teacher Training and also Bikram's goals. It leaves many of the best students deeply unhappy with training and many other yoga traditionalists scornful of the process.

In Bikram's eyes, the ideal instructor is a mouthpiece. They give instructions. They hold a standard as only a flesh-and-blood human can do (hence no actual tape recordings or video conferencing): but they do not actually teach. They never demonstrate. They never ever adjust. Instead they disappear behind a script. Mary Jarvis has her teachers stand in a back corner alcove, completely invisible to the practicing student unless they go searching for him or her. To the student, there is freedom in this disembodied instructional voice. The brain can focus only on listening, aligning, and adjusting to the blitz of commands. To the teacher, there is safety. After millions of classes, the imperfections and hiccups have been stilled. Instead of requiring critical thinking, the dialogue becomes a mantra of sorts, its drumming recitation a catalyst for teachers to slip into a different sort of meditation.

And of the text itself? There is poetry ("Open your chest like a flower petal blooming"), there is lovable but clumsy phraseology ("Grab your elbows each other"), there is precision ("Then left hand down, grab left heel, thumb outside, fingers inside"), and there are a myriad declarations that make no coherent sense within the confines of the English language ("I want three-hundred-and-sixty-degree angle backward bending for gravitation!"). As a whole, the dialogue reflects Bikram's genius for teaching a class that successfully gets inside the head of a struggling practitioner. It gives precise advice for otherwise minor-seeming details (the alignment of a grip, the tuck of a chin) that force major changes to overall muscle use. It is, in short, the distillation of a really good yoga class.

Which is, of course, explicitly the point. Bikram has a document that gives him both quality control and flexibility to expand. It answers his 1970s dilemma. He can spread his yoga with no screwups and with completely mediocre teachers. He can teach millions and ensure that at the end of the day, nobody ever knows more about the yoga than him.

And for that last reason, for the true practitioner, the dialogue pierces the industrial into the spiritual. It is the central transmission. The codification of the guru's wisdom. Even foreign students who will never teach a day in English must learn it in English. Their mechanistic atonal recitations a testament to some need beyond the practical. Throughout the training, the actual text of the dialogue is referenced, dissected, and parsed for meaning in a tradition that would make the most midrashing of rabbi proud. Why we ask during this nightly lecture, does the dialogue specify kicking before stretching? What does it mean that the dialogue specifies one must "roll like a wheel" in a stationary posture? Repeatedly we will ask for clarification about the alignment in a specific posture, and instead of answering, even extremely experienced, otherwise personable and knowledgeable teachers will respond by simply reciting the words of the dialogue back despite the fact we have heard them endlessly before. The need to adhere to Bikram's broken, often counterproductive phrasing becomes an end in itself, an effort to ensure a continuity of tradition, a seminal instinct: it is a gradient for the hierarchy to flow, of senior teachers over their juniors, of juniors over the newbies, and of Bikram over all—replicating himself ad infinitum, alighting like a Xerox flash in his followers' brains each time they teach his class.

Problems versus Weird

And this is Posture Clinic. We are in a tiny room in the Town and Country. Bland green Town and Country carpet on the floor. Oil portrait of feverish girl on the wall. All us trainees crammed in the back, all sitting on the floor, knees bent up and hunched over, mumbling at the copy of dialogue between our legs. In the very front, just like a low-budget *American Idol* audition, a panel of certified teachers sits with a giant binder. One by one, students either volunteer or are called up. They take a last look at the section of dialogue we are performing for the day, stand in the center of the room, and then spit up the words they have just been studying. As they recite, three students demonstrate the postures in accordance with their words, providing visual feedback. Many times, those demonstrators become those poor demonstrators, left dangling in between movements, trapped in a difficult posture while the presenter's mind goes blank. Their legs quiver; their legs fail. When it is over, the panel of certified teachers makes various cryptic notations into the binder. Then they offer feedback on delivery. Then the next presenter is called.

Tonight, after dispatching with the first two-thirds of presenters, we go off on a tangent about the problems typically faced in the yoga room.

"The biggest problem is that men are gross," a female teacher says.

"I'll second that. Lot of balls . . . Soccer shorts with no underwear is not proper yoga gear, gentlemen."

"Biggest problem I see is maintaining your own practice. . . . If you are teaching ten to fifteen classes a week, that is a lot of time in the hot room. It takes a physical toll."

"Yeah. And the first thing to go is your own practice. You become one of those: the undead, the yoga teacher who doesn't do yoga."

Someone in the audience asks what the weirdest thing is they have encountered.

"Everything is weird! This is Bikram, darling."

"Your first fainter will be weird."

"Or how about the people who show up and then absolutely refuse to do anything you ask them. They are weird."

"Oh god. How about the people who sneak cell phones or watches. It's ninety minutes, darling, you can make it."

"Or the couples that try to hold hands during the floor series. Weird."

Then the lead teacher in the room inserts herself. "You will see a little bit of everything. Teaching is a great big perspective shift. You are going to see things from offstage instead of being one of the actors. It is a new yoga for you to do. You will begin to understand why people come to class in the first place. You will understand how fragile people are and how important this can be for them."

She continues: "I've had a seizure during class. That was weird. . . . The girl had these great big googly eyes, then she stumbled. I knew it, I could see it happening, and so I stepped up and caught her. She went into a seizure in my hands, and I just kept on with Eagle posture dialogue, holding her. The girl just needed to shake. Not so many people in the class noticed.

"And I'll tell you what, my mouth kept moving the whole time, I knew the dialogue that well . . . which is where you need to get to. . . . When it was over, she lay on her mat. I crouched down to check on her, and she said: 'Please, please, don't make me leave.' She was desperate. So I said okay. And she continued to lay out. When she got back up, she did the best Standing-Bow in the class."

There are a few follow-up questions on the seizure and the fainting. But this is the fourth week of Teacher Training, so we are well inured to the possibilities of fainters, seizers, criers, yellers, and other potentially extreme reactions to the yoga mainly because we have seen them all in the hot tent. So we drift back to reciting dialogue.

More trainees rise and recite, another and another. Everyone goes back to studying their dialogue.

Finally we get down to the last few presenters. At this point, the volunteers have stopped. The lead teacher scans a list of names in the binder and calls people up at random. These are the unprepared, the ones who never volunteer. They are made equally of people who are chronically anxious, foreigners who can't speak English and are essentially memorizing a series of sounds, and people like me, who simply suck at memorizing anything.

A name is called and a shaky woman I have never met before gets up. She has long brown hair and softly says her name. She is in her forties, certainly older than the majority of the room, but not atypical. The lead teacher asks her to repeat her name louder and with more confidence. She repeats her name identically and before she can be interrupted goes right into reciting her dialogue. It is halting, slow, atonal, and therefore totally par for the course. Then she stops in media res. Her arms are limp by her sides, but her fingers are chewing against her palms.

The lead instructor interrupts the silence. The abbreviated performance was not good enough, and so she asks the woman to begin again. This time, she suggests, the woman should smile more while she is speaking the dialogue. The lead teacher tells her this will make her more confident even if she doesn't feel more confident.

The woman begins again. But instead of smiling, she starts crying. The words of the dialogue are coming out in the same halting manner, but are half swallowed by sobs. Most of the room is still staring at their dialogue, trying to memorize the language they'll need for tomorrow's recitation. The lead teacher stops her again and asks her to start from the beginning again. The woman stays frozen. Her palms are open and shaking like jazz hands.

Then she starts really crying. A younger teacher from the panel gets up to offer a hug, but the lead teacher stops him.

"Why are you crying?" she asks the woman in a calm voice.

The middle-aged woman continues crying, shoulders hunched, arms still oddly straight by her sides. I find it terribly moving, like watching the secret life of my mother.

"Why are you crying?"

At this point, everyone in the room has looked up from the dialogue and is watching. The woman has her head turned down, staring at the floor. She wipes her hands against her cheeks, but keeps crying. The silence grows and I'm convinced the teacher is about to ask for a third time, when suddenly the woman chokes out: "You know the yoga saved my life. . . . I just don't want to just go through a posture without knowing it. It's disrespect-ful to the yoga.

"What's that?" The lead teacher asks almost hungry, "Who saved you?"

"The yoga saved my life," the woman repeats, wipes her cheeks. "You know doing the yoga, coming every day."

"No, who did this? Who saved your life?"

"The yoga," the woman begins.

"Who?" says the lead teacher.

"The yoga," the woman begins again, but by this point the audi-ence, now completely engaged in the scene, is shouting out, "You!" and "Yoooooooooo!" and "You you you!" The lead teacher is smiling but in-sistent.

"Me, I guess. I saved my life. Me and God."

"No. You saved your life. You did it." There is a pause. "Not God, not—"

And then from the back of the room, a lone guy shouts out: "And *Bik-ram!*" Everyone laughs, and a chorus of affirmation ripples around the room.

When the laughing dies down, the woman who is no longer crying but kind of smiling and sniffling says, "I mean yeah, God or Bikram, it's all the same. . . ." Then she sniffles a few more times and laughs and then bows to us weirdly.

Just as I am processing it all, imagining a future twenty centuries ahead where history has given Bikram his most fondest wish and he's been deified, the door pops open. It is the head aide of teacher training. He pokes just his head in the room. "Good news, bad news, people. No late-night lecture to-night. But I need one of you to massage Boss. If I can get eight people to agree to massage Boss in his room, then the rest of you can go to sleep."

He looks around the room. "Any takers? Just a massage?"

"I will!" It's my friend Katie in the back of the room. She is raising her hand and leaning forward like she just won the lottery.

"Perfect." The head aide looks relieved. "Don't worry, I will be with you the whole time."

He closes the door to move down to the next room to canvass for more volunteers.

Then, with the sniffling-crying-smiling woman still standing in the front of the room, arms still straight by her side, hands wringing against themselves again, we go on with our night.[31]

I quickly discover that although Janis will never tell me that class is difficult for him, his stress levels are directly correlated to his spending habits. When things get really bad, Janis goes shopping.

I come back from Posture Clinic one day to find him laid out on the bed, surrounded by open tins of wasabi nori crisps, computer propped on his stomach, eyes zoned out on the currency fluctuations of the ForEx market. He barely acknowledges my arrival.

"What's wrong?" I give him a long glance.

"Too many idiots," Janis mumbles.

Apparently, Janis got in a confrontation during his Posture Clinic. He was reprimanded for not knowing the dialogue. Then asked to recite a passage again and again, which he felt was designed to humiliate him and his poor English. He cursed the room, stormed out, and headed to the mall.

For the first time during our stay, I sit down on the edge of *his* bed. I agree that there are too many idiots. I tell him about my troubles with dialogue. Janis's mood rebounds considerably. Soon he has put aside the ForEx market and is standing on his knees on his bed.

He pulls up his shirt to reveal a weird electronic bandage. "I buy! The best!"

The bandage is a Slendertone belt, which seems to bridge the surprisingly narrow gap between late-night TV and the Sharper Image catalog. It

---

[31] Reference point to the emotionally vulnerable place we were at during teacher training: That night, three other people also burst into tears delivering dialogue. Follow-up point to Katie and her massage: "It was so weird because it was so normal. I went up to Bikram's suite, which was just a larger version of the crappy suite we are all staying in and sat next to him, massaging his ankles and calves for two hours. It was completely unremarkable, like a college hangout, people walking around eating, visiting teachers schmoozing with each other. Eventually Bikram decided he wanted to see a Bollywood movie, and half of the room exchanged glances and left. . . . What was amazing was being so close to him, watching his effect on people. Big, tough, tattooed, agro-looking guys coming up to him and just staring in his eyes and saying, "I just love being around you. I just love being in your presence."

electronically stimulates the muscles in the abdomen, causing pulses of contraction and relaxation. Janis pulls a little dial from his pocket. He twists the knob, and his face contorts into a grimace of concentration and pain. Then it releases. He sighs in relief.

"Really, really good. Much better than sit-ups, I think."

I wave off his offers for a test run and go to study dialogue on my bed, listening as Janis sighs rhythmically every ten to fifteen seconds.[32]

Later that night before going to sleep, he tells me: "This is very good. But I think it is too much. We overtrain. The women here are not very good quality, all broken. Otherwise, why they here? Bikram is very, very smart. But I think only smart for idiots. Do you see them staring at him during lecture. Like dogs at food . . . I do not quit now. But I think I make mistake. I miss my Latvia, my women, my clubs."

Many Sides of the Diamond

The Advanced Demonstration arrives to remind us how little we have actually learned. This is the very last week, when we are the most exhausted, but also finally feeling a bit triumphant. The demonstration consists of ninety-one postures performed at a breakneck pace. These postures

---

[32] In addition to the electric stimulation belt, by week five, Janis will have bought: two Brookstone electric back massagers (for exchanging massages after class) two MiFi WiFi devices (to circumvent the T&C's terrible Internet), a second MacBook Pro laptop (no clue), a third camera (this one waterproof), a cool-looking electric thermometer to track the heat fluctuations in the tent, a heart rate monitor, a scale, a sixty-dollar bracelet with magnets that he was told would help with balance, a giant red bouncy ball for additional postclass abdominal crunches that never really happen, and, in a fit of fear after this freakout Posture Clinic, a tiny Bluetooth earbud that Janis decides he can use (with a confederate at a remote location) in lieu of memorizing the dialogue (plan never enacted). Note also that the above clutter doesn't count the legions of supplements, pills, algae, herbal joint remedies, protein powders, and horribly stinky liquid whole-food vitamins, all whose desperate purchasing speaks to the pain and exhaustion he, like everyone else, is going through. The greatest of which, in size if not sheer awesomeness, is his gigantic canister of X-Treme Lean Black Label Weight Loss Diet Pills purchased to ensure he wins his bet, but which he dares take only once— albeit in double dosage—because "Two hours later, I worry I never sleep again. Heart becomes very funny. Hard to walk, only want to run, run, run."

represent the entire Bikram–Ghosh universe, the sum total of the lineage's postural offerings. Within them you find the twenty-six postures that Bikram selected to make his beginners class, but also postures that no beginner could ever even attempt. The biggest reason the Advanced Demonstration reminds us of our collective ignorance is that aside from the twenty-six beginning postures that we have repeated ad nauseum by this point, most of us have never even seen the bulk of the advanced postures, much less been given the opportunity to bend into them. They are largely off-limits, not only to beginning students but also to beginning teachers.

For the demonstration, the best of the best—or at least those best who can afford the time and expense, or those best who need validation or favors from the guru—fly out to Teacher Training to perform for the trainees. It is a stunning opportunity to see where the yoga can go. Without lecture and Posture Clinic, it is also a vacation from the grind—and the mood among us cadets is beyond upbeat. It's like the circus has come to town. Cameras are out in force. Gossip about who will be attending is circulating. Jaws are ready to be dropped. Adding to the intrigue, the Advanced Demonstration is the only time during Teacher Training where Bikram actually performs his own yoga. Instead of teaching, he practices in the group alongside everyone else while Emmy leads the class.

The actual setup is yoga in the round. A little after noon, everyone crowds into the hot tent, and we trainees ring the smaller cluster of advanced demonstrators in the center. In the center of the center is Emmy, eighty-three and leggy, in one-piece leotard with a headset microphone. Standing on the sidelines as the heat rises, I am amazed how disgusting the room feels. It is sticky and stinky, the plastic carpet hairs filled with raw-looking crud that has exuded from our bodies over the last eight weeks. There are ants. There is a filmy layer on the tent siding. When you practice the yoga, all that is blocked out, extinguished by the meditation; when you sit around as a spectator, it is just kind of gross. The whole place evokes the hygiene of a worn-out Band-Aid.

Finally, after everyone else has assembled, Bikram arrives, striding in to join Emmy at the center. There is no swagger in his entrance, it is a beeline purpose, a hyperserious intention, like he has girded up his loins for this event for a while now, and wants to broadcast that gravity to the room. His mask of intensity is completed or undercut (probably depending on whether you are Bikram or merely one of us watching him) by a singularly goofy headband he has chosen to wear. The headband bobs as he walks, reinforcing, to me at least, the image of the middle-aged athlete, weekend warrior charging out to do battle in a pickup basketball game. Regardless, for the first time all training, Bikram is absolutely and completely silent despite wearing his own headset microphone.

The crowd, of course, goes completely nuts at his entrance.

With Bikram at her side, Emmy begins the advanced series by initiating a rapid breathing exercise. Bikram stands next to her, bobbing his head in the hyperrhythms of the respiration, clearly game to the fact that this is Emmy's show. He follows her instructions, accepts her corrections when she offers them, and isn't cracking endless jokes.

As the first posture concludes, Esak sprints in. He brings only a single towel and wears only a modest pair of black shorts. The towel goes on the floor to serve as a mat. Naturally no water. His minimalism is more impressive because almost immediately his postures separate themselves. In a room of the best of the best, he is visibly stronger, visibly stiller, radiating amidst the radiating yogis. As the demonstration enters some of the more dramatic postures, Janis leans into me and points at Esak while he is balancing on one leg: "That is the master." Then, "You think he comes to Riga to teach if I pay?"

By the ten-minute mark, Bikram is clearly lagging. Soon the lagging turns into lollygagging, then a dramatic collapse onto his back to sit out a few postures. When he returns from his rest, the mask of seriousness falls right off. Like many an underperforming student, he begins to act out. First joking into the headset, moaning about his back pain, then pulling out a bright red Coke bottle and swilling while others bend. Finally, chattering all the while, he gives up on the postures and scampers up to his throne, where he basks in the cold air vents that pump on his head. It's behavior that is antithetical to everything he teaches. A friend comes over to me and says, "Uhhhh. Just so embarrassing. The man cannot stand not to be the center of attention for even a second." The demonstration continues, and Bikram eventually descends from the throne to join back in—but he has definitely moved from being a demonstrator in earnest to class clown.

The advanced series ends with a series of abdominal contractions collectively known as nauli. They are not actually postures, instead belonging to the class of hatha exercises known as kryias or purification rituals. In nauli, each band of the abdomen is isolated separately while the rest are relaxed, churning the stomach, creating an oddly hypnotic pattern not unlike a sidewise version of a bellydancer's ripples.

To perform nauli properly, you must be able to variably relax and contract muscles that are typically either interconnected or under involuntary control. It is an example of the mind controlling body at its best, right up there with reversing persistalsis and slowing the heart rate. It is also not taught in the modern Bikram studio, largely because nobody really knows how to do it. As we approach nauli, Emmy asks the advanced practitioners if anyone is capable. "Come on, who has a good nauli? Esak?" Several people attempt it, some approximating the motion, but nothing even verging on the impressive. In response, Emmy clucks a few times and summons Bikram. "All right. You've had your fun. Now, get up and show them nauli," she prods. "How else will they know what it looks like?" But Bikram is dead to the world, long since collapsed and on his back. He waves her off several times without rising. Too exhausted even to think of a quip. But Emmy continues pushing, and the room begins cheering, so he finally pushes himself upright and wobbles to the center.

Bikram takes a moment to gather himself together, places both hands firmly on his pelvis, and suddenly his abdomen disappears. His gut has contracted to a single braid. The rest of his torso is sucked in so tightly, it looks like it has been shrink-wrapped. It is an eerie and ugly position, completely unnatural, nothing you would ever see in a gym class, nothing you could imagine human flesh doing without CGI. It is everything that hatha yoga represented, as it emerged from the jungle, every mystery that Bikram as yoga master should possess.

He churns the braid several times. The room explodes in applause. His face is a contortion of exhaustion and concentration, and when he exhales he stumbles directly toward the door, headband bobbing. Halfway there,

his knees give out, and a loyal aide rushes to his side to prop him up. Together they walk to the fresh air outside. Emmy calls after him, "What?
You can't stay in here and just breathe with us? Such a hurry."

With his exit, the room falls into silence as we watch the rest of the
demonstrators lie in final breathing for a few long moments. Then we are
told we can exit. As we walk out of the tent, it's so jarring that I almost
miss him. There is Bikram lying down in the cold, right along the side of
the tent. The man who disappears immediately into seclusion after every
lecture, who acknowledges vulnerability exactly never, has made it a total of
ten feet before collapsing. He lies there not even on a towel, totally gassed
from his advanced class, eyes closed, brown face a limp pudding, pale fingers by his side taking short quick breaths. One of his aides is crouched next
to him, telling him—the great master of prana—to "just breathe." Streams
of his students walk by their guru without noticing him, gossiping, chatting, discussing food options. I wonder whether this means the night lecture
will be canceled.

Two hours later, Bikram bounds into the lecture tent reborn. He is wearing all white, topped with a white leather cap. "Operation successful!" He
crows, "The patient dead! Doctor very happy. Paid by Blue Cross!" He
holds both hands up like Nixon's victory salute. "Today's class was very
hard for me. I think I kill myself very well. . . . I also must thank Esak—he
gave me the most wonderful massage after class. Without him, who knows,
maybe I won't be here." We roar with approval. The image of the guru
who has obviously not been practicing his own yoga, of the child acting
out moronically to hide his lack of abilities is gone. I catch Esak peering in
the doorway, beaming. His love for Bikram is enormous. I hear later that
he picked Bikram up from his corpse position outside the tent and carried
him back to his suite to give him a one-hour full-body massage.

And boy did it work. Bikram is floating, on a yoga-high nonpareil. It
derails everything. In a pause, just before the lecture, an aide comes onstage to make announcements, the last of which involves a Bikram Yoga
Calendar created by a local studio. "This one is a prototype," the aide
says, flipping through a tiny packet of papers. "I can only assume the images

will be a bit clearer in the final version, but here it is: a calendar! Buy one if you'd like. Support a good cause."

As he walks offstage, Bikram, eyes lit with energy, leans over and playfully snatches the calendar. "Let me show you something!"

He holds the flimsy packet up. "Let's have an auction. I will autograph this calendar, just my name." He looks out at his audience. "I want to auction this calendar, and we give all the money to my guru's charity in Calcutta. You will buy it." He looks around the audience eagerly, scanning faces. I try to hide mine. This offer of an optional auction of an absolutely worthless calendar to a room at least two-thirds filled with people who just emptied their bank account to pay for the opportunity to be present, who are returning to a career that pays subsistence wages at best, and who have zero opportunities for advancement within their profession without a bank loan, strikes me as absurd.

But all of a sudden, instead of lecture, we are in an auction.

Bikram stands center stage. "Bidding starts at fifteen dollars." He looks out at his audience, who like me aren't entirely sure whether he is joking or not. "Who will pay fifteen dollars for this calendar? A beautiful calendar. A calendar with pictures of my beautiful yoga and my beautiful autograph."

A sole hand goes up. I distinctly remember thinking, Well, there's always one.

"Good, good, good. Do I see twenty dollars? Twenty dollars for a beautiful calendar with my signature. This is a first edition! First edition calendar!"

Now a few hands in different parts of the tent. Everyone is still evaluating the situation. Bikram's enthusiasm, however, is growing on itself. He is getting jumpy. He claps his hands in pure joy at each bid, like playing "auction" is the most fun game in the whole world.

"How about twenty-five dollars?" A few more hands go up. But different hands. A woman next to me bids for the first time.

All of a sudden, we are at thirty-five dollars, and Bikram's intensity heats up.

"Come on, forty forty forty forty, do I see forty? Yes! Fifty? If you do fifty, I also come out to dinner with you to celebrate your auction win. It will be the best day of your life. Who has fifty?" The bidding now grows into a frenzy. And Bikram's energy blossoms too, his body bouncing around the stage like he is on the verge of spontaneous combustion: winking at his offstage aides, winking directly at the audience.

With the offer of dinner, we rise from fifty fast. Now half the room is bidding. Eminently sane people are bidding. And when we rip through one hundred dollars, even for those like myself, who have no intention of humoring the event, it's hard not to be a little excited. It's spectacle. It's a man excelling at what he loves. It's Bikram bouncing around the stage, pointing at outstretched hands, screaming nonsense enthusiasm into the mic. Soon we are past $150. But then, slow again at two hundred dollars.

"Come on, just a lousy two hundred dollars! Let's go! We were doing so good!" Bikram says.

Finally a hand shoots up in the back of the room. People stand up to see who it is. I know because I live with him that it's Janis. Of course Janis would have the two hundred dollars for a worthless calendar he doesn't want: especially because it just might help his studio-ownership aspirations. But when I, in my turn, stand to look at who this crazy bidder is, it's not Janis. Instead it's a man I have never seen before. And he is promptly outbid by a woman on the other side of the room.

Bikram immediately plays off the sexes. "You are going to let a woman beat you? A woman?" And when the woman bids it up to $350, he crows again: "I love women!"

At $350, there is a resurgence. Hands are flying up; new bidders are entering. Bikram is explaining that he likes big numbers.

At $550, something insane awakes within: For the first time, I get an undeniable urge to bid. But too late. The bid is six hundred dollars. I imagine myself at dinner with Bikram, all the questions I could ask him for my book. It seems like a not unreasonable price for access. Then we are at seven hundred dollars. I think how purchasing the calendar would show him that for all my authorial doubts, I am still sincere in my investigation. What better way to show that I'm an honest evaluator than to support his guru's charity? I sit and watch my hand twitch in curiosity—and realize this is yogic projection at its finest: Bikram has crept into our imaginations, sparking different fantasies perhaps, but somehow still inside each of us.

"Seven hundred fifty dollars? Come on, who will bid seven hundred fifty dollars! You must! There is only one me! There is only one Bikram! Who else could have done this to a calendar!"

Finally at eight hundred dollars, a new type of silence enters the room. There are four bidders locked in a death match, and the reality of the situation has sunk in for the rest of us. In place of the frenzy from $350 to $800, there is an exhausted, uncomfortable mood in the room: that familiar postcoital instinct, where we're all hoping to flee so we can evaluate what exactly happened in the privacy of our own thoughts.

What's amazing is how quickly Bikram feels this change in mood. His crowing stops. Instead of driving the price upward, he switches from salesman to mediator. He calls the top four bidders up to the stage and announces that they will make a deal. Instead of one copy, he will give all four of them signed copies, and instead of a dinner one on one, they will all go out to dinner together. Never mind that this undermines most of what made the calendar desirable in the first place, the four caucus as directed. In the pause without either Bikram's enthusiasm or the crowd's curiosity, a visible case of buyer's remorse sets in. They return uneasy to offer a collective two thousand dollars as a group. The auction ends. Bikram reminds us he is amazing and unique.

We step out into the calm San Diego night. My friend Anna finds me. "Did you see how happy he was? Did you get that! It was amazing, watching him do what he does best. I mean, would that even have occurred to you? Auctioning something? And if it did occur to you, would it have brought you joy? It's crazy, but I think watching that made me love him even more."

Janis will win his bet, eventually achieving the brass ring of the naturally pudgy: visible abdominal muscles. He strides around our room with his shirt off. But it comes at a cost. Yoga is no longer just an adventure.

"Is it possible I feel this good?" he bounds in postclass during week eight. "If someone tells me, I don't believe it!"

Then he looks at me. I feel like he is about to beat his chest like a gorilla. "I love it! We are strong. We are yogi!!!!"

The Joys

The last few days, there are no lectures. Instead we discuss the postures.

Here is the full joy of Bikram. He moves from posture to posture, describing each contraction, exhalation, or quarter inch of torque. He describes the anatomical benefits, braying like a tonic salesman. ("Spine twisting? Good for life, good for health, good for mind, good for sex, good for spirit, good for business!") He describes his own experiences within the postures, identifying movements that caused him trouble. But mostly he jumps around the stage, adjusting the postures of volunteers.

And with the volunteers he is masterful: cutting the knees out from the valiant and cocky who get up to demonstrate their already perfect poses, ministering softly to the damaged and injured, exhorting the shy to join him onstage. For everyone offering tiny modifications that correct major alignment problems. The effect is of unconscious expertise, not unlike a chess grandmaster walking through an open exhibition match, making moves against twenty simultaneously opponents. At some bodies he is casual, widening a stance, straightening a foot. At others he is brutal, pulling on a ponytail to yank back a neck into a deeper bend. Occasionally he will find himself in front of someone who requires deeper scrutiny. "Banged-up boy," he will ask a man, "how you hurt shoulder?" Buying time to assess the situation, before pulling the shoulder in question to the exact place it needs to be.

The entire time, Esak stands quietly at the back of the room, scribbling at his notepad. This is the part of Teacher Training he flies out for every year.

In many ways, the biggest lesson to learn from his corrections isn't in the details. It is his natural, almost unconscious attitude of compassion to those who need it—completely different from his rhetoric while teaching. Watching Bikram make individual adjustments, you realize how much the dogmatic approach that defines Bikram Yoga in many studios is simply a limitation of knowledge. There is only one way, because teachers know only one way. Bikram Choudhury, on the other hand, will adjust a single posture in a thousand ways or, if the case warrants it, throw the whole thing out.

The flipside to this compassion is brutality for those who can handle it. Again, here his instinct is deft. One night, a man is literally "pulled apart" after performing a lackluster backbend. Bikram orders a volunteer to pull his arms backwards while another holds his torso in place. They yank, and the man jerks back in an ugly motion. When he gets up, the man, shy with his long hair, is left shattered, weeping from either the pain or the humiliation.

I spend the rest of the night wondering if I would have had the social strength to object if Bikram had ordered me to be one to pull him apart. Or whether, full well knowing my Milgram, I would have caved and participated.

But by the next day, my anxiety is revealed as amateur. When Bikram orders the man to bend before him again, he eagerly complies with a back-bend that is absolutely stunning. A curve deep and smooth and confident.

Bikram crows at the development. "Yesterday he was at zero. Today ten thousand times better. . . . What is my name? Bikram! Nobody can do that but me."

If I hadn't seen it with my own eyes, I would assume it was typical bluster. But there is no denying it. The man was touched. He improved epically at something he cared greatly about. The man knows it too, rising out of his new backbend excited, flushed, and bursting with pride.

The next day, Bikram searches the audience for a woman he remembers from class. She has a rod in her spine, a souvenir from a severe case of childhood scoliosis. Bikram places the woman on her knees, and then slowly coaxes her into a deep backbend—Camel posture. Her rod pokes against her skin. Bikram gently cups the back of her head. Finally the woman emerges upright with a huge flush and tears. In a flash, Bikram yanks her up to her feet like she just won a prizefight.

"That is nothing!" he exclaims. "I used to have a student with *two* rods in her spine. And when she does Camel, it is perfect. Most beautiful thing. I could do Crow [a balancing posture] on her chest holding the boobs. Nice boobs too. I have picture!"

Timeless at the 4 A.M. Movie Club

On the last night of TT, after dispatching some irritating business in his suite, Bikram forgoes lecture and instead leads us through a breathing exercise. It is an initiation almost, a meditation that Bikram explains he will teach us exactly as his guru taught him.

"When I was a young man, I used to do this a lot," he says, sitting cross-legged on his throne. "But I stopped. I want to live among humans, not in some cave in the Himalayas. This breathing is the most incredible thing, but you must be careful. Can easily fall into it, easily spend many hours in meditation, and lose all track of time. . . . No good if you want to live in the world."

It is an odd proviso, but with it he begins to instruct us in the technique. Patiently explaining how to wrap our tongues, which phonemes to pronounce on the exhale, and soon we sit and breathe together: completely silently, completely softly, in one rhythm, 381 people. I am very much moved.

After the breathing exercise, Bikram announces there will be a last movie. He tells us it will be optional, but he would like it if we stayed up with him. He says this like a child asking for a gift he knows he just might receive if he is good enough. And I decide, energized by the breathing exercise, joyous that this is our final day of captivity, that just once, I will.

As the rest of the room shuffles off to bed, I push some chairs together into a makeshift bed. Bikram sits with his legs dangling off the stage. Students file past him slowly on the way to the doors. Each and every student who passes says good-bye, some with a head nod, others with a handshake or a hug, sometimes with a suddenly embarrassed rush of tears. There is a realization that after nine weeks, after so much of him, this is the last time we'll be seeing Bikram for a long while.

When the last student has shuffled past and it is just us who are watching the movie, Bikram unclips his microphone. He loosens his hair from his topknot, and his face relaxes. It is a little after midnight, and the room, spacious in its emptiness, seems to soften in fatigue. Bikram stands up and stretches, then walks up and down the length of the stage by himself, drowsily, taking it all in. At his throne, he leans over to pick up a pair of slippers. With no assistance, he slides his feet into them and then sits again on the side of the stage: slippers dangling, shoulders slumped slightly forward, eyes closed, the loosest smile over his face.

A senior teacher, one of my favorite staff members, slips behind him and begins massaging his scalp, unasked for and unawares. Bikram's relaxed smile grows and he does not open his eyes or look up at who is massaging him. He knows. The staff member is smiling too as she rubs, first his scalp and then his shoulders. She has a warm, completely disarmed look to her whole body. Her eyes are half-closed, almost squinting from the pleasure of doing something she knows gives someone else really, really tremendous pleasure. Bikram finally opens his eyes and leans back, looking up at her. They exchange a few words of a conversation I cannot hear. Both laugh. Not the pointed laugh of a joke, but the soft laugh of enjoying each other's company. Everything in the room has decompressed. There are no students to impress. No stage antics being performed. No big gestures, no microphones, and no sound of his own voice for Bikram to react to. His throne sits empty. The fact that everyone is sleepy makes it feel a little hazy, like a dream sequence in a movie. And for a second, I allow myself to imagine that is what has happened. That we have slipped, not so much into a dream, but into a parallel universe: a Bikram in the here and now, but somewhere far away, a place where he is not a yoga god, nor adored, nor surrounded by adults who have surrendered to his personality—a place where he is not lonely, or angry, or betrayed. Just a man, sitting relaxed, getting a shoulder rub.

Eventually, another teacher walks in, carrying a box full of DVDs. He ask Bikram what he wants to watch tonight. Bikram paws through the box. Paws again. Finally he looks out at the ten or so of us remaining and says, "Well, what do you think?"

PART V

Sickness of the Infinitude

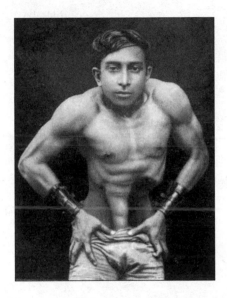

Nauli

A careful scrutiny of various schools of psychoanalytic psychology reveals general belief in the presence in the human psyche of what I call the "Great Self Within," a very real inner presence that is not the same as a healthy human self or ego, but can take possession of an ego and drive it to frag—mentation and total destruction. This "Great Self Within," also called the god—complex or the god—imago, has sometimes been equated with Satan or the devil, but it is very much more complex than the imago of Satan. It is not evil in itself, even though it does fuel the Luciferian tendency.

—ROBERT L. MOORE, *FACING THE DRAGON*

A Perfect Upside-Down Linda

Linda is laying out pictures for me on her dining room table. She has this section of her life preserved. In an otherwise aggressively spare house, she has a whole room devoted to her yoga memories. It is choked. There are shelves of photograph albums, drawers crammed with negatives, and shoe boxes upon shoe boxes filled with invitations, hand-drawn diagrams, scrawled notes, and other accumulations of yogic hoarding. At the dining room table, Linda whips through a few carefully selected items: opening lids, tossing chunks of photographs to the side. Finally, she gets to what she is looking for. Pictures from the earliest days.

"When I met him, he always dressed the same. White. He liked cleanliness. White pants, white shoes . . ." She lays out a series of pictures: Bikram at Disneyland pushing his daughter in a stroller, Bikram with his arm slung over another man's shoulder, Bikram wearing an orange life vest, gingerly stepping onto a boat. And sure enough, there he is in every one: wide smile, straight pants, all in white, looking like an Indian tennis pro.

Linda straightens a photograph. "You can't see this, but his lips were the softest lips you have ever touched. Because he took care of them . . . He was a man who kept himself in the most pristine condition."

Listening to Linda talk about her time with Bikram in the 1970s, I get goose bumps. To anyone who has read the Bikram dialogue, Linda is someone special. She isn't just any Linda, she is *the Linda*—"L like Linda"—mentioned in every single class as an example of how to do the postures, only the third person Bikram allowed to teach his yoga. She took her first class with Bikram at nineteen and studied with him for the next sixteen years. When Emmy would leave town, Linda taught the Advanced Class in her place. More important than her yoga expertise, however, Linda became someone Bikram clung to, someone whom he needed and loved. They traveled together. They celebrated each other's weddings. They raised their children together. In her words, she became his shadow.

In his words, he raised her. She says he repeatedly told her he taught her everything he knew.

Linda touches another photo on the table. "This is us on a hike. Maybe 1982. We went in search of a place called Shirley Lake. We called ourselves explorers." She opens another box, then lays out a series of photographs from the trip. In each, Bikram is grinning, mouth open, like he has just accomplished the most amazing, refreshing thing. "We had so much fun. I don't think he had ever been to the woods before. . . . We had to climb up this one hill on all fours. Just laughing and laughing as we climbed."

She pushes the collection of photographs aside. Paws through another box. "We'd make him presents of us in posture. Photographs. Nothing pleased him like seeing his students. . . ."

And there they all are, the Bikram regulars of the 1970s: Emmy looking like a young princess in a red one-piece; Tony Sanchez in Om posture, leg slung over his head like a middle school backpack; and in the center, Linda, looking like a young Jodie Foster, in full spine twist.

She opens another box. These are real family as opposed to yoga family pictures. There is a picture of her husband pre–wedding ceremony. There is Linda in a bathing suit, her stomach carved into eight clear abdominal muscles. There are pictures of cake and of Bikram pushing a little girl on a swing. He is in a small backyard at a birthday party for Linda's daughter.

Behind him there is a cluster of three balloons tied to a post. Bikram looks like the happiest dad on the planet.

"He promoted families back then," she says. "He was into saving marriages and lives. He counseled people. If he heard about a divorce, he met with the couple and took the husband aside. . . . He wanted people to value each other."

She stops to think.

"He would talk and talk and talk and give and give and give."

She stops again.

"I don't use the word 'guru.' He was my teacher. He took me under his wing."

For a second, she is lost to the room. In the silence, I stare at a picture of Bikram on the Shirley Lake hike. He is young and eager and powerfully strong. He is striding off to take over the world.

Then Linda comes back.

"It almost didn't matter," she says, "the part of him that was not perfect. It almost didn't matter, because what he did have was a perfect gift. I will always hold on to that. Because I got that from him. I earned it."

It almost didn't matter, but it turns out that it did. There is a point where all the boxes of photographs are out on the table, where all the memories are spread out and faceup, and where Linda suddenly stops wanting to talk. We stare at the pictures, thinking very different thoughts. Then she asks me if I would excuse her. She asks if she can get me a piece of fruit from her kitchen. She asks if I would mind if she takes a shower to clear her head.

Then there is a longer silence. Then I push her slightly.

"It got out of control. . . . And so I removed myself. I released myself. . . . I was dying. I was dying spiritually, dying physically. . . . This yoga saved my life. It made my life. But then all of a sudden, I was dying. . . . I don't want to say any more. . . . It got out of control and so I released."

The Sacrifice to Charis

A 1988 study investigating the personality traits of eighteen charismatic leaders in New Zealand—a wide collection of gurus, visionaries, eager saviors, and stentorian mongers of the apocalypse—found them, from a phenotypic standpoint, shockingly ordinary. "Indeed," notes the author and investigator of the study, Len Oakes, "a healthier, more normal-looking profile would be hard to find." When the numbers were crunched, only three traits stood out as places where the charismatic leaders differed even modestly from the general population: slightly higher creative expression, slightly lower deference to authority, and an elevated sense of personal freedom (called the "free child" subscale in the study).

Oakes goes on to explain that the combination of those three characteristics creates a personality profile of individuals who tend to be "head-strong and compulsive," delighting at the defeat of their rivals, and lacking in self-restraint. They are often overtalkative: humorous but self-dramatizing. Individuals viewed as "entertaining but aggressive," who are comfortable expressing their hostile feelings directly, "and prefer not to delay gratification."

All of which is to say, Bikram is less of an anomaly, than cut from the charismatic cloth.

Our word *charisma* comes from the Greek goddess Charis. Charisma was Charis's gift—the transmission of her grace to a human. To possess it, in the original sense, was to be touched by the divine.

This meaning of *charisma* speckles the Bible, both New and Old Testaments. It is typically used to describe a person "full of God's grace," "radiant with divine light," and/or figuratively plugged in and glowing. The biblical embodiment of this charisma is Jesus on the mountaintop amidst the transfiguration, bright halo of light spreading from his back, a visible merger of human nature with heavenly spirit. The Romans had a similar concept, using the word *facilitas* to describe a hero's ability to lead; *facilitas* too came as a gift from the gods, empowering a speaker, issuing out from the body as a force.

And while the religious origins have slipped off our modern usage, the feeling of an intense, almost physical talent remains. In modern descriptions, charismatics are imposing. They operate with an inverse square law like gravity. The aging, reclusive George Washington was dragged to the Constitutional Convention because the Framers believed his physical presence was indispensable. It wasn't enough that he sign off on the results or send a representative on his behalf. The organizers were relying on his body, on his largely silent but terrifically dignified presence to prevent infighting and squabbling by imposing its virtues on the scene.

The flipside to this charisma—like all things divine—is devotion. And here the physicality of the charismatic's appearance is matched by the physicality of his effect on others. And so we have 130 women fainting at a single Michael Jackson concert in Vienna—hyperventilating in tears as he walked onto the stage. We have a mere touch from Bhagwan Rajneesh described as incomparable bliss by a follower, "addictive as the strongest drug," compelling the lucky fellow who was brushed "to go back for more to try and regain that feeling of harmony and being at one with the universe."

Or consider the example of Mata Amritanandamayi—referred often as the "hugging guru." Mata Amritanandamayi's rites consist of a brief ceremony followed by hours of the guru simply hugging participants. Thousands attend, each patiently waiting as the Mata wades from participant to participant, giving a brief, emphatic hug.

If it sounds like harmless, if needy, nonsense to you, you are not alone. But consider this description from a real-life, stony-faced, balls-out investigative reporter, Lis Harris: "I was doing a story on a corrupt healer and wanted to ask the Mata to verify information pretty much only she could verify. My plan was to wait in the hugging line and then, when I got up to the front, ask her as many of the questions as I could, instead of getting my hug. . . . This, of course, proved totally absurd. . . . I mean, here is this little old lady, she barely spoke at all, let alone English, surrounded by a few thousand people all looking for hugs. So there was no way I was going to get anything like an interview. But by the time I realized this, I had already waited in line for a couple of hours, so I decided to stick around for my hug. . . . It was curiosity, nothing more. When I got up to her—honestly, I don't know what happened. . . . I felt this enormous energy all over me. My legs felt like they bent up into the splits from underneath me, all I could hear is her whispering 'ma ma ma' in my ears. Tears were everywhere. I was crying so much, my cheeks were slick. When she moved on, I was a mess, totally undone. Naturally, her handlers immediately swept down on me and stuffed all sorts of books in my hands. I mean, they knew they had a live one."

On this level, charisma operates almost as a lovers' bond. One man's guru can be another man's boiled rice. Pathetic. Transparent. But when it clicks, when personalities align and the moment is right, someone else invades us. It creates a powerful, almost anti-intellectual instinct toward surrender. We doubt it until it happens to us. And often when it happens to us, we deny it out of embarrassment.

The first attempts to study this interaction focused directly on the power dynamic. The great sociologist of capitalism, Max Weber, saw charisma as a revolutionizing force. To Weber, the energy between charismatic and follower was a social fuel. Unlike traditional forms of authority, the charismatic's "superhuman" qualities inspired an intimate form of obedience, a call to service in his followers, a "mission." Moreover, because this obedience was rooted to a single individual, it was unconstrained by the checks and balances and conservative anchors attached to institutions. It existed as an extension of the leader's whims—beyond ethics, aesthetics, or intellect—and accordingly offered a pathway for radical social change.

Weber saw charismatic leaders continually testing their followers, challenging them with feats of commitment and strength. He saw them rejecting economic and material goals in favor of humanistic and spiritual aspirations. He saw them as risk takers, blazing with confidence, often moving rapaciously forward without fear of failure. But ultimately Weber, firmly the sociologist, was never interested in exploring personality traits. His study of charisma was fixated on the relationship between follower and leader. The actual essence—the compulsive force, the divine gift—would remain mysterious for the next seventy years, until a rising star in the psychoanalytic community named Heinz Kohut found himself forced to deal with it.

Heinz Kohut did not set out to study charisma. Instead he spent most of his career grappling with a group of patients known in the 1960s as the narcissistically fixated. Many of these patients were semifunctional in the outside world: brittle, shallow, little men; the tyrants of petty authority; compulsive boasters; and snooty contrarians. Their condition was for the most part crippling—and under examination, many revealed lives of intense loneliness and sadness. These were men and women whose persistent need to be correct prevented them from asking for assistance or seeking advice. Whose insistence on being dominant prevented them from caring for or loving another person. Whose delusions of grandeur prevented them from admitting they were wrong even when presented with direct evidence to the contrary. Their behavior isolated them. In fact, many appeared for analysis only because they had been forced: they were often exhibitionists who engaged in fraudulent and sexually deviant behaviors.

But Kohut was struck not by the pathos each patient eventually revealed. He was stuck on their first impressions. And at first impression, many of these individuals enchanted. Despite knowing exactly who and what he was dealing with, Kohut found his narcissists could make him doubt his clinical diagnosis. Their confidence was infectious. They were often extremely clever, well read, and funny. Their powers of perception, especially when it came to reading him and his moods, were uncanny. And their conversational style—persuasive and assertive—made them appear not just competent, but extraordinary. They glowed.

But the charismatics Kohut was dealing with were deeply ill. There was no mistaking who they were. And so suddenly, after five thousand years of description, a link was made clear that in hindsight looks absurdly obvious: The magnetic exterior of the professional charismatic can be stripped away to reveal a desperate need for attention, a cold core of narcissism.

The Darkest Place Is under the Lamp

The story below is not the result of combining sources, but it might as well be. It is based on the specific words one person told me, although I heard variations of it so frequently that, at a certain point, it almost felt like a ritual of my interviews.

This was at a training. . . . Someone told him I had disrespected his yoga. Why? I don't know. Someone always wants to get closer, and Bikram rewards that. . . . Of course, the idea that I had disrespected the yoga is crazy. I have devoted my life to spreading his yoga. I own a studio. I teach free classes for the community. I had just flown, at my own expense, thousands of miles to see him because I loved the yoga and I loved him. I practice six days a week. When I go home, I bring my parents to practice with me. But suddenly it didn't matter. Someone had told Bikram I had disrespected his yoga—that I talked bad about it—and that was that.

The way it actually went down was this. . . . He finds me right before a lecture and pulls me out. I think the whole time he is going to thank me for flying out to see him. Instead, he pulls me outside and points at a chair: "Sit down!" So I sit down. . . . He puts his finger in my face and starts shouting: "You piece of shit. You scum. I heard what you said. Remember me! Remember who I am! You think I don't know everything! I know everything! I'm Bikram! Now, get the fuck out of my face. I never want to see you again." Anyone else on the planet I would have walked away and called the police. But this was the man I had devoted my life to. I loved his yoga. I still love the yoga. And so I sat there, totally blank, frozen, and listened as he just kept repeating it: "I never want to see you again! Get the fuck out of here!" Eventually he spun around and left. My eyes welled up. I called my partner, I couldn't speak. I had no idea what I would do, not just that moment, but with my life.

From here the stories diverge. Where one person slinks off, an erased member of the community, another will lurk on the periphery until they are reabsorbed. Sometimes the anger simply vanishes as quickly as it came, and the next time the person sees Bikram—sweating with apprehension, an apologetic greeting well rehearsed—they are met with an immediate hug. More often, a groveling process begins. Gifts,[33] charitable donations, direct

---

[33] The gifts that people use to worm their way back into Bikram's graces have their own special absurdity. I have heard a senior staff member grievously instruct a terrified young woman to "approach Boss carefully. Give him space. Then when he has cooled off, find something that he'll like, you know, like ruby red hot shorts, a leopard print something or other, a gold cap, and present it to

payments, indirect apologies, and their continued regret-filled presence at official events finally result in an opportunity to get back into good graces. For others, it is to no avail: I spoke to one studio owner who found himself abruptly cut off from the entire community. People he knew for years refused to acknowledge his presence.

There is a cruelty to many of these interactions that goes beyond the anger. A senior instructor deliberately kept around so he could be fired on his birthday. A studio owner who was invited over to dinner at Bikram's house—who flew into town for this dinner—and who arrived excited and honored, only to have Bikram use that occasion to publicly exile him. Bikram enjoys the setup. Balancing the vulnerable on the tee.

Or from my training, the story of Brian.

Brian was a tall, muscular, hyperfriendly, yoga-teacher-to-be. I loved hearing him give dialogue because—even more than the mechanistic blushing Japanese or the goofball Australians—his thick whaddaboutit Queens accent reminded me how diverse the yoga was. That it could cut across economic worlds and undermine every obvious stereotype. Brian was in my group for Posture Clinic, so I got to know him fairly well over the nine weeks. Which is relevant only because otherwise I would very likely never have heard any of this. It would simply have vanished like so many other interactions with Bikram.

On the very last day of Teacher Training, right before the Timeless 4 A.M. Movie Club, Bikram called Brian up to his hotel suite. Everyone else was off celebrating, discussing where they were going to teach their first class, sleeping past 9 A.M., or even skipping a class or two.

In his suite, Bikram asked Brian to sit. Then he announced Brian was not going to be allowed to graduate. That he would not be allowed to teach and that he would not be given his money back.

Brian asked what was going on.

Bikram spoke slowly and calmly, like everything was perfectly obvious.

---

him. Then tell him how much the yoga means to you, how much you love what he has done, take his class, take a seminar, and usually it will blow over."

Brian watched the hotel suite begin to blur into nonsense. Before coming to San Diego, Bikram explained, Brian had taken classes at a studio that also offered other forms of exercise. Regularly taken classes there. This studio was unsanctioned, Bikram explained, illegal, a cheat, stealing his money and his property, by which he meant his yoga. This was written into the contract everyone signed at Teacher Training, and Brian knew this. As punishment to that studio owner, Bikram had decided he was not going to allow Brian to graduate from Teacher Training, he was not going to allow him to teach his yoga, and he was not going to give him his money back.

Brian said: "Boss, I have done everything you have asked. I have followed every rule here. I have nothing to do with that illegal studio. I just took classes there. It was near my house."

Bikram explained that was beside the point.

Brian said: "I have never taught at that school and I will never teach at the school. I will walk away from everyone I know at that school. And I will do it for you."

Bikram explained that he had made up his mind. That the rogue studio owner had forced his hands. He explained that if Brian wanted to blame someone, he should blame the studio owner. A studio owner Brian barely knew and did not like. Then Bikram smiled at Brian and informed him once again he would not be refunding his money. He explained he had known about this problem from the beginning of training but waited until the final day to tell Brian. Then he asked Brian to get out of his suite.

And so no Brian at graduation.

And finally there are the women. You don't need all the salacious details to understand, so I won't belabor the point. Just to link it to everything else.

When I first got to training and watched him play favorites, it was hard not to be amused by how silly it all was. This was Bikram of a thousand dirty jokes. Who never misses an opportunity to push up his sleeve to show off a diamond-encrusted wristwatch. Or who offers to let a cute girl try his on if she'll let him wear hers. Who tells a stammering but statuesque girl delivering dialogue that she was perfect, just after ripping the heart out of a stammering but scrawny boy. Who discusses how slippery men can be and how it is a wife's responsibility to prevent her husband from cheating. There was something so transparent about it that it was disarming. He was a world-class ham, a flatterer, overt to the point of insecurity. But as training progressed, I learned that is what makes Bikram so potent: Authenticity is morality. Being open and funny is his method. Or as he might say: "The darkest place is right beneath the lamp." Bikram would eye the prettiest, blondest women in front of all 380 of us. He would begin from the very first moment he stepped onstage. He watched where they sat during lecture and how deep their practice was during class. He joked about them, teasing them on his headset microphone. His favorites were the big women, thoroughbreds, who hit the archetype of feminine hard, with long hair, proud legs, perfect figure. But if the big women were too proud, too married, he also knew exactly where to look next. The slightly smaller version. Still beautiful but two or three steps more insecure. The one who always made prolonged eye contact with other men, who made a point of sticking around and watching movies with him, who was always wearing short-shorts, and who was already so exceptionally comfortable with her body that it made you wonder what exactly happened to make her learn to be so comfortable. Bikram can pick out a weak ankle twenty years after the injury. Do you really think he can't pick out the few needy young women who believe his yoga has saved their lives and will do anything to prove that to him?

I learned in conversation after conversation with these women that Bikram is not all rhetoric. I learned because these women brought it up, angry and still trying to come to terms. He is not a world-class flirt, not a goofy ham. He might let you wear his wristwatch, but occasionally he wants something in return.

This is the ur-story.[34] Maybe you have the best postures. Maybe you are stronger than almost everyone else. Maybe you can make other people laugh, and everyone in the room naturally looks to you. You are a woman

---

[34] As the prevalence of *maybes* below makes clear, this isn't based on any one person. But the group of women whom it is based on might be forgiven for thinking I am taking personal details from stories they told me in confidence and making them public. That is understandable. But sadly, I heard the same story again and again and again.

who is noticed—whether at your training, at headquarters studio, or teaching class. Then you are noticed by Bikram himself. Maybe you dance with him at a party. Maybe you volunteer to massage him. The idea of service attracts you. The idea of honoring an elder attracts you. Bikram has given you something that made you. That transformed the way you see the world. He took a life that existed in pea green and colorized it. You also understand how important the role of guru was in Bikram's life. You want to show him that you get that, and that he is similarly important in your life. Maybe he personally invites you up to massage him. Maybe this happens only once or maybe it goes on over the course of many weeks. The fact that you are noticed builds. Maybe he gets off the podium and stands behind you in class. Maybe he mocks your postures and pushes you harder than anyone in the room. Amidst the 380, he has seen you—and now every interaction with him in the room builds your relationship. Whether he calls you up to the stage or he ignores you and flirts with someone else, he has you on some level. Finally, it is late at night and you are mostly alone in his suite. Just you with the senior teachers, the chosen few. He jokes with you. He makes an amazingly accurate uncanny bird noise for you. He makes fun of someone else in the room and then looks back at you for a reaction. His attention, usually divided up among 380 bending bodies, is focused just on you—and it is enormous. You see how human he is, how needy. When people leave his suite, he explains how lonely he is, how nobody understands him. He explains how similar you two are. He tells you he is going to make you famous. And although you are usually savvy and would normally be impervious to this idiotically clichéd line, you indulge the fantasy as he repeats it again: He can make you big in the yoga world. He whispers he will take you to the *international level*. He invites you to massage him in the bedroom. Just so he can lie down. This kills the fantasy, and you don't know what exactly went wrong, what messages you sent, and you blame yourself for letting the situation get to this point. He invites you into the bedroom again, but this time turning directly toward you, placing one of his hands on one of your thighs, and then his other on your other.

You tell him firmly no.

You get out of there and then you really freak out.[35]

Of course, maybe I have it all wrong. A senior teacher, a woman, looked me deep in the eye and said, "Don't make any mistake, they want to sleep with him. They are women. Don't devalue them."

I can't speak for anyone except myself. And Bikram certainly never tried to sleep with me. But I am not making a mistake when I say the women I spoke to did not want to sleep with him. All of them expressed discomfort or disgust. I am also not making a mistake when I say, they described pressure, games, and promises that sound like the manipulative, abusive, and ultimately self-destructive behavior of someone who has found himself atop of an empire and will continue pushing boundaries until he is stopped. They described a man who was punitive when he didn't get his way, who was aggressive in his pursuit, and who would bully past their objections when he sensed weakness. A man with a financial and spiritual stake in their lives who was unafraid to use that leverage to manipulate them. These were not women telling stories out to ruin Bikram. Almost all expressed reservations that their comments would ultimately damage them financially because Bikram Yoga was their occupation as well as their life. Many of them are still active in the community. Some still interact with him at formal events. But every single one said, I don't look to him for anything spiritual anymore. I don't really respect him.

"I'm not sure exactly when I realized," Chad is telling me. "You are surrounded by people who are in silent compliance, acting like everything is okay, when the situation is totally out of control."

Chad Clark, the heat specialist, is telling me about his time working for Bikram as his superintendent in Los Angeles. "I didn't even blink when he asked me to spy for him—it was an honor." Bikram sent Chad out to studios across the country as his "policeman," investigating studio owners who were cheating him: which translated less as a financial issue and more in terms of

---

[35] At least that is how it turned out for most of the women I talked to. They also all seemed certain it turned out differently for other women.

control. Cheating Bikram was failing to do what he asked when he asked it: teaching with words beyond his dialogue, refusing to put carpet on the yoga room floor, keeping the heat too low, renting a space too big or too small, or disobeying any of the other hundred tiny byzantine regulations he insisted upon when someone opened a studio in his name.

"There were other spies too," Chad says. "Obviously, my work put me in a special position, going in and out of so many studios. But reporting on someone else is a way to prove you love him. Having a network of 'spies' goes right along with his whole gangster fantasy. It builds him up. Bikram on the top and everyone else below and uncomfortable."

The spying didn't give Chad pause. Neither did Bikram's frequent requests for Chad to work for free. Neither did the constant screaming, the petty tantrums, the casual insults to women, the insane boasts, or the refusal to consider Chad's personal needs on the rare occasion he voiced them. What eventually pulled Chad out was a growing belief that Bikram was driven to hurt the people who were around him.

"I was superintendent, so maintenance fell on me. And his personal studio was a death trap. I don't say that lightly. Bikram refused to pay me to make basic repairs. And any construction that I was involved with used illegal untrained labor. He had the money, of course. He was swimming in money. But he just wouldn't spend it on something that didn't benefit him." Chad pauses. "I went through this slow realization that he really and truly does not give a shit about other people. Not about their lives. Not about their safety.

"And so I was working in a death trap. We got over twenty-seven violations from the fire department in a single year. The enclosures around the windows were electrified hot where the wiring was put in poorly. The cleaning staff would complain to me that they couldn't close the laundry door or they would 'go to sleep' from the carbon monoxide that collected there. Light lenses would fall out of the ceiling and crash onto the floor. Dryers were constantly catching fire because they were overused and needed to be replaced." As Chad is listing these grievances, it feels less like the details matter, and more his way of expressing a greater outrage. This is just the one area he has a firm grasp on. "This was normal life. Another fire in the laundry room! Bikram screaming at another girl until she cries! And for a long time, my attitude was, it's his business. He can run it however what he wants. And then one day, he demands that I help him expand the studio. He wanted me to cut a hole between two buildings, with two different landlords, without informing either one, in a seismic zone. It was totally illegal. I told him I couldn't do it."

And so Chad was out. Exiled from the community, banished from Bikram's presence.

"But that hole is there today," Chad says. "Right through two buildings, right in a seismic zone . . . And at the end of the day, that's why he is still where he is. Someone will always step up and do exactly what he wants."

The Hole

Eleanor Payson began studying narcissists out of necessity. She was working as a marital therapist in Michigan and noticed a sharp spike in the number of her patients struggling with a narcissistic partner. "But at the time, the literature on narcissism was almost unreadable." She explains to me, "It was a dense overacademic tangle. Completely unhelpful to someone actually dealing with an abusive relationship in their life."

She decided to fill the void. The book that resulted, *The Wizard of Oz and Other Narcissists,* became a runaway hit: spreading first among therapeutic professionals hungry for a resource to give to their patients, then by word of mouth as their patients reported back to their friends and families. It is written with a casual, direct tone, an expertise earned in the field rather than filtered by academic theory.

"You don't have to be particularly clever to remark that we are living in an age dominated by narcissism," she says. "So much of society rewards that behavior, and so many social pressures help form it. It is held out as a virtue."

Narcissistic personality disorder is tricky precisely because of those social pressures. It takes qualities we all strive toward and carries them to warped extremes. Confidence is stretched into delusion, passion is converted to ruthlessness, drive to obsession. Self-love prevents love of another.

But because we all must possess a healthy form of these qualities to thrive, recognizing the narcissistically disturbed often feels like a queasy mix of jealousy and self-indictment.

When we talk, Eleanor begins by addressing these concerns. The narcissist, she explains, is in desperate pursuit of a need we all have: to feel valued. Unlike healthy individuals, however, the narcissist is unable to satisfy this drive no matter how much admiration, money, sympathy, or status he receives. Instead he builds an idealized, grandiose self—an image of himself that is special and magnificent and therefore justified in pursuing his own needs, regardless of the effects on others. The charismatic narcissist hungers, above all, for adulation. It is his greatest need; and like all creatures that hunt to survive, he has learned from a young age a number of strategies to feed himself.

As a result, these narcissists are often extremely charming on first impression—laugh-out-loud funny, persuasive, and energizing. "They intoxicate, they tell stories of this amazing life, and although they might feel overwhelming—perhaps a little too self-referential—it is very easy to brush that feeling aside." If he is surrounded by codependents, the interaction might end with an eye roll and someone explaining "that's just Steve being Steve."

Later as the scales begin to fall, the introduction seems less of a one-off performance than a mode of being. "A narcissistic relationship is a one-way street," Eleanor explains, "Once you engage the narcissist, the dynamic increasingly takes place on his terms—each encounter dictated by his moods and whims, and inevitably serving his agenda." Indeed, the narcissist's pursuit of his own needs are so overwhelming that he has a great difficulty seeing other people as humans with separate needs and wants. He might give—indeed he might shower attention, love, and gifts—but only to receive in response. He will impart knowledge but withhold crucial information so nobody can rival his expertise. The narcissist will seize on trivial details as weapons. Corrections become a method of establishing dominance. Friends, coworkers, sons, wives exist only to serve his purposes. Indeed, in the most extreme cases, the world itself—the fabric of reality—exists only as an extension of the self.

And until something—or someone—acts to disprove their delusion, everything can move merrily along its way. But when the world deviates from their expectation—when things do not go their way—the narcissist will often react catastrophically. Alternately becoming outraged or wounded, overtly domineering or covertly engaged in sabotage as they work to manipulate the world back to their self-obsessed image.

Eleanor points me to the *Diagnostic and Statistical Manual of Mental Disorders* (DSM) criteria for diagnosing narcissistic personality disorder:

1. Has a grandiose sense of self-importance (e.g., exaggerates achievements and talents)
2. Is preoccupied with fantasies of unlimited success, power, brilliance, beauty, or ideal love
3. Believes that he or she is "special" and unique and can only be understood by, or should associate with, other special or high status people
4. Requires excessive admiration
5. Has a sense of entitlement, i.e., unreasonable expectations of especially favorable treatment or automatic compliance with his or her expectations
6. Is interpersonally exploitative, i.e., takes advantage of others to achieve his or her own ends
7. Lacks empathy: is unwilling to recognize or identify with the feelings and needs of others
8. Is often envious of others or believes that others are envious of him
9. Shows arrogant, haughty behaviors or attitude

According to the DSM IV, a narcissistic disorder is indicated if five out of the above nine descriptors are present in an individual. In my opinion, it offers a description, in bullet point, of Bikram.

At one point during our conversation, apropos of nothing, Eleanor cuts me off. "So is this a cult?"

The question catches me unawares, leaving a full two seconds of silence.

I had been giving background on my book, rattling off my professional history while her mental gears were clearly still grinding over something I'd said previously.

"No." I scramble. "I mean, I don't know. There are a few people within the community who might have a cultlike relationship to Bikram the man. But I think they are the minority. . . . Also everything is out in the open."

Eleanor responds with her own moment of silence.

It turns out, not surprisingly, that people who experience a certain type of wounding in childhood are more vulnerable to the charismatic image of the narcissist than others. In a community, these individuals may be em- powered by the narcissist to act out their own needs—seeking adulation, status, and control.

Or as Chad says, "The biggest lesson that being close to Bikram taught me is dark energy attracts dark energy. At a certain point, Bikram became a magnet. The image of the student flows from the guru. And so if you wanted an excuse to be abusive, you had Bikram acting as an example. If you needed to be a petty tyrant to feel good about yourself, here is Bikram glamorizing being a control freak. . . . There are plenty of extremely won- derful people in the Bikram world—definitely the majority—but most of them are very frustrated and sad by the fact that there is a whole different set of people running around, acting like mini-Bikrams, screaming and ranting and in general acting like sociopaths."

Eleanor points me to the psychoanalytic literature. Here the narcissist and codependent are fully intertwined.

Both are children who are not "seen" for who they actually are: who learn from their parent's reactions that their natural instincts are unwanted or unwelcome. In both, this becomes a wound or inner vulnerability, where a healthy ego just isn't good enough. Instead, both as compensation and in an effort to prove worth, these children develop strategies to gain the love denied.

In the narcissist, this becomes the quest for grandiose achievement. In the codependent, this is turned inside out in a grandiose vision of an ac- cepting caregiver or perfect learner. One child chasing admiration, the other desperate for approval. Two sides, same essential coin.

As this need for validation grows into adulthood, the codependent becomes steadily more vulnerable to the narcissist's greatest seduction: the flattery of mutual admiration, a needed infusion of self-worth. The charismatic narcissist, long practiced at making other people believe he is extraordinary, hooks his audience by making them feel special too—either overtly through compliments or an inspirational message ("you are a gold mine of infinite potential"), divisively by pointing out someone else's flaws, or more insidiously, simply through the decision to grant his attention. Later, if the narcissist's power allows, this can extend to creating inner circles where codependents can be rewarded or shunned—where proximity itself is used like a drug—and where ultimately moving closer to the center means allowing deeper hooks like financial dependence, sex, or position in the community to be inserted and used to dominate.

Eleanor ends our conversation by cautioning me. "I know very little about this yoga community, but if you are dealing with a community of individuals who have surrendered to a narcissist, you will find yourself very isolated very fast if you explore this with them. No matter how rational you feel you are being, a person in the thrall of a narcissist has lost all sort of reference point. You can't talk him out of it, or make him 'see the light.' This is a person with a false center, who will tend to react just as hysterically as the narcissist when challenged."

Yogi-Raj Light of Yogic Learning

One only needs to read the title of Alice Miller's *Drama of the Gifted Child* to come to a weak hypothesis. In that work, Miller posits that a child raised by narcissists is denied true love and rewarded only for his or her accomplishments. The child aches for love, and works to get it in the only way the narcissistic parent awards it: by achieving external success. The parent in turn sets up an addictive cycle: Success is rewarded with great beaming displays of joy when the child performs, and love is withdrawn when the child fails. On the outside—clean, quiet, pulling perfect grades—the gifted child gains some relief from all the praise they earn, but the inner self—denied any affection, desperate for love for love's sake only—grows increasingly needy, insecure, and tormented.

In that book, Miller writes:

> *It is one of the turning points in analysis when the narcissistically disturbed patient comes to the emotional insight that all the love he has captured with so much effort and self-denial was not meant for him as he really was. In analysis, the small and lonely child that is hidden behind his achievements wakes up and asks: "What would have happened if I had appeared before you, bad, ugly, angry, jealous, lazy, dirty, smelly? Where would your love have been then? And I was all these things as well. Does this mean that it was not really me whom you loved, but only what I pretended to be?"*

Accordingly to Eleanor Payson, the golden age for narcissistic development is three to five years old. It is when a child is most vulnerable emotionally and biochemically.

Three years old is, of course, precisely when Bikram was first introduced to yoga. It was when his inner worth became synonymous with his postural depth and self-denial. When he lost his mother for an indefinite apprenticeship that involved fourteen hours a day at the hands of a mad, charismatic sometimes sadist who punished his imperfections with burns and who extremely rarely—when Bikram was at his absolutely cleanest, best, least lazy, and most dedicated—rewarded him with slight praise. A man whom his absentee parents revered, who with his overmuscled physique and legion of overmuscled followers was almost a superhero figure of powerful male dominance. This was Bikram's formative experience. This was how he learned to value himself.

And so now when I hear him say to his wealthy clients: "I'm not going to be your American momma."

Or: "I *hate* lazy people."

Or when he sneers: "No, sweetie, don't push yourself. . . ."

Or: "You know biggest problem in your life? You never work. You always have big American momma saying, 'Take it eaasssy, baby.' "

It's hard for me to hear anything except a form of wishing, almost prayer: his lectures endless and repetitive tirades against comfort and love because if repeated enough, perhaps those sentiments could become true. Like all good critiques, Bikram Yoga began primarily as a self-critique: If only I could rise to this ideal. If only that ugly whining internal voice fell in line with the sentiments my external self is vocalizing.

Bikram found a home in America. Beverly Hills loves an orphan. All those movie stars intuitively recognized one of their own. They grabbed on to his critique because it was the one they had been giving themselves. Who is more insecure about the love, praise, and adoration they receive than the Hollywood starlet? Who has a valuation as transparently false as the silicone gel in her cheekbones? And then all the AAs, NAs, the abused, the damaged, the chronically ill, the borderlines, all of us seekers, all with our holes to fill, we came next. We couldn't help ourselves. I'm not talking about most people who step inside a Bikram Yoga studio. I'm not talking about the ones who can walk away. Just us, the hell-bent.

An hour and a half of staring at ourselves in the mirror, of self-critique being masked as self-improvement, of being told we were healing because we were punishing ourselves. It was and is irresistible.

Listen again to Mary Jarvis describe the present moment, her goal for practicing the yoga: "In the present moment, you can't feel pain, you can't be snotty, you can't be sad."

Which is of course why Bikram—by being hopelessly damaged—is exactly the doctor we needed to get the message. He is the guru the living curriculum conjured up for our damaged egos. He is perfect and sad, and we needed him to explain to us how to be perfect within our sadness too. This is precisely where for me it gets complicated and self-referential. Where the tragic flaw is also the key quality that enables the success. A "better" guru would never have been our mirror. A "better" guru would never have given us this yoga tool.[36]

---

[36]Bikram always says that "yoga makes you, you" a claim I have never found accurate. Instead, I have always felt my essential nature—my sense of self—has remained fairly consistent through my yoga practice. Almost like a song melody that contained my most personal characteristics. Yoga never altered this song, never even tweaked the notes, but what it did do—and what makes it, in

And so I can't help but think that this is the last truest requirement of Bikram. A special opportunity. In part because of Bikram's dedication to truth as he see it, in part because of his recklessness, we have a legitimate chance to kill our guru. Kill him just as he explains we need to kill ourselves during every class. And once we have done that—really done that, in an open, thorough, and probably horribly difficult process—once we have sacrificed our notion of him completely, maybe we can love him again. I know the community will be stronger. I also know, just as with a single class, a half-assed approach isn't going to work. We can't skip directly to the "love him" phase without doing the hard work first. Ignoring things, looking the other way at disturbing, dangerous tendencies—those attributes we are complicit in, which are in fact fueled by our adulation. We can't continue explaining to other people as well as ourselves, that, well, I can see him as a flawed man and I can take the good with the bad or I just gotta love him, I mean, he's Bikram, one of a kind, without ever honestly dwelling on the really bad parts, or the fact that uniqueness and charm are no inoculation against sexual manipulation and sociopathic greed. To do anything less is the community equivalent of walking out of a class because it's just too damn hot. And for those who must see every quality of Bikram in a positive light, perhaps see this as his greatest gift of all. See him as a perfect guru because he is so thoroughly imperfect and thus all the easier to discard.

---

my opinion, fairly incredible—is act as a tool, raising or lowering the volume. It can amplify my ego as it already exists. Or humble me to my knees. One of my best friends at training, Anna, always said, "I don't know how the yoga works, but I do know that I started practicing and I grew a pair of brass balls. I kicked my alcoholic husband out of my life. I got a better job. It's a power tool for taking responsibility." I couldn't agree more. Like all power tools, however, if used improperly, it can be dangerous. And as a community, we need to step up and realize that when this aspect of the tool does not get addressed, it gets abused.

PART VI

All Lies Are Aspirational

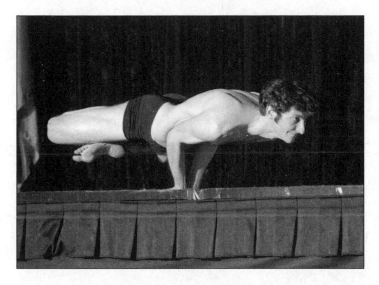

The author, competing in the 2011 Yoga Asana Championships

The true opponent, the enfolding boundary, is the player himself. . . . The competing boy on the net's other side: he is not the foe: he is more the partner in the dance. . . . [In tennis], you compete with your own limits to transcend the self in imagination and execution. Disappear inside the game: break through limits: transcend: improve: win. Which is why tennis is an es— sentially tragic enterprise. . . . You seek to vanquish and transcend the limited self whose limits make the game possible in the first place. It is tragic and sad and chaotic and lovely. . . .

—DAVID FOSTER WALLACE, *INFINITE JEST*

The Song of Solomon

Before our first class, we meet in the locker room.

Without his shirt, Sol has the sad body of a circus bear. An exhaustion of grayish flesh, lumbering and emotive in itself. Pocked and microcreased, whole sections giving way like an overstretched plastic bag. It is amazing how much depredation clean baggy clothes can hide. I see the incision from his gall bladder surgery where the little bag that collecting his drippings interfaced with his body.

We set up on opposite sides of the room. We clasp our hands under our chin for the opening breathing exercise, and class begins.

As in all classes, I quickly lose track of myself within myself.

At a transition between postures, I sneak my only glance at Sol. He is lying flat on his back, chest heaving up and down, eyes locked on the ceiling, terrified—this massive respiring clump of flesh: just a few gulls away from a beached marine creature. I think of Ashley. At least from that position, he isn't going to hurt himself. Then I resolve not to look over again.

I never ask him about class. Instead, we conclude in the locker with a ritualistic swilling of vitamins and electrolyte powder I have decided we need to take every day. Sol very formally shakes my hand and then staggers out; instead of heading off to his office, he decides to go back home "for a while," which I think sounds safe enough for Ashley's purposes. Later, we talk on the phone, and he describes himself as sore but excited.

Day two was a success in that Sol showed up; it was worrisome in that he fled the room at Camel posture. He explained later he thought he heard his cell phone alarm ringing in the locker room and decided he should leave to turn it off. I nodded and just hoped he would return for day three. He did. Day four, Sol announced he was having trouble walking. His legs felt like they were on fire. Day five he said he hurt all over and was cramping up while sitting at his desk. But he kept coming.

As per our agreement, Sol took the first Sunday off to rest. That night, the city was hit with one of the worst snowstorms of the year. School was closed. The subways struggled. I called Sol to discuss skipping class. But he dismissed the offer without consideration. "As long as the teacher's there, I don't have much excuse."

The teacher made it. And then we were off. By day fifteen, when I expected Sol to be struggling the most, he declared he loved the yoga. He actually used the word *love*.[37] He told me he was getting the best sleep of his life.

---

[37] Love! And a word about its use herewith: I am sure the more socially aloof have been snickering along with my heavy-handed use of the term. I certainly know that between the time I first arrived at Backbending and when I left, my cynicism was just as bruised as my backbones. But the experience of love—the euphoria, the cravings, the earnest sincerity, and full-bore absorption—is an extremely real part of the whole yoga experience. Among new couples, new mothers, and the freshly fucked, significant attention has been paid to the release of a hormone called oxytocin. Oxytocin is a neuromodulator intensely associated with both the maternal instinct and sexual bonding. (Hello, Freud.) An injection of oxytocin to a mother boar will cause her to bond to an orphaned young piglet regardless of providence. Similarly, when at play, oxytocin levels increase with arousal and crest at orgasm. A sudden injection into a rat will cause a sudden erection. Both yoga in particular and vigorous exercise in general have been shown to flood the brain with oxytocin. The rapt emotions Sol feels toward the yoga are neurologically probably not too different from the rapt emotions he felt toward his wife Ashley when they first started courting. Important too is the growing understanding that a major role of oxytocin might be to *decouple* neurological links (i.e., when you fall in love with someone, it is actually very helpful to first fall out of love with your previous partner, lose all those old memories and associations). Thus the blast of oxytocin during a yoga binge might actually be a key part in the self-transformation process: the powerful feelings of

The Super Bowl coincided with a rest day, and Sol got atrociously drunk—but he showed up for the evening class of day twenty-one anyway. By day thirty he declared he was done with rest days. The studio offered a free month of unlimited yoga to anyone who did thirty days in a row, and Sol announced that he was going to earn it.

Friends kept coming to bend with us. Two came from out of state, each staying for a week. Another dropped in for a single class and ended up buying the monthly pass. But instead of acting as pit crew, pushing Sol forward, they were an audience to his performance.

Return of the Jedi

I arrive at 1 A.M. to another Backbending. In another oversized suburban home, after driving through another webbed private community of cul-de-sacs. This time in New Jersey. This time it's snowing.

Once again, I find the front door unlocked. Now, however, I thrust it open with a honey-I'm-home confidence. The first person I notice is Fiona from Ireland, and I feel relief with her gigantic openmouthed smile. She wraps me in a bear hug. Then while still hugging, I hear yelled only slightly sarcastically, straight past my ear: "Are you guys talking about yoga??" And she darts through our hug off into a conversation in another room.

I drop my bags and look around. Every time I walk into one of these—inhaling the squalor of protein mixes and supplements, scanning the stacks of cucumbers and bananas, the dorm room scampering of women in boxers—I have a flash to some late-night docudrama on meth labs. The kind that always reminds you that secrets lurk behind every ordinary home. Nobody rolling down these suburban New Jersey streets in their Audis and Infinitis would guess that behind those quiet hedges and tall white doors there lurked a full-blown yoga refugee camp.

---

love erasing old neural connections and decoupling those ugly relationships (to food, sex, drugs, pain, sleep, etc.) that aborted so many other nascent health kicks in the past.

Our host is Brigit, a young local studio owner. Brigit is also organizing the New Jersey Regional Asana Competition, and a key superficial difference between this Backbending and Charleston is we are training specifically to culminate in the New Jersey competition.

Under the surface, there are other differences. As soon as I see Esak, he slaps a surprisingly soft purple shirt against my chest. "Check it out!"

It is a more professionally designed incarnation of the Backbending shirt he was given at the end of Charleston. On the front, there is a series of extreme yoga poses. On the back, written in the style of the upward-scrolling *Star Wars* prologue:

JEDI FIGHT CLUB:

CHANGE YOUR MIND.

I decide I love it.

So does everyone else, I realize quickly as it ends up being pretty much the only top anyone wears for the rest of the week. Beyond the shirt, there are other improvements. The DIY mentality is here but streamlined. A schedule has been produced so we know what we are doing ahead of time. Esak has convinced a masseur-friend to tag along, and he is occupying a room in Brigit's basement doing brisk business. There are fresh juices prepared for us after class if we want to buy them. Then protein smoothies after the morning workout. Even crazier, there is a small crew of yogis who are practicing half-time. In Charleston, it was apostasy to sit out even a single workout. But now there is a whole crew who do only morning work with the Backbenders, then go off to prepare the juices, smoothies, and dinner that keep the rest of the benders bending.

All these services demand separate payments, so Esak has assigned people to collect money, and one of the big themes of the week is people coming up, trying to collect dues. Dinner dues, juice dues, smoothie dues, seminar dues, T-shirt dues. The experience is still pay what you can—now there is simply a lot more you can pay for.

But in-house masseur and post-class smoothies aside, in all the essential ways, all the ways that occur inside the hot room, Jedi Fight Club is still identical to Backbending. It just got an upgrade.

Given the opportunity, I quickly fall into the group doing half lessons. This is not out of weakness so much as because of finances. I still have a nonyoga job. And, as this incarnation of Backbending/Jedi Fight Club is located within the reach of my New York home, the lure of work proves more powerful than the lure of endless back pain. Every morning, I wake at 6 A.M., get in my car, and drive the two and half hours to Southern Jersey. Then I take class with the group, do the morning workout, take the second class, and drive back to New York to hunker down in front of a computer monitor. Or I do the reverse—stay the whole day, do the night workout too, and find myself awake until 2 A.M. with implausible backbending energy, only to have to wake up four hours later for the reverse commute back to New York City in order to gingerly slide my sore shoulders into a suit jacket to attend a meeting.

My yoga becomes not falling asleep on the New Jersey turnpike.

Unlike Charleston, where I would have killed for this type of relief, I find I am annoyed by being unable to participate fully. My body has changed. The backbending itself, while not easy, is no longer crippling. In fact, a set of thirty backbends begins to feel almost inadequate. Just a bite. My spine never achieves more than a mild discomfort rather than the barbed wire bruising from before. Best of all, instead of being the grumpy old man, I get jacked on the backbending energy too.

Unlike Backbending in Charleston, where I was just trying to keep up, in New Jersey, my mind is set on competition the entire time.

In yoga, David Foster Wallace's self-competition—what my favorite teacher, Courtney Mace, calls "the battle between the ego and the soul"—is intensified even further. There is no opponent, there is no dance partner, before Bikram there wasn't even a mirror. Yoga is just you: attempting to disappear inside yourself, break through the limits of your own conception, match your body's actions to your will. The mat, the mirror, the instructor, your fancy quick-dry attire, even the postures themselves are all only useful as guide rails. They channel you toward this meeting of the self.

Or as Linda put it to me, "No bats, no balls, no nets. Just you—yourself and yoga."

This is one of the reasons we intuitively distrust ostentation in the yoga room (and why nonpractitioners have intuitively decided it is ripe for derision and claims of hypocrisy). If you want to avoid the self-competitive aspects of most sports, you can dodge it by focusing on an always salient external manifestation: beating your opponent. It's an easy escape, one where buying a three-hundred-dollar tennis racket, a pair of two-hundred-dollar sneakers, or a three-thousand-dollar bicycle will always be justifiable. They help you win, after all. On the other hand, if you feel overcooked by the competition with the self in a yoga class and, in a desperate attempt at steam release, decide that a glossy pair of eighty-dollar ass-defining shorts will help, you end up looking silly and materialistic.

Unlike David Foster Wallace's "tragic enterprise," yoga pulls out a happy ending. In the end, yoga has a goal of union. Instead of vanquishing the self, Courtney's battle between the ego and the soul yields an unfolding definition of self, the living curriculum as autobiography: you acknowledge all that you are, all that you were, and all that you can become and then get to work integrating those three selves into something like a cohesive person.

To fully understand, I return to Courtney. Esak may be providing the quickest route to a backbend, and he may be filling me with helpful techniques for stage presence, but Courtney represents—inside out—the competitor I want to be.

"I'm a great loser," she says. "World class. When it comes down to it, I've never felt like I have to be better than anyone else. Never wanted to beat them. What I do care about is knowing what my best is. It almost sounds corny when I say it like that, but it's true. I've never stepped onstage thinking about winning or losing. That's not part of my preparation."

Courtney continues: "That's not to say I don't get nervous. I don't want to disappoint myself. I don't want to disappoint all these people watching me. But nervousness can also be this great teacher. You get up on stage, and your mind says, 'I'm not nervous.' But your leg is shaking all over the place. What type of yoga is that?"

In those situations, Courtney tells me she focuses on creating unity. But not by demanding her brain control her leg in some trance-focus. "I've always felt that competition, like any demonstration onstage, is a shared event," she says. "Everyone is there to create this event. I don't want to be a performer, I want to be a role player. I try not to feel separate from the audience and if I do, I try to push myself to connect."

For Courtney, this is an internal shift. "As a competitor, you are the center of attention, but your role is to serve. I think one of my best qualities is that I can see that. I can step onstage and see that we're all part of this one thing. . . . Suddenly, it's not about you. It takes all this pressure off."

And then, just in case I can't connect the dots, Courtney moves from the internal struggle for self-transcendence to the out-through-the-in-door revelation of the *Katha Upanisad*.

"You know, that pressure can really capsize people. It requires a lot of strength to deal with. And when you practice any discipline that requires this level of strength, you quickly discover that it requires you to forgive yourself.

"The discovery is really sink or swim. If you don't figure it out, you can't continue. You'll quit or you'll burn out."

"And to forgive, you have to go outside of yourself. Forgiveness, surrender, the ability to see your actions without being at the mercy of those actions, being able to detach from your own expectations . . . It's all the same. I think of my yoga practice as a way to go within myself to get outside myself. I assume a posture, but I am tapping into something greater— into source—and then concentrating on expressing that. People call it many things." Courtney stops and tries to vocalize. "Although for me it is usually love. Love or the possibility of love."

The only source I've tapped into at the moment appears to be the air-conditioning system. My entire body is in goose pimples, no doubt screaming some Braille message about fear and anxiety. Which is unfortunate because I'm basically naked in the central rotunda of a shopping mall. The

2010 NJ/PA Yoga Asana Championships have arrived. Instead of a stage, Esak decided to bring the yoga to the people—and on a Saturday in New Jersey, he figured that meant performing in a mall. There is a buzz of ambient noise, escalators rolling up and down. Mall walkers on their weekend rounds give long up-and-down glances over my pasty body before continuing off to attend to their needs.

Esak is prowling around the center of the rotunda, microphone in hand, exhorting the benefits of hatha yoga. It is a rebirth of sorts, a window back to Bishnu Ghosh on the dusty Calcutta streets. Esak is dressed head to toe in a highly professional urban gray, his gleaming black loafers in stark contrast with the bare feet of the performers around him. He looks up at the crowd gathered on the second-floor balcony,

"A yoga competition might seem odd to many of you. But the decision to compete is simple. It means 'I am not afraid to be my best in front of other people. I am not afraid to inspire.'"

He explains the rules of the competition. He explains the sequence of postures. He tells everyone and no one we are here to choose a champion.

"And by champion," he says, "I mean a representative. We are selecting the single person who will embody the best of the beauty, skill, and dedication of the collective here."

Esak keeps his attention skyward. From there, no doubt, it's a great scene. But standing amidst it, on the ground floor, knees knocked and my arms self-hugging in my instinctual position of semi-nudity, it's harder not to feel the social yawn at the core of the mall experience. On the ground floor, most shoppers barely give us more than a glance. The doors of the Body Shop, Godiva Chocolatiers, and Go! Games continue to swing open and closed. Esak is naturally undeterred. And so, with the escalators continuing their ambivalent scroll in the background, he calls up the first competitor.

In yoga, all lies are aspirational. Public prayers to our better selves, mission statements set in the weird liar's tense of *I have done* instead of *I hope to*. I learned quickly in my yogic interviews that it is very difficult to call a completely earnest liar out. It's unclear where the line between self-delusion, self-deception, and outward trickery lies. Especially when the lies are completely mundane and harmless (a wakeup time, the extent of an old injury, the number of days a week they practice). At a certain point, I give up trying to understand these. I take them all as broken gifts and think of Viktor Frankl's Goethe: "Treat people as if they are what they ought to be, and you help them to become what they can be."

Which doesn't quite explain what I was doing the night before that chilly over-air-conditioned Saturday in the mall: sitting at Brigit's dining room table, lying my ass off.

Desperately saying things like: "First of all, regardless of where I file taxes, I consider myself—spiritually—a resident of New Jersey."

Or, "I have roots in New Jersey! My parents met in Newark."

Or, "Actually, when you think about it, I've been living in New Jersey for the last two weeks."

Primarily, I was trying to convince Brigit and Esak to let me register last minute for the New Jersey Regional Competition despite the fact that for all intents and purposes, I live in New York City. As local studio owner, Brigit was organizing the event; and Esak, being Esak, was the voice of senior authority and wisdom. Either one could get me in with no trouble.

On a different level, like I said, I was lying my ass off. From the bottom of my heart, I can tell you I hate New Jersey. I associate the I-95 stretch through New Jersey with death itself. I once got a dick tick while camping in the Pine Barrens. And with the possible exception of "Thunder Road," I think Bruce Springsteen is an overrated blue-collar hack who needs to take a long USO tour full of short sets. So yeah, me and New Jersey have no love. But I wanted into the New Jersey Asana Competition. I had a book to write. I had an editor who wanted a story. And god bless my cowardly unyogic sex, there were no men competing from New Jersey. As in zero. Which was in striking contrast to New York, where "I" "lived" and which had something near twenty male competitors. Male competitors whom I knew and who were very good. In other words, competing in New York represented a difficult gamble, and competing in New Jersey represented a craven ticket to the nationals level.

To me this was a no-brainer. The New Jersey competition was happening now. I was here and ready, coming off two weeks of Backbending. And most important, there wasn't anything in the official rulebook prohibiting me from competing. After all, yoga teachers—especially Bikram Yoga teachers—are an itinerant traveling bunch, many floating from studio to studio for years. Enforcing residency requirements would be madness.

In fact, as I saw it, there was only one problem of any consequence in this scheme: Esak and Brigit hated the idea. It made them visibly uncomfortable and twitchy. Quite correctly, they saw it as going against everything the yoga stood for. A central Bikramism is the understanding that if something feels hard, that is where you need to do the most work. And competing in NJ was certainly not hard, nor where I needed to do work.

"But let's be serious," I say to Esak. "This would not be about what's right in terms of yoga. This would be about what's right for my book."

"I hear you. I get that," Esak says. "But for me to be comfortable, it has to be what's best for the entire community. . . . This feels bush league. If we want the competition to reach the Olympics, we need to structure it around fairness."

"I totally agree. But since this is following the letter of the rules, aren't we actually doing that? Wouldn't it be more unfair for you to shut me out just because you know my situation?"

"No. It would be called thinking about what's best for everyone, not what's best for you. Which is hard for you to do. Because you are you and inherently self-interested. Which is why I am here . . . But I'll tell you what, it's not my call. If you can convince Brigit, I'm open to it."

Brigit was completely against the idea, although she wouldn't say that to me, because she is exceedingly polite. Instead, she said she wanted to talk about it more tomorrow. Which was the day of the competition. When I asked her what that meant for me, she suggested I register. Then she took it back. Then she suggested I register again. Then she took it back again.

Of course, sitting at the table, hashing out the extent of my allegiance to New Jersey, the ethics of competition, it was pretty hard not to laugh at the whole situation. I mean, just what type of yoga did we think we were practicing? This was Bikram Yoga, led by a guru who insanely declared he wrote the script to *Superman* once during a lecture and then—just to be clear about the fact that he wasn't making some type of weird metaphor about his superhuman abilities—followed it up by claiming he wrote specific scenes for the Peter Sellers drama *Being There*. A man who routinely claimed he didn't need sleep, despite being unable to rouse himself to teach a single morning class my entire nine-week training, excepting the one week where we had no late-night lectures. If anything, a New Yorker competing in the New Jersey competition for entirely self-interested reasons was the rational path in the absurd yoga we practiced. It was an homage of sorts.

But the longer we discussed the matter, the more I turned down the volume on my internal sneer: I realized their refusal marked a proud point of departure. To someone like Brigit, the yoga was not about Bikram. Nor was it absurd in any way. It was about her health. And my appropriation of some of the obnoxious qualities of Bikram the man was not cute. It was an ugly coincidence. It flaunted an aspect of reality that she accepted—because it was, after all, reality—but refused to celebrate.

But that was because Brigit's relationship to the yoga was forever unlike mine. At age sixteen, Brigit had five tumors removed from her thyroid. The procedure robbed her of three-quarters of the gland and almost all its functionality. She was put first on a synthetic thyroid hormone, and then a host of immunosuppressants to stabilize her condition. Related or not to the thyroid, she also began experiencing arthritis and her doctor began medicating that as well. By eighteen, Brigit began her meals by counting out pills. Her body was saturated with prescription medication, and instead of young, she felt sluggish, depressed, and grossly unhealthy.

At nineteen, she found Bikram under her windshield wiper. A stuffed flyer led to a single class, which led to more. Within six months, her fractional thyroid had resumed enough production that her doctor took her off her Synthroid. Over the following six years, she shed the rest of her medications. To me, sitting across from her at the kitchen table, her medical history was essentially invisible. She was a beautiful, strong yogi. In fact, I would probably never have found about it at all if her husband hadn't mentioned it casually one day in the car when I was going on and on about my interview with Joseph and his triumph over his childhood heart attack.

Regardless of the dining room table, I am here now. During one of Brigit's waffle moments, I registered, paid, and am on the list. The fact that she subsequently reneged only adds to my tension. After the introduction, I retreat with the other competitors to a temporarily vacant storefront across from the rotunda that we are using as a green room to try to stay loose. In a somewhat private corner, I lean my head back and drop down the wall for my first wall-walk of the day. My face skims along the wall as I count the little holes where the now-defunct store used to hang its shelving. At the bottom, I hang in the moment. I breathe. Then come up for my first head rush, observe the electric crackle up my spine. A groggy early-morning backbend is like waking up and shaking hands with the day, only to find the son of a bitch is wearing a joy buzzer.

Despite knowing I have nothing to lose, I am deeply uncomfortable. Brigit isn't making eye contact with me. The cold dry air has roused my nipples into attack mode. They stick out from my chest like the bug eyes on a crab. The other competitors walk by with stiff spine assurance, the blond highlights in their hair almost flaunting the fact that they are legitimate denizens of New Jersey.

Worst, my yoga shorts feel impossibly tight. The elastic pinches inward at the tiny amount of fat remaining on my waist, producing a furrow, making me aware of that flesh all out of proportion to its reality. A rational glance in the mirror indicates I am emaciated. Doing a forward bend in a shopping mall in short-shorts makes me feel like a cow. I imagine this awkward, inadequate cow-feeling at age thirteen and swear eternal war against the women's fashion industry.

Names get called. People leave the green room looking exhausted, do their routine in the rotunda, and return looking refreshed. Finally it is my time. I am on deck.

Bare feet against the mall floor, I walk to the center of the rotunda to demonstrate. I bow. The lead judge tells me to begin. I scan the room and I lower myself into the first balancing posture. Just as my standing knee locks into place, I watch as my whole structure tips forward and I very slowly, with a gentle inevitability, fall out. The rigidity of the rest of my body almost enhances the effect, like there was a fatal swing of the ax and someone to yell "Timmmmbeerrr!" I feel a flush creep up my face. I turn into my next posture, but my brain stays behind with my imbalanced posture on the floor. I worry so much about falling out of my next posture, also a balancing pose, that the result is so feeble, I might as well have fallen out. I hit the floor and make the mistake of looking directly at the judges. I make eye contact with one and watch as she shakes off the moment by scoring a deduction.

As the judges tally the results of the competition, Esak's wife, Chaukei, steps into the center of the rotunda for a demonstration. It's a yogic half-time show of sorts. She has competed on the international level regularly, but her demonstration begins slowly with a few gentle warm-up poses.

Then, from a seated position, she slips both legs behind their respective shoulders, and—with feet pointing in a straight line over the top her head, her hands pressing deep into the floor—she slowly raises her body parallel to the ground. Her arms straighten, her body stiffens, and she hits her note of disturbing stillness: this floating arrowhead hovering above the mall's poured epoxy floor. She stays there, mastering the moment, until, almost magically, her levitation increases another two inches as she pushes up onto her fingertips.

And although I've seen the posture—Crane—hundreds of times, I am still transfixed. Behind me I hear the kind of jaw-dropped "fuuuuuck" that signals someone's neural fuses were just blown. I turn toward the source and find a middle-aged man with his young daughter perched on his shoulders. His jaw is indeed hanging loose. His daughter is clapping excitedly into his hair. Behind them another women stops, her trademarked Big Brown Bag in hand. Behind her, a young couple. Suddenly an overlapping audience four or five deep rings Chaukei. Above us, the balcony overlooking the rotunda has filled out too. This is a spontaneous crowd of four or five hundred people drawn to silent attention by her postures. Cell phone cameras are out in force, held in front by straight arms like weird religious icons to ward off evil or, in this case, trap a small moment of perfection.

As Chaukei morphs from posture to posture, it is as if she is casting a spell over the place. Creating a central focus, a single object for a communal meditation. The spell is so deep that when an elderly man next to me turns to his wife and says, "I take it back. This really could get to the Olympics," his wife refuses even to turn toward him to collect her vindication, instead putting a single finger in front of her lips to reinforce the room's silence.

Chaukei lowers herself down. She is upright, legs still behind each shoulder blade. Then slowly like she was opening a pair of scissors, her legs split off her back and come down on either side of her.

The most clichéd riff on yoga competitions asks the question, "Competitive yoga? Well, what are you supposed to be judging them on? Karma? Purity of soul?" Which, cliché or not, points to the entirely reasonable fact that much of yoga is devoted to cultivating intangible and immeasurable ends. And more, that judging those immeasurables feels not just impossible, but contra the entire spirit of the enterprise. But in reality, the nuts and bolts of a yoga competition don't go near those ends. They are purely physical affairs. A subspecies of gymnastics crossed with the sequined leotards of the Ice Capades. But watching Chaukei, feeling the weight of the silence descend on a shopping mall rotunda, it is hard not to feel that something more is on display. Done at the highest levels, a yoga posture will move you. Chaukei is not prettier, stranger, or sexier than many of the other participants. But her postures are different, and that difference has brought the shopping mall to attention.

This effect isn't limited to yoga. If you ever sit courtside at an NBA game, you understand instantly why people are willing to pay the otherwise demeaning markup for those tickets. The humanity of the players is restored by proximity at the exact same moment their magnificence is amplified. You can feel all the intangibles that Chaukei is expressing. Sportswriters trying to convey the experience usually end up submitting abysmal copy. The sheer *tonnage* of abysmal copy, however, attests to the power of this spell. The difference in yoga—which alternately attracts and repels people—is here these intangibles are emphasized. They are an essential part of the whole enterprise, so chances are, you are paying attention to them in a way that doesn't usually happen in the NBA.

Before the judges announce a winner, Esak gathers the contestants in the center. He orders us to pose for the crowd gathered at the balcony. We obey with smiles and bend. When we stand straight again, we shiver and clutch our skinny bodies awkwardly.

Brigit wins! In her jubilation, she jumps over to me and tells me if I can get this straightened out with Headquarters, she'd love to have me represent New Jersey. A few days later, she sends an email telling me, "I just want you to know I think what you are doing is wrong."

But at this point, I don't care. I realize how fun it is to play Bikram with the truth. Neither, as it turns out, do the competition's organizers in Los Angeles. When I explain the situation in an email, they enthusiastically invite me to nationals, excited to have a male representative from New Jersey to further expand the competition.

Beyond Sixty

After Sol's sixty days, a funny thing happened. By day forty, it was clear the effects were real. He had dropped twenty-four pounds without any conscious change in his diet. His insomnia disappeared. For the first time in his adult life, he was going to sleep without the TV on in the background—and when he did conk out, it was continuous and deep in a way he had never experienced. Everyone we hung out with noticed the changes. He had a freshness that was palpable. His face had tightened. His pants size had reduced several times. He had a habit of cornering people who didn't know much about his challenge or the yoga and talking to them about his progress with the slightly depraved eyes of a ten-year-old discussing video games. When waiting for the subway, Ashley caught him bending over to practice his grip for Standing Forehead to Knee on the platform. The alcoholic curmudgeons he played darts with stopped ridiculing him for going to yoga and started asking what exactly he was doing to look so good.

In the midst of this day-forty enthusiasm, I left the city for two weeks on an extended business trip. When I returned on a red-eye, I went directly to our 7 A.M. yoga class, the last place I had seen Sol, excited to hear about his progress. But when I looked over the mats and the other groggy-eyed

7 A.M.–ers several times, there was no Sol. He had slept through. I put my mat down and sprinted back to the locker room to call him. But it was too late even for his thirty-second commute. The teacher had locked the front door. It was the first time I had been stood up by Sol. I trudged back. We had emailed a few times during my trip, and Sol had claimed to be going every day, but it suddenly occurred to me that it had all been going too perfectly. That Sol, just like every other yogi, was capable of—if not driven toward—lies of kindness. That my expectations and public pressure made it not just possible but likely. As I straightened my towel, waiting for class to begin, I said good-bye to his month of free classes and began wondering exactly how many classes he had skipped over the last two weeks, and how I would write about Sol cheating on his sixty-day challenge.

Then the guy directly in front of me, picking up on my anxiety, broke the pre-class silence by demanding to know "What's with all the shuffling today?"

I looked up. It was Sol. In my two weeks away, he had transformed to the point of being unrecognizable to my brief scan. It was day fifty-four, and it was no exaggeration to say he was halfway back to that picture on his student ID. Looking at him sitting calmly upright on his mat, I realized this wasn't a dramatic change of any one aspect; an agglomeration of microchanges had made him invisible to me. The heuristics I used to identify him—audible sighs, awkward chunky legs, restless shuffling, hunched shoulders—no longer fit. His body, still big, had streamlined. It was a weight distribution more than simply a weight loss. His skin was clearer. His wedding ring was loose on his ring finger. His body had an ease to it. It simply didn't look like a burden anymore.

As we bent together during that class, with Sol directly in front of me, I saw how much these changes to physical appearance matched his progress in the postures. Sol, who had opted to lie on his back motionless for the bulk of his first class, now made the postures look effortless. Between movements, he stared straight ahead, never flinching or fidgeting, his spine straight even during the most difficult standing postures. In Camel, the posture that had sent him running from the room on his second day, he leaned back deeply, almost basking in the elevated heart rate. When class was over, he took a long savasana and then, while I was still recovering, bounced up, tapping me on the shoulder to tell me quietly he had to get going.

We finished out the challenge like that: Sol growing stronger each day, me amazed by the yogi who had replaced my tired friend. On the final day, Sol claimed his month of free yoga and announced he was going to celebrate the accomplishment by going to class the next morning even though the challenge was over.

But then the funny thing happened. After his celebratory class, he stopped bending. Abruptly and completely. He just quit. Of the thirty free days he had earned, he ended up using two.

Sol still proselytized. He still told people how wonderful it made him feel, how radically it had transformed his body, but after the challenge, his only relationship to the yoga was verbal. When I would ask him about it, he would shrug. *I know I should go. I'm meaning to go. I want to go.* But something had changed, and we both knew he wasn't actually going to go. With a free month of unlimited yoga sitting waiting for him—a month he had earned through a seized back, through two months of shitty coffeeless early-morning wake-ups, through self-doubt and self-triumph—he couldn't be bothered. The transformation started creeping backwards, like a jungle creeping back in over cleared land. The weight came back first. He bumped into his favorite instructor while walking his pugs, and she reached out and pinched his newly re-forming stomach in anger. Sol assured her he would be in soon, but never made it. When we were out drinking, he was open about the fact that he wasn't sleeping very well again. We made a doctor's appointment to track the physiological changes from his sixty days, and Sol blew off his first appointment. By the time the reschedule came along, he hadn't been practicing for three weeks. The yoga glow we wanted his doctors to try to measure had faded into an ember. The whole exercise had been both a resounding success and a complete failure. I became grateful I had made the challenge so public; otherwise, I would doubt my own memories.

It would be exactly what I feared most, the oldest story in the history of binge exercising—the Duncan of yo-yo weight loss—except for one thing: Sol didn't return to form. Not all the way.

Instead, he started running.

Within a month of stopping yoga, before the weight had completely resettled on his frame, Sol—the single most inactive man I knew prior to his yoga binge—decided to train for a 5K. After successfully completing that, he began training for a half marathon. He made a regular schedule and stuck with it. And that is where he is now Monday, Wednesday, and Friday: a big Mexican doing loops around Prospect Park, becoming a somewhat less big Mexican by the day—a yogi in sneakers, never bending much more than in a few post-run stretches against a tree, but undeniably touched by change.

Strong Medicine

I arrive in Los Angeles for the national competition and head directly to Bikram's central studio, "International Headquarters," for class. It is a ritual of sorts: the day before the competition, all the competitors gather and take Emmy's Advanced Class.

I arrive at the studio just as the preceding class is flooding out. Bikram taught. And he killed. The world's best are stumbling into the lobby, gasping for air. The floors are instantly slick with sweat, and soon the whole studio feels like we are standing on the edges of an indoor pool, right down to the heavy scent of chlorine. When the exodus clears, a short guy with a mustache comes out and mops the floors down, pushing the standing water/sweat/drippings toward a drain in the cement floor.

I am not keen on putting my luggage down in this muck, and so I head to the locker rooms despite the fact they assuredly are jammed. Inside is a similar jungle, every surface slick and crammed with bodies stripping off or replacing clothes. It is a mash of familiar faces and bodies, a giant yoga family reunion. Everyone gets a head nod, more than a few hugs.

As I search for a spot to stow my gear, I feel a firm clap on the shoulder. It's Hector, my teacher who had the stroke.

"Been looking for you, buddy," he says before grabbing a towel and heading out. "So has Rajashree. She's been asking about you."

This is fascinating news, but before I can completely process it, the locker room begins to thin out, which is a sign Emmy's Advanced Class is about to begin. I rush out, towel in hand, in the straight-legged run that I use over slick surfaces to avoid slipping. Once inside, I spot Hector and take a position as near to his mat as possible. I haven't seen him in months and want to impress him with my strong practice. I am, after all, in the best shape of my life.

At this point, I've been on continuous yoga overload since Backbending in Charleston seven months prior. The climax was no doubt the two classes a day throughout teacher training, but I have continued a similar frenzy since returning to civilian life, cramming as many classes and extra home-work into my week as I can manage. A fancy little scale that shoots elec-tricity through my body tells me my body fat is down to 8 percent. A week prior, when a meeting for work keeps me from the hot room, I go on a brief jog and end up going nine miles without ever feeling taxed. When my sister visits, she immediately announces I'm emaciated. Which prompts the immediate retort in my head that I'm on the right track.

Best of all, when away from the city on work and I drop into a new studio, the teacher there asks me—me!—to demonstrate my floor Bow for the entire class. During class. So that new students can see what a floor Bow looks like in its advanced form. Since demonstrations like that almost never happen in the tightly structured Bikram room, it becomes quite the feather in my hat.

I want Hector to notice all this. I want all my work to be validated by appearance. Which turns out to be unlikely for two reasons. Primarily be-cause relative to everyone else in the room, I am still nothing to be noticed. The room is filled with people who may or may not be 8 percent body fat, and may or may not be able to dust off lengthy runs, but who have bodies that are far more toned up and in tune than mine. They flow. They focus. I am still a collection of static movements that only occasionally conjoin.

The second reason I realize that it is unlikely that Hector will notice my superb physical condition is that I am about to faint. Really. Almost immediately, from the first sequence of Emmy's Advanced Class, some-thing weird and awful has been operating on my system. It is like being in

Headquarters is exerting a gravitation pull on my energy. Rajashree's image implanted by Hector's offhand comment is stuck in my head. My heart rate rises. Then I'm down on one knee. I close my eyes and worry about what Rajashree wants to talk about. When I rise, the unthinkable occurs: After seven months of preparation for this single Advanced Class, I head for the exit. The impulse to leave is like a biological commandment. It is the first and only time I have ever left a Bikram Yoga class.

The cool air of the lobby does nothing for my condition. My body feels faint, and there is the first sign of an ugly knot rising in my stomach. With a fawn's legs and addict's determination, I stagger down the hallway toward the locker rooms. The closer I get, the more clear it becomes—and by the time I am inside, I am frantically searching for a stall. Then I drop to my bare knees on the disgusting wet floor and puke my lungs out. I don't even have time to put up the rim, and for stability end up gripping it with both hands. I come up for air after a heave and find myself eye to eye with a few droplets of urine. Disgustingly dehydrated cheddar cheese–colored droplets. This prompts a few more pukes. It is a low moment.

When it has passed, I sit in the locker room on a bench for what feels like an eternity. Tamping a towel against my mouth leaves a nice purple ring. I grab two bottles of water, which I had been saving for after class, and muster up all remaining intention for the plunge back into class. Then I am back to staggering down the hallways, back toward the heat, when out of nowhere Rajashree appears.

Her face is perfectly calm.

"You are the man from New Jersey yes."

A statement to which I can only stare at her and say: "Thank you."

It hangs there for a moment while I wake to the situation. With the sudden embarrassing taste of acid around my mouth, with my face still pale from the puking, with my brain wondering if Rajashree can tell I was just absolutely shattered by her husband's yoga, we study each other's faces intently. I am not actually sure if I have ever stared so intently at another person's face without a pillow as backdrop. Emmy's class is still going on in the background. I can faintly hear her voice. Rajashree is very beautiful, and while we look at each other in this completely odd frozen moment in the hallway, her perfect calm drops into something much nicer—it becomes something perfectly calming to me. I almost wonder if we are going to have our conversation right here in the hallway now.

Instead, I break our gaze. I have a class to attend, after all. I smile softly and leave her with my best thoughts mid-hallway to stagger back into Emmy's class.

I drop one of my bottles of water by Hector's mat. He looks up, never quite making eye contact, shaking his head mournfully: a combination of shared adversity, total gratitude, and friendly reproach for leaving the room. I understand completely. Then as if to emphasize the total gratitude and shared adversity, he slumps out of a posture onto his back and guzzles the water.

After class, in the locker room, Hector tells me I look cross-eyed. It becomes a theme of the weekend. Every time I see him over the next few days, he repeats this, "I'm not sure Ben was really there. He looked like he was knocked out."

So much for being in the best shape of my life.

After drying off, I split a cab back to the hotel with some other competitors. It is driven by a seventy-nine-year-old man who looks like he just turned forty. There are four of us yogis splitting the cab, so I end up sitting in the front next to the driver. He is easily the most handsome, fit, and generally attentive cabdriver I have ever ridden with. He tells me his wife is in a convalescent home. He visits her every day after work. He tells me he loves being a cabbie. He talks about his daughter, about serving in the military, and about gardening. I feel completely empty from the class, and he talks into me as if I were a conch shell that he is blowing to make a sound. Suddenly there are tears as he explains his daily ministrations to his wife.

We talk yoga only briefly at the very end of the ride when he asks me suddenly why I am in town. His eyes widen, and instead of the typical questions demanding to know why competition isn't antithetical to the spirit of yoga, he asks whether I would recommend it for him.

Recommend? Given that I am writing a book on the topic, the question seems so portentous. And given that I now know more about this cabbie than about most of my relatives, I take a long time considering it. It is like at different points in the cab ride we have become angels to the other. Unaware but helping each find answers. I tell him he looks fantastic for seventy-nine. I tell him I wouldn't change a thing. He smiles at this, and when I exit he shakes my hand with both of his. I get out feeling very dizzy.

Two hours later, I am shadow boxing in my room.

The United States Yoga Asana Championships are a production of USA Yoga, which is Rajashree's organization. They are her baby. She is in charge of organizing the regional competitions, attracting press and sponsors, and in general, transforming an otherwise drab convention space into a cathedral for appreciating all things asana. Which, poking around the Los Angeles Westin, I see she has done to superb effect. The hotel looks like a bona fide Yoga Expo, filled with booths and tables, all hawking specialized hot yoga supplements, berry-of-the-moment rehydration drinks, and rack after rack of synthetic quick-dry yoga gear. Yogis—competitors and voyeurs alike—flit around in bare feet, greeting, hugging, and collecting free samples. The Backbending purple shirt is out in force. Although I notice the circle has expanded yet again; Esak has joined the vendors, hawking the shirts to nonbenders as well.

Striking in absence amidst this cacophony is Bikram, as man, if not brand. The competitions are consciously trying to become more than a hot yoga affair. The stage itself is room temperature, and other lineages are hungrily welcomed. USA Yoga's stated mission is to push yoga's physical practice into the Olympics, thereby making it into a serious, perhaps even hip alternative for middle American children to consider when choosing an after-school sport. I arrived with doubts as to whether this was possible, but Rajashree goes to great lengths to preserve the separation. At nationals, Bikram does not MC or lecture or even get onstage, save for a quick wave to the crowd. He is subdued when present, but mostly—probably because he is almost impossible to subdue—he stays away. In fact, the only time I really feel Bikram's presence at nationals is when, as an official competitor,

I get a gift bag upon checking in. The first thing I pull out: my very own pair of tiger-print Lycra hot pants! You can't make this shit up. Nor I discover, when I try them on in the mirror, would you want to.

I awake the morning of the competition and begin backbending almost immediately. My computer is playing Michael Jackson's "Stranger in Moscow" on infinite repeat. I inhale and stretch backwards. The world goes wavy. I rise, inhale again, and pushing again, slowly let my upper deltoids relax. I do this again and again, passing each time slowly in front of the hotel emergency exit plan framed on the door.

When I stand straight from my final backbend, body opened, thin stream of sweat covering my skin, I'm fully awake. I look out at my hotel window at my view—some gigantic white-concrete parking garage. It is shimmering in the pollution-enhanced L.A. morning light, and I decide it is the most beautiful parking garage I have ever seen.

Strolling into the green room, I stiffen from all the nervous energy on display. Yogis in handstands; yogis off by themselves, stretching out on headphones. And just a few feet away, the cavernous ballroom and audience staring in darkness. We queue in a giant line, each one stepping up and off through the stage door in their turn. As we wait, we listen. There is the regular calling of names and the announcing of time. There are occasional jokes from the MC. But mostly there is silence. As we get closer to the speakers by the stage door, the huge amounts of gain from the various microphones in the room provide a diagetic soundtrack to the event, as if the energy into the room has been made audible. The line inches forward, three minutes at a time.

And then I am standing in the doorway, staring out. Then I am kissing Mary Jarvis's hand. After that, it is only scattered memories.

I remember trying to do like Courtney and project my love. I remember giving myself several vicious reprimands not to look awkwardly and terribly at my ankles. Not to hunch my upper back. Just to smile and let everyone in that great big room know how grateful I was to be there.

Then all of a sudden: "Start please." Had I bowed?

And smiling, I turned to announce my first posture, Standing Head to Knee.

I remember jiggling all over the place like I had just jumped out of an ice bath. I remember thinking to myself proudly that I'd remembered to breathe, and immediately realizing that—*shit!*—if you are thinking about thinking about breathing, you are not in the present moment.

But crazily, I was already in the second phase of the posture at that point. And my head was slowly lowering. I could see my little toes squirming to keep my balance, but I couldn't feel a damn thing. The lights were so white. My lower body was so absent. It was as if I had softly pressed a mute button on it. My brain was alive, but my body completely detached. This, I decided, wasn't good. I was supposed to be in meditation, not some closed-captioned version of my own life. Especially because my standing leg wasn't straight at all! And with that, all of a sudden the world rushed back in. My lower body unmuted itself. I was at war. My standing knee straightened, my knee locked. I heard the burst shutter on the high-res camera purr like someone shuffling a deck of cards. My face was flush and hot and pressed up against my lifted leg. Which meant I had completed the posture. Who knows how long it had been there? My lower body was now not just unmuted, but on the verge of populist revolution, every cell ranting in its own bug-eyed outrage. And so I came out, took a huge breath, and turned to say:

"Standing Bow Pulling."

The rest of the routine just flowed. In floor bow, my back arched up like the ceiling itself had reached down and pulled my legs taut. I don't think I did a thing. Rabbit, Stretching, I barely remember those when I do my routine on a normal day, but onstage as far as I'm concerned, they didn't even happen. Neither did Pigeon. Not for even a second. None of it is there. Nothing is, in fact, until, as if dropped abruptly back into this world, all of sudden I found myself motionless, levitating perfectly parallel to the stage in one of the best Peacocks of my life. I wasn't remotely tired, I was humming and smiling and thinking of Courtney thinking about expressing joy for all the people watching. I rose from the Peacock. I bowed. I thought of all the other competitors behind me, and I almost sprinted off the stage, giddy with the realization that although I didn't win, I didn't come in last.

At the end of the day, all the competitors are invited back onstage for a group photo. As the front of the second level, I am standing on my knees, back straight. Much to my surprise, Bikram and Rajashree plunk down right in front of me during the group photo. They both stare out into the live feed of the international simulcast. The room explodes into a frenzy of pictures. My knees are killing me, but I keep smiling. Bikram is yammering away— "Do I look good in my suit? Do I look like a gangster?"—in a free flow of nonsense chatter that continues for two or three straight minutes.

Rajashree without flinching from the camera or breaking her smile, speaks like a ventriloquist to him: "The world is watching us."

Bikram ignores her, continuing to free-associate about gangsters. Then suddenly he is finished. "Is that enough?" he asks the room as he stands. "I think that is enough." He waits for Rajashree to rise next to him, and together they walk offstage, drifting apart as soon as they are back in the audience. Although he has been on best behavior all weekend, the farther apart they get, the more Rajashree seems to relax.

Stranger in Moscow

Three months later, I am at the international competition, in another hotel wasteland: more competitors scampering barefoot over carpets, more vendors selling even slimmer yoga gear, more free samples of coconut water. This time I am not competing. And this time there is another Bikram in attendance.

Instead of the restrained, humane Bikram of nationals, content to play sidekick as Rajashree ran the show, at internationals, Bikram is determined to be front and center. The result is a sustained and unpleasant tantrum.

The weekend kicks off a little after 11:30 A.M., at the Los Angeles Airport Radisson, when a young man from Australia comes out, bows before the judges, and promptly falls out of his first posture. At this point, everything is set. The great room is dark and silent, the stage lit by three beams of white. Great energy and expense have been spent to transform the vast hotel conference room into a more regal venue. With its overblown chandeliers, its seating for the press, its elegant stage—dripping with flags and live-action video-projection screens—the room looks the part. The elaborate rigging for the international simulcast, with monster camera atop derricklike tripod, feels impressive. The audience is hyperalert in its stillness, projecting collective silence as a badge of respect. There are ushers, MCs, programs, and heaps of third-party vendors. But despite it all, the event reeks of the amateur. A multimillion-dollar operation with the soul of a high school musical. I am trying to figure out exactly why, when Bikram shouts into the silence.

"Need to move the X! Need to come forward!"

Apparently, the spot where competitors perform is too far recessed for Bikram's liking. A competitor—on deck and nervous stands awkwardly on the edge of the stage, unsure what is going on. Then to make sure things get changed, Bikram stands up, cutting through the lighting to start ordering people around. It is perhaps 11:45 A.M. The now-terrified contestant is ordered onstage to perform a few postures on the now-moved X. He dutifully complies, and when everything has been adjusted to Bikram's whim, the competition proceeds. The competitor retreats offstage and waits to be called officially.

This moment more than any other defines the rest of the weekend in my eyes. But it is only the beginning.

Soon after, a woman from Canada does an extremely difficult handstand variation—Lotus Scorpion—that is not found in Bishnu Ghosh's ninety-one postures. With the room still in silence, Bikram shouts "Wrong!" at the judges. "Should be zero points."

Another contestant, one of Bikram's favorite students, falls out of his posture before holding it. There is no stillness. No grace, no gut-check moment, no demonstration of control. And almost to emphasize the fact that it is his show, and that he can therefore bend it into his reality, Bikram exclaims loud enough for the judges to hear: "Very good posture. Perfect. Just like it should be done."

His restlessness grows as the competition proceeds. The outbursts become more juvenile. Corresponding rumors of his fickleness sweep through the audience. Contestants might be disqualified for performing a posture on their fingertips instead of their palms. Others because they entered or exited a posture in an as-of-yet undefined improper manner. There are more outbursts. All prompted by Bikram's burning urgency to inject himself into the scene. My lasting image of the morning is not a performer onstage, but rather Bikram in an ink black suit with a red tie, standing up just as a contestant is walking off. He is furious about god knows what, trying to track down exactly who or what is responsible for failing to carry out a request. "At least he confess," I hear him tell a circle of aides, trying, I think, to be hushed, but instead appearing even more teeth-clenchingly angry. "From now on, nothing moves here without my sign. Nothing without my okay. Like check signing. Get it?"

Finally, when the competition is over and all the beautiful asanas have been performed (and they are beautiful, as always, still and majestic, representing years of dedication), the judges file out of the room to tally the scores and discuss in private. In the meantime, photos of Bikram with various celebrities flash in a slideshow on the stage. Soon a chatter of well-intentioned awkward exchanges fills the room: "You looked so beautiful up there." "I love your outfit." Conversations so sincere and superficial that for the most part, they are dead on arrival.

After an extended break where we're all given plenty of time to peruse the vendors and collect free samples of various soaps and supplements, the judges file back in. Rajashree takes the stage to announce the winners. There is suspense; there is applause. A runner-up shrieks just like it's a beauty contest; the female first-place winner looks completely stunned. Then Bikram charges the stage.

With Rajashree frozen, looking like she is trying to increase her smile from 1,000 watts to spontaneous combustion, Bikram strides to the front. "I learn just now, no cash prize for shopping." He pulls out his wallet. "So I look into my wallet and find some cash. For winners, one thousand dollars. I think I give it to each of them." He laughs and waits for applause.

Which is tiny. He points at the first-, second-, and third-place female champions, all of whom are Asian. "Can you believe all three have triangle eyes?" There are titters. "And man"—he points now to an Asian male, just in case we didn't get it—"has triangle eyes too." More titters. Feeding off these weak laughs, Bikram continues on, stomping over the awards ceremony, rearranging the contestants around the stage, demanding they assume poses for pictures, and generally asserting his ability to do anything he wants anywhere he wants. There are still some people, the most loyal loyalists, who are laughing at these antics. One of them is sitting in front of me, snickering—and I can see him giddy as he rises to his feet to take a picture of Bikram with the winners and their slender scalene eyes. But I'd like to think most people in the room, like me, are past sad with the sudden devolution of the event, well into what Bikram fears most, boredom.

The next day there is a judges' meeting. It is held in another well-carpeted hotel room, with low ceilings and accordion partitions compressed to open an awkward array of adjoining rooms. The judges' meeting is ostensibly for training judges for future competitions. Competitors and coaches, however, are also invited, as obviously an understanding of how postures will be judged is crucial for training. To further both these ends, the room is full of flat-screen TVs running loops of competitors performing routines as demos for discussion.

We, the die-hards who are interested in this sort of thing, sit fifty deep in folding chairs arranged around a mini-stage.

The meeting begins by attempting to tackle the issue of how variations will be judged. There is no set procedure. At the moment, it is every judge for themselves. The hope is to create a more consistent system. It is not a small issue. The Olympics are the driving force, and if the competition is ever to get there, it must be something more than just a Bikram Yoga competition. It must be open to all lineages, all styles, and they must be able to receive a score.

Soon, as with all large group discussions led by a highly tolerant moderator, the discussion gets lost. The specific tangent has to do with how to score a non-Bikram posture like Lotus Scorpion. Should contestants submit the name of their postures in advance, so judges can determine a score? Should they be limited to a predetermined list? Should it be left to the individual judge's discretion? The conversation winds in and out politely, different yogis standing up, sharing their view, sitting down. Nothing is recorded, and good ideas are lost with bad ones. It reminds me of a hundred dysfunctional staff meetings I've tried to sleep through during my professional life.

Then Bikram intervenes. He has been sitting anxiously in the front row, but now he stands up. "No. No. No. We must have borderlines." Suddenly the moderator is sitting down and Bikram is bouncing from foot to foot in his place. "We must have borderlines, and to compete you must accept them. This is the way we do. You like it, you welcome. You do not, good-bye."

A teacher seizes on the pause after that last statement, "What about other yoga communities? How do they participate? What about the Olympics?"

Bikram stares at her. "Who cares? I control ninety-eight-point-five percent of yoga in this world."

He says this in front of everyone, and unlike most of what Bikram says, it is easy to tell if he is joking. Because he is not. He is defiant. And in his defiance, he repeats it again. "Ninety-eight-point-five percent of yoga is Bikram Yoga."

It's a moronic statement. One of millions he's rattled off in the last forty years, and as always, the sensible people in the room decide they don't have the energy to argue. And so they ignore it. The difference here is this particular moronic statement directly undercuts something every single person in that room has worked for. Something they have poured their weekends, vacations, cash, and passion into. Something embedded in the mission statement of the competition they just participated in. And yet, as always, not a single person raises their hand to mention that this isn't true. That, *No, Boss, you don't control 98.5 percent of yoga.* That, *The real figure is just under 8 percent.* And that, *Actually, Boss, that is a delusional and destructive statement that will guarantee your wife's goal of the Olympics goes unanswered.*

Instead, a senior teacher interjects, saying, "So it seems like what you are saying is the Olympics are no longer the goal." Bikram grunts at this. The room remains silent. Then Bikram continues speaking, rambling forward on an entirely different issue. The discussion is over. Now it is just Bikram talking and an audience to listen to him speak.

I wonder what would happen if I stood up and said something about any one of his totally false claims. I wonder how the room would react. But instead, I make eye contact with a Backbender across the room. She makes eyes back at me and then rolls them deep in the back of her head. I nod toward the door. She shakes her head no. As if to say, I know this is silly, but I want to stay. I smile back. But I have had enough of Bikram for one life, and so I close my notebook and walk out.

Later, and as a fitting coda, I find one of the judges from the competition. She is a woman who has taken the entire process perfectly seriously—embraced Rajashree's idea of an open, fair competition; a gymnastics for yoga; a meeting ground of different lineages and styles.

"I couldn't take another moment. It was madness in there. Everything being changed just as it is decided . . . And yesterday was worse! Nobody ever told me to change my score exactly, but they also made sure we got the message." The woman is not angry, but very focused. Staring off like she is working through an important calculation. "We were gathered in a group and instructed. It was all very clear. You know, stuff like, 'You're an idiot if you scored her more than a zero,' things like that."

I listen and tell her that sounds very tough and a little sad. I say I hope someday Bikram Yoga can grow into something beyond Bikram's Yoga.

She looks at me a moment. "Sad? I just wish they would make it clear, so we knew exactly what to do."

Making It Clear

And then, two months after internationals, Esak is out.

With the ineluctable logic of narcissism, the true disciple—who did everything right, who submitted and fetched Coca-Cola after Coca-Cola, who massaged and preached and built an entire life for himself that was incased within Bikram, within the community, and within the yoga—is out.

Bikram banishes him. His exile is announced with a quick note on the official website:

To My Dear Studio Owners,

It is with much sadness I share this message that Esak Garcia has left his wife, his son, me, and the Bikram Yoga Community. As he has joined another weird organization and is with another woman. This is reason why nobody can invite him to do any kind of seminars, lectures or anything whatsoever in a Bikram Yoga school or in our family.

Thank you,
Bikram.[38]

It is a note whose paternalism and clumsy attempts at sincerity indicate all the contempt they are trying to hide. Esak didn't want to leave the Bikram Yoga community. It was a community he helped build, that he gave himself into, that he expected to sustain him when he needed a web of support, and that provided a substantial income. When I spoke to him a few days after reading the note, he told me it felt "completely surreal."

He was indeed separating from his wife, something he had discussed with Bikram in confidence. But he in no way wanted to leave the Bikram community.

"There isn't too much for me to say at this point. I can't help but feel there has been a huge misunderstanding."

It is a misunderstanding only in the sense that it was always a misunderstanding. That this is exactly how it has to end. Exactly how it has always ended.

The banishment came just days before the latest incarnation of

---

[38] All spelling and grammar mistakes here are from the original; and although there is no way to know for certain, I suspect it means Bikram pecked this particular note out with his own two fingers. Silent testament to Esak's place in the community: for this killing, Bikram had to do the wet work himself.

Backbending—now officially and resolutely named Jedi Fight Club—was set to start in Lawrence, Kansas. This was the first clinic where Esak was going to charge a flat fee instead of accept donations. No more scrounging for meals at midnight. No more vague and unpredictable schedule. He had hired a vegan chef to prepare restorative meals after the day's practice. He had retained a masseur for endless hours of professional-quality bodywork, and he had arranged a Mary Jarvis seminar to kick off the two weeks. It was going to be the best Backbending/Jedi Fight Club ever.

But Bikram was getting left behind. The exact reasons are lost between Bikram and Esak. Maybe Esak was unwilling to put up a high-enough tithe. Maybe Bikram, like Emmy, thought repetitive extreme backbending was unsafe and poorly represented his yoga. Maybe he was sick of seeing Esak's purple Jedi Fight Club shirts at every one of his events. Maybe he realized that Esak, the one man who never told an aspirational lie, who never made an excuse for anybody including himself, simply had too much integrity. Or maybe Esak just got complimented one too many times in his presence. But for whatever reason, Bikram decided Esak had outlived his usefulness to him, he decided the best, most responsible way to handle this was public banishment, and suddenly Esak—who had months of seminars scheduled in advance, whose career, life, son, and mother were rooted in the yoga—was left to try to levitate when the rug was pulled out from under him.

The community was shocked.

"I just don't understand."

"Terrible misunderstanding."

"Best not to talk about it until we know all about the details."

"Just something that makes me very confused and very sad."

But there was one man who wasn't confused at all. Jimmy Barkan, Bikram's head of instruction for the late '80s and early '90s. A man who devoted himself to Bikram with almost the same passion as Esak.

"Of course," he says with a laugh. "The only reason I got to become a senior teacher was all my predecessors had a falling out. . . . Bikram is very threatened by any career uprising. . . . And if I'm going to be completely honest, it was only when I moved across the country that I became really close to Bikram.

"If you do exactly what he tells you, you'll get along fine for a while," Barkan says. "That was the key to my relationship with him. And—relatively speaking—I lasted a long time. I was extremely deferential. I was there to learn."

But eventually, even the three thousand miles of space separating Barkan's South Florida studio and Bikram couldn't stop the inevitable.

"He kept cutting me down every time my career would take off. I started running a yoga retreat in Costa Rica, and then he told me to stop going because Emmy didn't like the place. Then I got a book deal—fitness yoga for golfers, with the potential for sequels planned for other sports—but Bikram forbid me from continuing with the project. The publishers were completely baffled.

"Then, I was teaching private lessons to Dan Marino and the Dolphins, and got a chance to make a video with them—NFL players doing yoga in the early '90s way ahead of its time—an amazing opportunity. But Bikram put a stop to it. He forbid me from doing the video. . . . Finally he made demands that would have financially ruined me. I was opening a second studio in Florida with his permission. Six months after opening, Bikram decided he didn't approve of the layout and ordered me to close. . . . It was impossible. So I didn't do it. I didn't bow down. And so I was out."

Just like Esak.

PART VII

Finding Balance

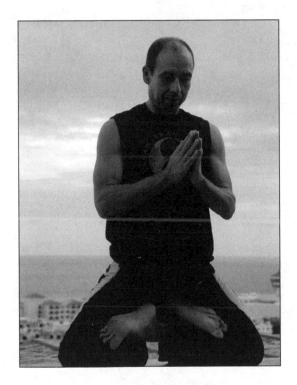

Tony Sanchez in Montain Posture

Patricide: Patricide is a bad idea, first because it is contrary to law and custom and secondly because it proves, beyond a doubt, that the father's every fluted accusation against you was correct: You are a thoroughly bad individual, a patricide!—member of a class of persons universally ill—regarded. It is all right to feel this hot emotion, but not act upon it. And it is not necessary. It is not necessary to slay your father, time will slay him, that is a virtual certainty. Your true task lies elsewhere.

—DONALD BARTHELME, *THE DEAD FATHER*

Everything is an evolution. To believe that yoga is different is an incredible act of denial. We must improvise, we must modify, and if that doesn't work, we must be willing to throw the system out. . . . If you want to learn yoga, spend some time asking yourself why. Then do yourself a favor and take a cooking class. That will definitely improve your life.

—TONY SANCHEZ

The Wise Old Man on the Mountain

n almost every Bikram studio, there is a poster of an elegant dark-skinned man completing every Bikram posture to absolute perfection. Many assume it is Bikram himself as a youth. It turns out the man is a Mexican-American named Tony Sanchez, who studied with Bikram from the age of eighteen onward, living with the guru as family. When Bikram traveled to India to meet his bride-to-be, Rajashree, Tony accompanied him as best man. Bikram called him "my greatest creation." He asked Tony to demonstrate endlessly. He put photographs of Tony on the walls of his guru's school in Calcutta. But ultimately, as with all his creations, Bikram grew threatened. And so, on Tony's birthday in 1984, Bikram had his accountant drive him over to the studio Tony managed to have a talk. For the occasion, Bikram choose his most impressive car at the time, a Daimler limo, complete with toilet and wet bar.

At the studio, as everyone else made preparations for a birthday celebration, Bikram asked Tony to step aside for a conversation. Among other things, he demanded Tony break up with his girlfriend—soon-to-be wife—Sandy. When Tony said no, Bikram fired him.

The last thing he said to Tony, greatest creation and best American friend, was "No hard feelings."

Their separation grew outwardly hostile a few years later when Tony decided to produce a line of yoga videos. The videos featured a series he created using the ninety-one postures Bishnu Ghosh compiled. They were not the series that Bikram taught, and they included postures that Bikram could not begin to do. "I called Bikram to tell him about the videos. My business partner, the guy who put up all the money, thought we should try to get his blessing." Tony explains, "When I called, there was no discussion. He ordered me to stop. He started yelling hysterically. He told me if I proceeded with the videos, I would 'die soon.'" Tony laughs. "I told him, 'Guess I better get on with it then, before I die.'"

Tony's name comes up at Teacher Training exactly twice. Both times feel achingly sad.

The first time, Bikram is sidetracked during a lecture, talking about the early days. A student asks him about his marriage to Rajashree, how they met. Bikram responds with his typical mixture of irreverence and dismissive charm. "Oh, that. Same old story. Arranged marriage. Took seven minutes. Fly to India. Fly back. Nothing special."[39] The room laughs, and Bikram moves on to talk about the party his students threw for him when he returned. Quincy Jones and L-Like-Linda had organized a reception. Linda raised forty thousand dollars from students in two weeks. Quincy provided

---

[39] When Rajashree is asked the same questions, she takes several seconds longer to answer before offering the exquisitely parsed: "I think our marriage spreads yoga. I think of it as a universal marriage for our students."

the house. Bikram gets lost in the memories from that period. He talks about the students he loved; he talks about how he helped each one of them open a studio of their own, each in different cities. Then he starts listing names.

In the middle of the memories, mid-name, he stalls out. "Ton—You know, that Chicano guy, whatever his name was . . ."

An older teacher in the audience shouts out helpfully, "Tony Sanchez!"

Bikram ignores her. He repeats, "Whatever his name was . . ." Then his voice trails off. He shakes his head, there is a tiny silence, and the memories are over and the lecture moves on.

The second time, Bikram is not in the room. Neither am I. I hear about it later from a senior teacher. Rajashree is talking about her yoga practice as a youth. She talks about her demonstrations, her concentration competing. She explains a difficult stunt she performed as a child, where she would dangle her stomach over a sharp knife while her guru broke a brick over her back. "I really don't know how it was done," she says. "You know, he wouldn't let me do it all the time, so I think it must have actually been dangerous." Then she talks about an injury she got, early in her time in America, when she pushed herself too far in a backbend during a demonstration. A teacher asks why she doesn't demonstrate anymore.

Rajashree pauses and considers the question. She seems pleased with the notion and laughs: "I think the only way I'd demonstrate again is if Tony was up there with me."

After his exile, Tony opened a nonprofit yoga studio in San Francisco. It grew quite successful, classes packed and Tony charging three hundred dollars per hour for the private instruction he squeezed in between. Tony rooted his instruction in the yoga Bikram taught him, although instead of relying on the Beginning series, he incorporated all of Bishnu Ghosh's ninety-one postures. There was no heat. When Bikram students would come and ask about it, he'd tell them, "You mastered the heat, now let's try mastering the cold."

He was regularly featured in *Yoga Journal*. A program he designed to bring yoga in the classroom won the first prize from the San Francisco Education

Fund for Most Creative Learning Environment. Soon he crossed into the mainstream with articles in the *New York Times*, BBC, and *Los Angeles Times*. When scholar Gudrun Bühnemann wrote her book *Eighty-four Asanas*, examining historical representations of hatha yoga sequences, she sought Tony out because he was the only modern practitioner she could find at the time who practiced a complete eighty-four-asana sequence, and could demonstrate it in full.

But one day Tony realized he needed to get out. His studio was still financially successful, but his newer students were treating him differently. He was no longer just their yoga teacher. People would smile at him, but they wouldn't talk. Others would talk incessantly, seeking endless validation and advice. One night a woman filled up his entire answering machine with different messages about her anxieties. A man sought him out and calmly explained he just wanted to be near him. Then a former pupil announced he had created a shrine, complete with candles, pictures, incense, and one of Tony's old T-shirts.

And so Tony decided to leave. One week, he stopped giving out business cards. Three weeks later, he donated everything in the studio to charity. He did a last interview with a reporter from *Self* magazine, and then, on the final night, locked the studio doors and climbed into an idling car; his wife had filled it with all their most important possessions and was waiting for him. Together, they drove the 1,500 miles down the California coast to the tip of Baja. From there, Tony disappeared. He went into what he calls a sabbatical. He continued a daily practice, growing even stronger—occasionally resurfacing to teach private lessons at the local resorts—but for the most part, he disengaged from the yoga community, withdrawing into a period of study and practice.

Tony's life in Baja feels like a myth. The type of urban afterlife that exists as a promise, the deliverance awaiting all our shitty commutes. He wakes at 6 A.M. on a house overlooking the Pacific Ocean, bedroom window facing the waves. Then, on a small section of his living room, between a coffee table and a couch, he begins a personalized posture sequence. It is just over one hundred positions, and Tony moves slowly and meticulously through them, stretching the sequence to four hours. Afterwards, he has two eggs, a slice of toast with butter and jam, and a cup of green tea. Then he begins his day.

He cultivates his talents. He has apprenticed himself to a Qigong master and traded yoga with several gourmet chefs for cooking classes. His kitchen has the manicured look of a *Food & Wine* photo shoot: the counter arrayed with little bowls of onions, bundles of scallions, a plate packed with tiny red cherry tomatoes. When he cooks, he always makes a tiny version of whatever he is cooking for his dog Rex, whom he calls his sous-chef. This includes his experiments with duck confit. When he sits down to eat, he will pull up a stepstool to the table, so Rex, a cairn terrier, can hop up onto the middle step to observe the proceedings.

After breakfast each morning, he drives a quarter mile to his former house to feed four wild cats. The cats dart off when approached by anyone else, but make an exception for Tony. They move toward him with the stretched-out sensuality of feline affection, and he will sit on his old stoop and rub their bellies in the sun until they tire of him. I have heard students of four different ethnicities describe Tony as reminding them of their grandfather. And somewhat abashedly, I will admit he reminds me quite a bit of my own. He is legitimately funny, often a little raunchy, but his humor is always slightly self-deprecating, never offensive. There is an unconscious courtesy in his movements. He opens his wife's side of the car first. He will not speak if you are speaking. His margarita orders have the same exacting precision as his postures. "Only the juice of a single lime and one hundred percent agave tequila, please no sugar, no premade mix."

Tony's biggest indulgence is watching bodies. It distracts him during conversation. He is endlessly assessing the obese Canadian tourists who parade around Baja in the winter. "I look at everyone and imagine they were a client," he says. "I think how would I adjust them. Do they have an imbalance in their walk? How could I make their life easier?" The waiters at his favorite restaurants all know and love him, because he offers them free one-on-one instruction. "No one has more aches and pains," Tony explains. "And although I think the waiters here are quite grateful now, at first they were very suspicious. 'Oh, you! When you come around, I want a warning. Who knows what you are going to ask of us?'"

In a kryia-like attempt to maintain his dog's health, he spends a half hour cleaning Rex's teeth with soft cotton cloth each evening. Rex, who is fifteen years old, responds by patiently submitting. When they are finished, he jumps off Tony's lap, stands waggling his tail, looking upward for more, before bounding up the spiral staircase to the roof deck where Tony and Sandy eat most of their meals. When Tony eats dinner out at one of Cabo's many resort restaurants, he always buys a rose for every woman at the table, much to the exasperation of his wife. One night when we are out, Sandy rolls her eyes, clutching the rose close to her chest, "Do you know how many of these I have back at home? He's impossible, I tell him, No, no, no, I don't want another. . . . But it's useless. It's like a talent of his. If there is a rose out there, Tony will find it and buy it for you."

And so this is Tony's urban afterlife: buying roses, teaching himself classical guitar, eating meticulously prepared meals on his terrace overlooking the ocean with his wife and fifteen-year-old dog. The day typically ends around midnight, with him squeezing in a last few postures before sleep, the ones he really wants to work on: Tony in handstand Scorpion, toes lowering toward his head while Sandy watches *CSI: Miami* on the bed above him.

I meet Tony and Sandy for lunch in Baja. Tony is dressed in tennis shoes, blue jeans, and a rugby shirt. The only hint of his profession—aside from his preternaturally calm demeanor—are his forearms, rippling with muscles when he makes small movements, such as shaking hands with the waiter who serves us.

After looking over the menu, Tony orders an espresso. He holds the tiny cup softly, bringing it to his lips.

"When I first met Bikram, he was a wonderful person. He was very new to L.A., and he would literally take the shirt from his back and give it to someone who asked for it. He didn't have so much money back then, but he was always giving. Very excited. Very idealistic."

Like everyone when talking about those days, Tony's body relaxes. "We used to do the Advanced Series together, sometimes eight hours in one day. Bikram had a beautiful practice at that point, and we would just lose ourselves in the yoga. He was strong, eager, and patient. It made him a fantastic teacher. . . . And when we were done, he would drag me off to the movies. If it was a Saturday, we'd stay all day—three movies back to back. In between, when the lights went up, we'd talk yoga."

It was the perfect time, but it couldn't last. "As Bikram got bigger, the stars walked away," Tony explains. "And instead of new stars to replace them, more everyday people came. The stars wanted private classes. They didn't want to be ogled. Bikram couldn't understand this. . . . At one point, Elvis was begging him. But Bikram wasn't convinced the yoga would help someone who wanted it on a silver platter. So he always said no.

"Having the stars leave hurt Bikram in a way that it might not hurt you or I." Tony says, "He gets mesmerized by fame and wealth. It's almost innocent, like a little boy fascinated by the fire truck. . . . Even back before he had the wealth, he wanted to buy the same Bentley that Howard Hughes had. Or the same Aston Martin that James Bond rode. This is the stuff he would talk about. We would stay up late, go dancing at a disco, end in a diner, maybe five A.M., and Bikram would be talking about the cars he wanted to buy. It wasn't greed. It was what he wanted from the world."

Raquel Welch represented an important moment in this exodus of celebrities. Bikram loved Raquel. He taught her like a daughter. She in turn became one of his most dedicated students. But then she decided to profit from the experience. She came out with a near identical yoga series, put her name on it, and sold the whole thing as an exercise video. For Bikram, it was a huge betrayal, the first time he sought legal counsel, and brought a lawsuit.

"Bikram believed Raquel taught him about America," Tony says. "This was his student, but she had no obligation to her teacher."

The food arrives. Three fish tacos for Tony and Sandy. Tony very carefully splices the middle taco down the center. Then he slides the plate into a slightly more centered position, and they both begin eating off the same plate.

"Bikram's idealism fell apart. When I met him, he truly believed that yoga was *the way,* that he had the responsibility to train people, to help humanity.

"But by the mid-1980s, he was really very different. He got pulled over for speeding at one point and spat on the cop who gave him the ticket. There was a notion that he was untouchable." The confidence that had made him such a powerful idealist was turned inward. "He could still turn on the charm when he wanted. If you saw him work with Martin Sheen or Kareem's father, it would pull your heart apart, just how compassionate he could be. But at a certain point, that compassion wasn't for the regular people anymore. . . ."

"There was an equality in the early relationships. The stars didn't need anything from Bikram. They enjoyed him as a peer. They all had other focuses to their lives." Tony pauses. "The next generation of students were chasing that relationship. And when they became his students, they made him their focus, they surrendered to him."

"I watched the changes. I went from being his very best teacher to hearing, 'Tony, you will never be a good teacher because you aren't loud enough. You don't make them afraid.' He would tell me, 'Just make them fearful. You will have them in your pocket.'"

"Now his teachers have it much worse, I think. They are meant to be used and spit out. . . . They believe his contempt is his love."

When I ask Tony if this was all there from the beginning, he is slow to answer.

"It was a metamorphosis. We all change. But we also have some control over the path. We choose our surroundings; we choose where we put our energy. Bikram—one of the most powerful forces to spread yoga—chose his road of materialism and control. He chose to surround himself by very needy people who gave themselves to him. Was it always there from the beginning? Of course it was. But so were many other possibilities. . . ."

The Negative

After six years of his sabbatical, Tony reemerges to offer a teacher training program. It isn't for the money. He has a private client list that includes multiple—as in several different—billionaires. Tony is teaching again because he finally feels he has a coherent system to offer.

"I needed to become a recluse to evolve. It is very tempting to keep forcing information into yourself, but you never get a chance to see the bad habits that develop, the big picture that surrounds you. Without the breaks, I could not choose how I was developing. It would have been a very passive process. This might not be the path for everyone, but for me to grow and choose how to grow, it was essential to disappear."

In preparation for the training, Sandy designed a small flyer announcing an "advanced instructors workshop," which they sent to a few old friends. It was quickly forwarded widely.

While there are students with many different yoga backgrounds at his training, by far the biggest group are senior Bikram studio owners. They have come secretly, risking their jobs and place in the community.

The hotel where Tony is holding his training is not Club Med, but it is close. The practice space itself is a small unheated room overlooking the beach, with huge windows cleaned to the highest degree of transparency. Below us, blue pools spill out onto a sand beach, which in turn fades into the even more blue water of the ocean.

There are no mirrors; there are no mats. Just a towel on the floor marking your space and Tony moving slowly around the room, giving individualized adjustments.[40]

After an initial breathing exercise, the first thing Tony does to me is walk over and whisper in my ear. "Please do not go one hundred percent. Today is your first day with us. Try fifty-five percent. Tomorrow maybe sixty-five percent."

When I ask him later, he explains, "One hundred percent is an illusion. Why do you think so many people in the Bikram world have a beautiful practice for a few years and then slip away? One hundred or even ninety percent is impossible to maintain. You will become exhausted. Mentally if not

---

[40] There is also no skin. His students are all dressed in T-shirts, leggings, or baggy shorts. "This actually produced the most fighting the first few days on the training," Tony tells me. "People did not want to give up their yoga gear. But I'm a man. With a wife. I don't need you bending over in front of me in something skimpy. I don't need a roomful of young men clenching their abs, trying to show their six-packs to each other."

physically. Terrified of practicing the yoga you love because it is draining you not replenishing you . . . But even if you could practice at that intensity—even if you were so strong, you would never become exhausted—it would be undesirable. You can't make adjustments at your edge. You can't listen to your body. For regular practice, seventy-five to eighty-five percent is fine—you will never tire out and in the long run you will grow much stronger."

In almost every way, his class is like a photo negative of a Bikram class. The room is cool. Tony moves from person to person, offering individualized instruction. He focuses on stillness within a posture rather than the pushing to get there. There is no humor to distract you from the discomfort. Where Bikram emphasizes the stretch on one side of the body during a posture, Tony will focus on feeling compression on the other side. And when we do balancing postures, Tony walks up and taps my knee.

"You don't need to 'lock the knee.' There are only two places where you lock the knee, ballet and Bikram Yoga. Both are aesthetic decisions, and both end up hurting people."

After we finish with the three-hour class, people rise off their mats, buzzing. Conversation picks up. This being a meeting of Bikram studio owners outside of the usual fearful Bikram space, there is a lot of gossip to be exchanged. Everyone has formed into four-person pods of chatter.

When he is ready to discuss the class, Tony stands in the front of the room silently. Nobody pays him any attention. Then he says, "Can we discuss?" and the room hushes out like a blanket thrown over a flame.

Without any pause, Tony launches into an explanation of several modifications he made during the morning's class. All eyes are on him, notebooks out, scribbling his every word.[41]

---

[41] The nuance and depth in Tony's teaching are quite simply unrivaled in the Bikram/hot yoga world. My jaw dropped when I watched the routine manner Tony's students approached postures like One-Armed Peacock, Mountain, or Dancer. Postures I had been taught took years to master and were simply unavailable to the 99 percent. His ability to step inside your personal body and analyze your approach—which feels absolutely supernatural as it occurs but which is actually the simple result of his four-hours-of-daily-practice-for-forty-years hyperconsciousness about all

. . .

Just as with Bikram's Teacher Training, the second half of the day is spent learning how to teach in small groups. However, instead of memorizing and reciting a script, Tony has his students lead a mini-class of their own design. Each group is asked to select a section of asanas from the Ghosh advanced series, not unlike what Bikram did when creating his Beginners Series, and then teach that section to the rest of the class. Tony will usually watch the instruction, but occasionally bend along as a student.

When he does, even these mini-classes become special. Despite being surrounded by students half his age, there is no doubt whose postures are the most advanced. At fifty-six, Tony has a body that looks preposterous, computer-enhanced, especially when juxtaposed with his crinkling face and balding hairline. During one afternoon series, I look up to find him holding a lone handstand in the room, body perfectly still, like an arrow shot straight into the ground, long after everyone else has collapsed out. His shirt, slipped down by gravity, reveals back muscles like six-pack abs.

After the students teach, there is a public debrief. Discussing the advantages and disadvantages of the sequence, what additions or rearrangements could make it more powerful. The student-teachers are often put on the spot, forced to justify their choices, the specific wording of their instructions. It is surprisingly aggressive, closer to a third-year law student's lawyering class than a yoga training. During the exchange, Tony sits silently

---

things related to the human form—allows him to teach extremely daunting movements to rank beginners. Moreover, Tony teaches the meditation, mantras, breathing exercises, kryias, and other components of hatha yoga that Bikram once taught but no longer shares with his students. They give an intellectual succor to his training that the Bikram community is craving. Most tellingly, Tony explicitly teaches the limitations of yoga. "Most yogis believe yoga is a total solution—that yoga will cure all their problems. If you tell them that you run or lift weights, they'll act like you are betraying them. . . . This is utter nonsense. . . . Actually, it is worse, it is fraud and will end up harming people. Yoga is a system for maintaining one aspect of your health. I have practiced for almost forty years and I have pretty good postures, but I would never rely on yoga alone. Bikram certainly never did. Even when his postures were in top form, he would go lift weights at the Santa Monica gym. Most of our students in those days—especially the actors and athletes—had other exercise programs to supplement as well. . . . Selling anything as a total solution is unrealistic. And buying it is a sign you have stopped questioning and learning and decided to give those qualities over to someone else."

on the side, maybe you think even drifting off, until suddenly, he interjects to correct an explanation or tweak a recommendation.

When this period of public feedback has been exhausted, there is a break. Paper is handed out, and students offer the student-teachers a private, anonymous reflection.

Tony reviews the instructions for me, "We score everyone on the basis of Projection, Confidence, Knowledge, Timing, and Clarity. Be honest. Be harsh. But be descriptive so that nothing you say comes off as cruel."

Later he will tell me, "There is a phony code of ethics that has developed in the yoga world. It says you can't say anything bad about another yoga teacher or a different yoga class, unless," he laughs, "—unless they were trained by someone else. . . . If yoga is going to evolve, it needs to change that. I want to encourage freethinking and individuality, but that comes with debate; it requires rigor and well-thought-out decisions. Sadly right now, we are at a time when neither of those attributes are really emphasized in the yoga world.

"Most teachers rely on humility because they are ignorant. They surrender to someone else who calls themselves an expert or a guru, and they never gain the knowledge necessary to critique or grow."

He pauses. "Do you know why yoga teachers get sued by Bikram? Because they don't know anything else. They only know the crumbs that Bikram has fed them. So that is all they can teach."

In between classes, the trainees sit around on their towels, gossiping. The atmosphere can feel a little like a Bikram support group.

"The first few days were basically just throwing up Kool-Aid for me," a current Bikram studio owner tells me.

"I honestly became addicted," a former studio owner chimes in. "I always wanted to be in the hottest spot in the room, I wanted to push my self further, drink more water, go deeper into stretching. . . . For me, Bikram was the Source. I was addicted to his authenticity. And I got off on practicing with three hundred people, the feeling of community."

"I was addicted too," a second Bikram studio owner says. "When I found

Bikram, I was in finance, I needed to be reached constantly. And within a few months, I put all that aside. I was doing two classes a day, every day. I would take a weekend and do a triple."

"This training," a current Bikram teacher says, "is the first time I haven't tried to go one hundred percent. I mean, it's no secret most of us are type A. We like the struggle. And I came here really worried that I would lose my postures. I would lose muscle mass. But the exact opposite has happened. Every day I grow stronger."

"The hardest thing for me," the second studio owner says, "is how to transmit this knowledge to my students. They want the heat. They demand it. It produces this huge rush of energy, but at the end of the day, it is just like a sugar rush. . . . And it may be in my head, but I think the Bikram name adds a lot to my bottom line. I can't just walk away."

The teacher nods understanding. "But you know what? This is what it should have been like. Tony is who Bikram should have been. I don't mean that in the sense of what a yogi is supposed to be. I mean it in the sense that Tony knows the yoga better than Bikram. He still practices. He is unafraid to modify it if he finds it hurts him. . . . If you look at all of the dogmatic senior teachers out there, none of them have a strong practice anymore. . . . How can you trust them?"

"I was so angry the first few days I was here," a third studio owner says. "We were cheated. I learned more in one day here than I did at Bikram's entire Advanced Training. And no one was belittled here. No one was yelled at once. We were empowered. We were helped and taught to help."

"And watching Tony with Sandy. It is so inspirational." As she is speaking, this studio owner begins crying. "At my training, Bikram would knock on doors, looking for women. Here Sandy comes here every day and supports Tony. I don't know if they have a dark side. How could I? But he checks on her, he cares for her. I can see that. I imagine them going home after the morning class. She makes him lunch, they talk about how it went, and he comes back to teach us. . . ."

And as she is saying this, Tony has walked into the room. He is standing on the far side of the room, leaning against the door, listening to his student crying and smiling and detailing her personal fantasy of his lunchtime domestic bliss. As the teacher continues on, I glance up at Tony again. He has turned away, and I think he is going to walk off to give her some privacy. But when he turns back briefly, I notice it's because he has tears in his eyes too.

On the afternoon of the penultimate day of his training, with everyone in a great mood, the last small group of student-teachers teach their series. It is very non-Ghosh: covering a tangle of different styles—flow yoga, Qigong, calisthenics, Bikram—all jumbled together with choppy directions. Portions of it work, but many represent the sloppy extreme of eager individuality: an imbalanced, poorly planned class where you could hurt yourself. I take class along with the rest of the trainees and find myself thoroughly confused the whole time, craving the precision and stability of the Bikram dialogue.

During the debrief, Tony remains silent, watching as other students express their confusion and as the student-teachers defend their decisions. Although everyone in the room looks to him for a reaction after they speak, he never interjects once.

His response comes the next day. Tony simply teaches. Or rather, he reteaches. Instead of his normal morning series—an enhancement of the ninety-one-posture Ghosh advanced series—he leads the room in a series that while not identical to the day before, clearly addresses the same aspects of the body. The overlap is quiet but explicit, respectful and firm. It is also tremendously clarifying. Through the juxtaposition, I learn more about which commands are critical for getting into and out of a posture than I did the entire Bikram training.

The experience is nuanced and respectful and treats his students like adults: it strikes me as something Bikram is simply incapable of producing under any circumstances.

Then, when the class is over, his training concluded, Tony does something else Bikram is incapable of: He invites everyone out for margaritas.

Once, almost as if out of a dream, Tony bumps into Bikram on the street. They haven't seen each other in fifteen years. Bikram is in San Francisco for a seminar. He is sitting in his Rolls-Royce at a red light when Tony walks past. They make eye contact and Bikram jumps out of his car, leaving it idling. He rushes to Tony and hugs him. Bikram mentions nothing of their falling out. He tells Tony only that he needs them to be friends again. They go out to a series of dinners; they catch up. They examine X-rays from anatomy books and debate the potential dangers of locking the knee. Bikram asks him to demonstrate for his students and Tony agrees, modeling several non-Ghosh postures for the group. After two weeks, Tony decides this is how he wants to leave their relationship and withdraws. He has not spoken to Bikram since.

Don't Stop Believing

When I finally sit down next to Hector to talk yoga, it is after an Advanced Class. Both of us have the well-drained, well-polished look that comes after smearing your face against a sweaty carpet for two-plus hours, struggling like a man in a straitjacket against your own limbs, and then taking a nice long shower to wash it all away.

We shake hands awkwardly. Hector has been my teacher for a long time; I have spent hundreds of hours bending half-naked in a room with him, listening and respecting his every command, but we have zero social relationship. Which is, generally speaking, perfect. But it does leave me wanting: to fill in the gap between the professional world where we interface and the more defined world in my head. I want to let him know the job he does routinely is a treasure to me.

Instead, I drum the table between us. Make a joke about the slow service.

Hector looks impressive. His face has the broad proud lines of a charcoal etching. It is ruddy from the yoga we just practiced, but otherwise looks ready to be bronzed. I study his jaw while he talks; there is no trace of his stroke.

"Yoga came into my life right when I needed it," Hector tells me. "I was at the end of a twenty-year dance career—Broadway, off-Broadway, traveling companies—when I tore my both my ACL and MCL in my left knee. It was a total ego injury. I was teaching a class and tried to model a jump. Just landed wrong."

I've stopped listening, however. A twenty-year career?

Which leads to the first monster revelation: Hector is forty-eight! This is almost disturbing to me for some reason. I had him pegged in his mid-thirties.

Hector shrugs. "The yoga keeps you young."

We talk about his introduction to yoga ("I thought I was in great shape—and ten minutes in, I was down on my mat, watching this one-hundred-ten-pound girl next to me up in the standing splits"), we talk about Teacher Training ("Holy shit!"), and his old injuries coming up ("They will come back. They will hurt. You are never finished healing."). Finally I ask him about his health.

"At first, it's a leap of faith," he tells me. "You learn by watching other people go through the same process. But at this point, having taught thousands of students, I simply don't believe you can get hurt practicing this yoga. Maybe in the hamstrings, if you are very reckless with your body. But for the most part, the range of motion in the Beginner Class is so gentle. . . . If you compare to something like running, there is no contest.

"I actually don't think you should be teaching," he says, "if you feel differently. That strikes me as very cynical."

When I ask about his stroke, he nods.

"There are a lot of people who walk away when it turns out the yoga hasn't made them immortal. They think the yoga has let them down. They have poured so much effort into their practice that they feel like they have been betrayed.

"But it is not a promise. It is a practice. . . . If you do it for long enough, maybe it gives you the self-compassion to deal with your mortality. Maybe it makes you more accepting."

Then he holds out his index finger. It looks oddly bony and wrinkled, not unlike a hot dog left to dry out in the sun. "Guess what this is."

I don't say anything, but I imagine it is dehydration left over from our class.

"I have a very serious kidney ailment. It turns out my body doesn't make a certain protein. And because of that protein, I have trouble regulating my water balance. I store it. I lose it. If I go without medication, I become a balloon. It's a small thing now that I have the right treatment."

He looks me in the eye. "The first time I went to the hospital for this problem, when I was diagnosed, they had to drain the water from my body. I eventually peed out ninety pounds of water. Can you imagine?"

I can't.

"The yoga is not an immunity card against disease. At best, it can help us deal with that fact." Now he drums his hands against the table. "The previous owner of my studio was a woman who got breast cancer. She left very disenchanted. She felt betrayed by Bikram.

"And I understand that mentality. I get it. But the truth is, if I wasn't doing the yoga, it might not have been a survivable stroke," Hector says. "If I wasn't doing the yoga, who knows what would have happened with my recovery. I have my face back now. . . . You know, when I went to the doctor with questions about what turned out to be my kidney disease, the doctor couldn't believe it. He told me I shouldn't be walking. By the numbers in my blood work, I should have already been in the hospital."

"They started me on seven drugs for my kidney; today I take one. I pin that on the yoga. Afterwards, when I was lying in the hospital, I asked the doctors what caused it. It was frightening. I wanted to know what to change. I told them about the heat. I told them about the yoga. I was terrified it might have been the ten Advil a day I took while I was a dancer. I've done my share of drugs too. Cocaine. I've made lots of mistakes with my health. I told the doctors all that, and I wanted them to connect those dots.

"And you know what they said? 'No cause.' Not the yoga, not the heat, not the Advil, not the drugs. 'No cause.' Just me. Just my life.

"I am sure there are people who would see it as failure. But I see the miracle. I see the strength the yoga has given me. I walked into that hospital when the numbers said I should have been comatose in an ambulance. I am forty-eight, survivor of a stroke and stronger than ever."

And sitting across from him, I believe it is all true.

One Point, Two Instances of Intersection

After talking with Hector, I go back just one step further.

I find Sarah Baughn living in a toy-strewn house on the edge of San Francisco proper, a little row house by the ocean in the Sunset District. We hug hello. Although I have met her only once, when she arrived at my studio in Brooklyn two years ago, I feel like I am connecting to something vital.

Sarah leads me through her living room. Her daughter Paiden plays on the floor, pushing multicolored pegs through multicolored holes. Her partner, Kyle, is at work at the bar he manages. Both are new additions since her tour as yoga champion. Theirs is a house with a Christmas tree clearly decorated by the whole family—complete with dangling homemade ornaments of stern-faced snowmen and crazy-legged reindeer. It is cozy in the way busy overwhelmed houses get cozy, a mess of overuse, not of neglect. We sit down at her country-kitchen table, high chair between us, and as I set up my notepad and tape recorder, I am served two thick slices of bread slathered in tayberry jam. Naturally, it is homemade. Paiden is laughing and splashing at her multicolored pegs in the background.

I wonder if it is all still a dream. Everything is exactly where it needs to be.

And as I make idiotic gestures, trying to convey my gratitude for the jam—which might contain an actual recipe for the divine—Sarah disassembles that notion completely. She does this without a trace of regret or pity while moving around in full multitasking mom mode: kissing Paiden on the forehead after a crash, pushing more raisin bread in the toaster for me.

"I hardly practice at this point," she explains as she moves around the room. "I'm still in significant pain. It all just slipped out of my control. . . . I became so skinny. I never saw anyone else. I never even saw my grandparents anymore. I was this tiny, obsessed, hyperbendy thing. My knee was the first thing to go."

Just after her first competition, Sarah had surgery on her knee.

"I was training too hard. I was already this superflexible girl, and I was pushing my body to the limits. . . . One day my knee just started locking as

I walked. It would make a *click click* noise when I bent it. You know, just felt slightly stuck. And when I went to a doctor doctor—not a yoga doctor—he told me that was an indicator of a torn meniscus."

She slathers my toast with jam so briskly, it almost feels like a reflex re-action. "I was young and flexible and full of arrogance. . . . Looking back, it was almost necessary for me to be humbled.

"But it was hard," she says. "Not just the pain. I felt tremendous pres-sure when I returned. I wanted to practice more, but people would look at me and I would feel their disappointment. Like 'That's Sarah, my teacher, the champion.' And they would wonder why my practice wasn't very deep. It took a long time for me to get to the point where I could say in my head, 'Good! I'm glad you see me. This is me—this is my practice—it might not be as deep as it used to be, but it is mine. . . . Now stop looking. What you need to do is look at your own practice.'"

Sarah arrived at a Bikram studio at nineteen during her sophomore year of college. Within six months, she had dropped out to attend Teacher Training. Just like with Tony, when she talks about those early days, I feel like I am listening to her talk about an old, momentous romance.

Childhood was sad for Sarah. The death of a friend when she was twelve connected with a powerful predisposition toward depression, and she sank into a hole that she never quite crawled out of. "I spent my high school feeling like crap all the time," she says. "Just really depressed. I couldn't sleep. I couldn't even see myself—all I saw was ugly and fat. I thought that might change at college, but instead, here I was, walking around telling everyone I met that I hated life."

By the end of her third class, she had decided she wanted to become a teacher. "I took an evening class, and when I came out, it was raining and dark—basically, a perfect recipe for my depression. But I was singing. Singing and walking in the rainy dark. I felt so good. . . . And that was when I realized I wanted to teach this yoga to sad people."

And so at age twenty, convinced the yoga had just saved her life, Sarah arrived at Teacher Training.

Bikram was on her from minute one. "He called me his 'assistant.' He told everyone he 'created me.'" Her multitasking has stopped for a moment, and Sarah is sitting at the table with me flipping through the thick card-board pages of a children's book, running her fingers over the scenes in the book and their primary colors. "I loved the attention he gave me. I loved being the special one. But I was too young, and the pressure became diffi-cult to handle. . . ."

"In the end, it made me stronger." She is staring hard at the children's book. "Learning to separate the man from the teacher is one of those delicate balances. It's a yoga in itself. Really one of those things you look back and say, 'Thank you, Mom, thank you, Dad. You raised me right.'"

I click off the tape recorder and ask Sarah instead about competing.

"It became my life. It was the most valuable time of my life. My coach made it much more about the philosophy than the postures. Really nour-ished me, because it wasn't something I was otherwise getting. But it wasn't until I didn't win that it all made sense."

Didn't win?

"Yep." She laughs. "I came in second place, you didn't know that. . . . Bikram played a big part in judging back then." There is a pause. She moves onward. "It was crushing for me, I wanted to win so badly. Looking back, I probably needed to lose. It certainly taught me a lot."

Sarah had dreams of using her championship to raise money for chil-dren with cancer. It is a dream so big and so wholesome and so cliché that if I weren't sitting in her home eating her homemade tayberry jam amidst her homemade crayon-enhanced Christmas ornaments, I might not take it on face value. But I am here, so I do. Unconditionally.

She explains, the winner of the Asana Championship goes on a paid tour—as a yoga ambassador of sorts—and she saw the tour as opportunity to fund-raise. She didn't even know a child who had died of cancer; it just struck her as a something important. A way to give back for the time she had spent on herself. And so throughout training, it provided an all-consuming motivation to push into the next set.

"When I lost, there was this huge sense of failure. You know here is this thing, where I did everything I was asked to do. No, no, no—I did everything I was asked to do *perfectly*. I dedicated my life to it. I executed.

And then, it didn't work out at all. Coming in second is nothing. You get nothing, no tour.

"I went to class the next day, I dragged myself—one of those things you very much do not want to do, but do because everyone expects you to be there—and the woman who won was teaching in the next room. As I did my practice, I could hear her. And in the middle of it, I woke up. I was staring at myself in the mirror. Nothing had changed. Being champion had absolutely nothing to do with raising money for children with cancer. I could still do my routine. And if I wanted, I could still use it to raise money. None of that had been taken from me."

And so Sarah went on the tour where I met her. She asked yoga studios across the country to donate the space for single class. Then she packed the class full—in the one I attended, there were over forty-five people in a room that typically held twenty—and she taught. Then when we were all exhausted, dripping, and open, she concluded with the posture routine that changed my life. The tour was entirely self-funded and occurred without the blessing or encouragement of Bikram the man. It was Sarah's gift to the community. With the ironclad idealism of someone in her early twenties, she didn't reimburse herself for anything and took on a significant amount of debt during the process.

But it was necessary. "That tour saved my relationship to yoga," she says. "Everything I learned, every good thing it has given me, I tried to give back during that tour. And I came back having gained so much."

It also set the stage for her current life. She gave away enough that she no longer felt beholden to the yoga. "One thing I have to tell people is, I'm not the person I was on that tour. I do yoga to live; I don't live to do yoga anymore," she tells me. "Some of the studio owners I teach for, they want me to smile constantly. They want me to bounce around like a yoga cheerleader and sell it to everyone who comes in. Yoga is a tool I use when I need it. It is a certain pair of clothes I have in my drawer. I can put it on if I choose to wear it. Or I can save it for a special occasion. I don't depend on it anymore. I don't allow it to define me.

"You know, after my knee surgery, nobody from the yoga world came to see me. They were all too immersed in their practice to visit. . . . That was also a wake-up call too. Not because I blamed them. But because that was just where I had been—exactly who I was. The only difference is that now that I was on the sidelines, I could see it all clearly."

Paiden has been periodically running into the room to deliver different goodies to Sarah. A blue plastic block, a clump of red ribbon. After each handoff, she runs out of the room, giggling with energy. Sarah points into the other room at her. "You know what I still believe in completely? Yoga babies. I practiced all nine months with Mary Jarvis. No water in class. It was wonderful. Magic." When Paiden delivers her next goody to me, I give her little hand a little kiss. She is as excited and eager as I have ever seen a child, and my momentary puzzlement over Sarah's certainty, hopefully forgiven.

The Yoga Effect

All this leads me to one unavoidable question: How much of the yoga is the yoga?

If Joseph had taken kickboxing classes as a twelve-year-old, would he have regained his health? If Luke had decided to dedicate his life to rhythmic gymnastics, would he have kicked heroin? If Sol had done sixty days of Tae Bo, would he have lost the weight and gained the energy?

It's impossible to tell.

When selective serotonin reuptake inhibitors (SSRIs) hit the market following FDA approval in 1987, they represented a new era of neurotransformative medicine. Over the previous twenty years, our understanding of the brain had been radically updated, largely through advances in imaging techniques. The SSRIs were presented as the promised fruit of that research—our newest, best, and most promising weapons in the war against depression.

Unlike previous generations of brain-fuzzing and personality-bludgeoning antidepressants, the SSRIs were precise, targeted, and clear in effect. Researchers could document how they affected neural channels, measure the exact changes they wrought on the brain. Almost as soon as they hit the market, they were a sensation.

In 1987, prior to the introduction of the first of these drugs, Prozac, approximately 4.5 million adults were using antidepressants. Over the next two decades, that number increased sixfold, so that by 2007, approximately a full 10 percent of Americans over the age of six years old were regularly taking an antidepressant. And because pills sold equaled dollars spent, the SSRI-driven antidepressant market grew into a 19 billion per year superindustry within an industry. The brand names of the compounds—Prozac, Zoloft, Paxil, Lexapro—became household names.

It is no understatement to say that the new SSRIs changed the landscape of mental health. A paradigm that had been slowly drifting in one direction shifted suddenly and decisively: brain-based medicine was here to stay. Freud, long since dead to his field, was now relegated to the most insulting status for a scientific thinker: historical figure. Nature, not nurture, was behind most psychiatric disease. And with that disassociation, a whole culture of cloistering shame was lifted. Side effects were debated on the sidelines of high school soccer games. *Listening to Prozac, Prozac Nation,* and the *Prozac Diary* became unlikely bestsellers. The depressive personality was marked for such a rapid extinction that a whole new contrarian movement of melancholy poets and artists began to champion it.

Nowhere was this shift more present than the psychiatric community. Doctors long wary of the growing influence of the pharmaceutical industry were won over by the powerful results.

The Hamilton Rating Scale for Depression rates a patient's mood, sleep patterns, suicidal tendencies, and energy levels. It is a detailed exam conducted in a one-on-one interview with a doctor. For something as slippery as a mood disorder, the Hamilton Rating Scale represents a hard statistical measure to gauge progress. It is the gold standard. And bottom line, when patients swallow an SSRI, their scores on the Hamilton Rating Scale change for the better. Doctors see results, patients feel brighter, the world is literally a happier place.

The problem is, it is all built on a mirage.

As early as 1995, Guy Sapirstein and Irving Kirsch decided to pool the results of previous studies on antidepressants. What they found shocked them. Over 75 percent of the effects of the SSRI antidepressants were attributable to the placebo effect. The tactical nukes of depression were three-quarters tactical Tic Tacs.

When Sapirstein and Kirsch examined the specifics of the studies, they found something even more damning. Most patients could tell when they were given an SSRI pill as opposed to a placebo because the SSRIs came with a host of side effects (dry mouth, nausea, low sex drive). Patients could and did enhance the placebo effect by figuring out whether or not they were getting the "real thing."

Nowhere was this clearer than when the drug company Merck—to much excitement—produced an SSRI with no side effects. The drug failed miserably. Merck ended up voluntarily withdrawing it from clinical trials after only four months because it could find no differences between the drug and a placebo.

Similarly, in nine studies in which active placebos were used—"active placebos" being those placebos that produce side effects but that should not yield any relief—there was zero significant difference between SSRI and placebo in seven of the studies. And when you look at the results of a successful antidepressant, such as Prozac, you find a 96 percent correlation between experiencing a side effect and experiencing improvement.

My point here is not to argue one way or another about the usefulness of antidepressants (and there may well be circumstances where they are invaluable). It is to emphasize the enormous positive role the placebo effect can play when we give it room to operate.

In fact, the biggest problem the placebo effect has ever had is its name.

The term comes down to us from Chaucer. Like a liturgical version of those mariachi bands that won't shut up until they're paid, medieval "Placebo" singers would march into funerals and bray away, pretending to be mourners in order to get a share of the food and drink. And to this day, the term carries that weight. It is synonymous with "sucker": sugar pills, saline injections, and kissing a baby's bruised fingers after they get pinched. A mocking reminder that no matter what our literacy rates are, superstition isn't dead and the world is still filled with plenty of people who can be convinced into just about anything.

But that's a problem with the name, not the effect. The effect is 100 percent real. And it works on people whether they are Aspergian or avuncular, scientist or clergy. All those depressives weren't faking their relief. The SSRIs did slash their depression.

It's just that most of their relief didn't come from the pill.

In 2005, Dr. Jon-Kar Zubieta examined the brain scans of men as they underwent a painful injection in their jaw. The screen flared up as the areas of their brains associated with pain response activated. The men were then given a saline placebo and told it might suppress their pain. Results were immediate. Not only did the men self-report feeling their pain lifting, but their brain scans demonstrated a physical response: their bodies began releasing an opioidlike substance associated with painkilling. The saline placebo caused the release of real painkillers in the brain.

To put it another way, belief caused the body to create and release chemicals that stopped the pain.

The effects go far beyond depression and pain. Over forty-five diseases—from herpes to Parkinson's to peptic ulcers—have shown clinically significant improvements attributed to a placebo response. Which is not to say the placebo is a panacea. It will not cure cancer. It will not stop a gangrenous infection. But it might alleviate their symptoms as well as any drug.

So think about this again. There is a known, documented, extensively studied effect that involves people's beliefs mediating positive physical changes on their bodies.

What if it were called the willpower effect? Would we still scorn it?

This is in essence what occurs. Through an act of mind—not related to the physiological efficacy of the substance, therapy, or operation in question—our bodies change. We will efficacy. It is the stuff of miracles, everything a New Age medicine could ever hope for. Even in the briefest survey of the scientific literature we can find evidence for the impossible. Placebos triggering immune responses, lowering heart rates, raising energy levels, enhancing athletic performance, improving sleep, and boosting sex drive.

Sound familiar?

Right now, the placebo is associated with shams because it is dependent on trickery. It relies on ignorance in the patient, and in most cases diminishes when the subject learns it is not valid. But what if we could train ourselves to turn it on and turn it off? What if we could practice changing our minds? And what if, like almost every other physiological response, with training it could be enhanced?

This, I submit, would be the "yoga effect" as described so many thousands of years ago in the *Katha Upanishad* and developed into a series of physical movements by the Naths in the jungles of India. Yoga is the placebo effect made tangible. It is the steady training of the will to harness the body.

In study after study, the placebo effect is shown to grow stronger if the placebo given has side effects or if the doctors in question treat the patients with more "attention and confidence." Patients see the side effects, feel the doctor's certainty, and the combined reassurance causes increased efficacy.

And when you compare Bikram Yoga to other exercise regimes or to other yoga lineages, what do you have? Side effects and confidence galore. Rajashree joked at my training that "yoga therapy was medicine without a prescription, healing without a pill." Which got me thinking, if Bikram Yoga were an FDA-approved medicine, what would go on the warning label?

Bikram Yoga
Side effects may include:
  Acne
  Weeping
  Aches and sores
  Sudden weight loss
  Occasional puking
  Seizure
  Hallucination
  Irrational bouts of euphoria and/or horniness
  Diarrhea

Because what is clear is if you engage in a protracted Bikram Yoga binge, you will experience some very clear, very demonstrable side effects. They will convince you that something profound and active is going on within you.

This would also explain why people in the West, especially the most ardent supporters, become so obsessed with the authenticity and ritual of yoga. The five thousand years of silent open-eyed meditation, chanting, hand gestures, urine drinking, and rigid Sanskrit pronunciations enhance the placebo effect. They enhance our confidence.

This is not to say that the forces behind the placebo effect are responsible for all the benefits of yoga. It is to point out that there is an amazing ability in every human to connect beliefs and thoughts to the physical body on a very deep and nonintuitive level, which yoga draws out. People learn to control their heartbeat. People learn to release endogenous opiates to control their pain sensations. Processes we think of as automatic can be brought under something like conscious control.

Ancient yogis realized this and spent years studying it. They discovered this effect and instead of deciding it was sugar pills for suckers decided it was a sign that our minds and bodies were unified. They decided most of us lived in a world of delusion they called *maya,* where we believed these units to be separate. But they also believed that separation was fundamentally artificial and that through yoga we could overcome it.

It can be no accident that the first and most important of the *tapas* was breath control. Respiration is a boundary—at various times during our lives, it is both a reflex action and under conscious control: autonomic and voluntary. Perhaps as focus recedes deep into the brain during breathing exercises we can locate the area of the brain that mediates this control. It is the basis for all yoga practice. The first place to practice manipulating the master switch that all the great yogis—the Tonys, the Eskas, the Courtneys—eventually learn to throw: integrating the voluntary and involuntary, material and immaterial, the union of an individual body with the world surrounding it.

We Are Yogi

Reading about the placebo effect felt like a coming-out party. Janis's "We are yogi" became a private decree. A cross between a physiological extension of Hamlet's "nothing either good or bad, but thinking makes it so" and Ernest Shackleton's declamation that he had "pierced the veneer of outside things" as he navigated into Antarctica. It is Jack LaLanne swimming from Alcatraz in the 60-degree San Francisco harbor, arms handcuffed behind him with his legs tied via tow rope to a ten-thousand-pound boat. Or Denis willing himself to walk again after his motorcycle accident. It is not a lifestyle or a routine. It is not dependent on heat or a particular series so much as it is an ability to tap into an understanding about human performance. It is every freakish human accomplishment that stuns us into believing some people are really and truly different—walking, breathing superhumans. And then it is listening to those superhumans describe their accomplishments and choosing to suspend disbelief for a second and accepting what they say when they invariably describe it as Luke did of his methadone detox: "The first thing to remember whenever you see someone do the incredible—and this includes incredible suffering—is they have been working at it for a very, very long time and they started from a place very, very close to you."

It is also, I think, to swear vigilance to the other side of the coin: the critical memory that no matter what heights of accomplishment you ascend, you are precisely not a freakish superhuman, that your normality is what made it all possible, that you are equipped with a body capable of failure and brain driven toward hubris and mistake. That true balance means exactly 50 percent of the time, less is more. That we all have a fulcrum point in our lives we need to identify and study. Negotiating that line is the true edge. The men and women who go over it are lost to us. They may burn bright for a moment, they may amass riches and attract our envies, but theirs is the brightness of the supernova, the flaring right before the collapse, and their trajectory is written as sure as any star into the cold self-absorbed energy of a black hole.

Cycling of the Gunas

I continue to practice every day, growing stronger Tony Sanchez–style, in the cold of my apartment, in a small space between a couch and a bookshelf. I still sneak off to the hot room every once in a while because I love it. And when I'm there, I do it all just as Bikram would want and burn myself to the ground. Janis has opened his first studio in Latvia. He calls me out of the blue one day to tell me his son was drafted by a pro-hockey team and offers to fly me to Riga to teach with him. Joseph, survivor of a childhood heart attack, wins the international competition in 2011. It is his beautiful asana I am watching offstage in the prologue, his spine in a perfect O. Luke is living in small house on the coast of Auckland with his girlfriend, surfing at sunrise, keeping warm with donated lumber in the evening. Courtney Mace is still my favorite yogi of all time. She recently adopted a three-legged dog named Mona. Sol is still jogging. Still training for successively longer races. He recently tore something ugly in his knee. After the MRI, he decided to rehab it in the hot room. So after an extended hiatus, he's back to bending again. Esak remains out. He tells me Jedi Fight Club will endure. He tells me he loves Bikram and can't understand what has happened. He tells me, just like competition, just like pain, Bikram exiling him is a part of him, that he doesn't blame anyone, that it's his work. He laughs and tells me he's excited. It's all yoga, after all. Now there's just more to do.

Notes

A Short Note on Folk Singing and the Space Between Solutions

viii "My one goal was to accurately try and capture my experience . . .": This book is the product of hundreds of interviews, detailed handwritten notes, audio recordings, extensive follow-up conversations, and cross-referencing through multiple sources. It is also, like all nonfiction, the product of memory and word choice. For that reason, I want to reiterate the obvious, and make clear that this is just the record of one person's experience, not a bead on the Truth of Bikram (whatever that may be), or an attempt at a statement on the beautiful, chaotic, confounding community that has grown up around him. To protect privacy and condense narrative, a very few names have been changed and a very few details altered—although in no way do I believe these changes effect the material truth of the story or the integrity of my recollection.

Prologue: Bombproof?

1 "Prologue: Bombproof?": A reference less to the epigraphic quotes below, or Bikram Choudhury's famous description of his yoga ("I make you bullet-proof, waterproof, fireproof, windproof, money-proof, sex-proof, emotion-proof. Nothing in the world can take your peace away") but rather to an offhand remark by Linda, "L-Like Linda," two minutes before she trailed off in speech during our interview (p. 193)—a moment that was very much on my mind as I stood staring out at the darkness from offstage and a moment

that speaks to the almost definitional hatha experience, where an event can be both devastating and life-affirming at the same instant—an offhand remark where Linda explained, while visibly trembling from the memory, that she released herself from Bikram because all of a sudden she found the yoga she loved exploding all around her.

1   **"If the radiance of a thousand suns . . .":** Oppenheimer quoted in *The Decision to Drop the Bomb,* produced by Fred Freed, *NBC News,* 1965.

1   **"I have balls like atom bombs, two of them, 100 megatons each. . . .":** Quoted by Paul Keegan, "Yogis Behaving Badly," *Business 2.0,* Sept. 2002, and repeated by eager trainees at every Teacher Training since then.

Part I: It Never Gets Any Easier (If You Are Doing It Right)

7   **"This story expresses, I think, most completely his philosophy of life. . . . He thought of civilized and morally tolerable human life as a dangerous walk. . . .":** Bertrand Russell, *Portraits from Memory and Other Essays,* New York: Simon and Schuster, 1956.

23   **"The Man in the Mirror (Aka What I Learn about Bikram from the Internet":** To be sure, this includes information from more sources than simply the World Wide Web; however, what distinguishes it is the self-referential, unverifiable nature of the material—almost exclusively originating from Bikram himself, either via lectures, autobiography, or retellings from senior teachers. And although I list the sources for which I came across this information, it is important to note that this is in no way meant to affirm its truth any more than it is meant to affirm the funhouse-mirror way information gets bounced around when it can be used for self-promotion.

24   **"By the tender age of three . . .":** For confusion about dates of Bikram milestones in the Bikram world, see endnotes for page 30. Dates in this portion of the text are those given at Fall 2010 Teacher Training or his official autobiography. (Bikram Choudhury, *Bikram Yoga: The Guru Behind Hot Yoga Shows the Way to Radiant Health and Personal Fulfillment,* New York: HarperCollins, 2007.)

24   **"A guru himself so powerful . . . he would stop his own pulse, allow an elephant to walk across his chest, or bend a bar of iron with his throat":** Descriptions—and even images—of Ghosh's yogic "parlor tricks" (in the words of Tony Sanchez) can be found in many places on the Web, most prominently www.ghoshtrustfund.com.

24   **"Ghosh demanded total obedience from his disciples . . . subjecting those who did to screaming fits and Brahmanical tantrums. . . .":** Biswanath Ghosh, *Tribute to My Beloved Father Byayamacharyya Yogindra Bishnu Charan Ghosh,* Bishnu Charan Ghosh Birth Centenary Committee, 2003.

24   **"The easily distracted Bikram . . . when Bikram lost focus, Ghosh burned the preteen with incense. . . .":** Repeated at Fall 2010 Teacher

Training. According to Bikram, Ghosh would also "chase him with a sword" and "refuse to eat until I had performed a posture to his satisfaction."

24   **"At the request of head judge . . . B. K. S. Iyengar . . .":** Staff Writer, "Yoga Masters Unite: B. K. S. Iyengar Blesses Bikram Choudhury," *Yoga Tree,* January–February 2011.

24   **"He ran marathons with no training. . . .":** Todd Cole, "Some Like It Hot," *Australian Yoga Journal,* 2011.

24   **"He became a competitive weight lifter. . . .":** *Bikram Yoga: The Guru Behind Hot Yoga Shows the Way to Radiant Health and Personal Fulfillment,* 2007.

25   **"Slowing his heart rate until he could be buried alive . . .":** A claim Bikram has repeated in numerous forms at recent trainings, typically with reference to a news organization that supposedly documented the event. I could find no evidence of Bikram proper carrying out a live burial; however, there are examples of other yogis using meditation to slow their heart rates to imperceptible levels and submit to live burial. It seems more than possible that Bikram, inspired by their example, decided to appropriate their talent as an aspirational lie of sorts. (For examples of documented live burial, see James Braid, *Observations on Trance: Or, Human Hibernation,* London: Churchill, 1850; or John Ding-E Young and Eugene Taylor, "Meditation as a Voluntary Hypometabolic State of Biological Estivation," *Physiology,* 1998.)

25   **"Around this time, Bikram learned he didn't need to sleep. . . .":** While Bikram Choudhury circa 2011 clearly sleeps, and probably does so more now as a sixty-five-year-old than he did as a younger man, interviews with people close to him repeatedly validate the idea that he relies on much, much less sleep than the average person: perhaps two to four hours per night throughout the 1970s. Back then, when even his most die-hard acolytes would conk out at 3 or 4 A.M., Bikram would continue toward sunrise, making long-distance phone calls to family and friends in India, watching another late-night movie by himself, or heading off to the all-night disco to indulge in his passion for dance—always to arrive bright-eyed and bursting with energy for the class he was scheduled to teach the next morning.

25   **"Bikram slipped and dropped a 380-pound weight on his knee. . . .":** This is the essential origin story of Bikram Choudhury, master of yoga therapy. It has been repeated in many forms in many ways. The details here come largely from Bikram's autobiography cited earlier. It is interesting to note that at least one longtime observer, Tony Sanchez, doesn't believe it's the Lord's truth—and that the story, which in some retellings includes the doctors urging amputation—has been wildly exaggerated. "You know who else injured their knees?" Tony asks. "His guru. Bishnu Ghosh badly injured both knees after a motorcycle crash. It prevented him from walking late in life. And it doesn't appear that he could use yoga alone to heal himself it, does it?" While there is no way to know for certain, I will say Bikram's description of his injury

definitely fits an ugly pattern I observed whereby practitioners exaggerated old injuries in order to justify/sell/inspire outsiders about the power of the yoga.

25   **"Ghosh made Bikram swear an oath: 'My guru took my hand and told me . . .'"**: All quotations from *Bikram Yoga: The Guru Behind Hot Yoga Shows the Way to Radiant Health and Personal Fulfillment,* 2007.

26   **"There, in the wealthy Shinjuku district . . ."**: Peter Sklivas, "Hot Yoga in America," from *Yoga in America,* edited by Deborah S. Bernstein and Bob Weisenberg, Lulu.com, 2009.

26   **"Mirrors were added. . . ."**: This is an inference made from several sources. Rajashree has said mirrors were not used in Ghosh's Calcutta school to teach yoga ("I hated them when I first came to America"), but were used to teach weightlifters form. Many older teachers have affirmed the presence of mirrors in Bikram's first Los Angeles school.

26   **"When word reached the president about the young yoga master . . ."**: Nixon story as told on CBS's *60 Minutes* (*60 Minutes,* 2005, Mika Brzezinski, "'Hot' Yoga Burns Bright," New York: CBS News) and repeated in *Bikram Yoga: The Guru Behind Hot Yoga Shows the Way to Radiant Health and Personal Fulfillment,* 2007.

26   **"The president issued an open invitation. . . . Bikram . . . arrived on a chartered plane . . . welcomed on the runway by a phalanx of high-ranking administration officials. . . ."**: Overlapping versions of this story were told on *60 Minutes, Wonders of Yog* blog, and Teacher Training Fall 2010. (*60 Minutes,* 2005, Mika Brzezinski, "'Hot' Yoga Burns Bright," New York: CBS News; Ram Godar, "Yogi Raj Bikram Choudhury," *Wonders of Yog* blog, http://wondersofyog.blogspot.com/2011/03/yogi-raj-bikram-choudhury.html.)

27   **"In India, gurus prescribed individualized posture sequences. . . . But that wouldn't be necessary here."**: Richard Leviton, "How the Swamis Came to the States: A Comprehensive History of Yoga in the U.S.," *Yoga Journal,* March/April 1990.

27   **"You all grew up in California on a king-size waterbed. . . . If you feel dizzy, nauseous, you must be happy"**: Both classic Bikramisms, repeated during lectures at Teacher Training Fall 2010 and on his audiocassette class, *Bikram's Beginning Yoga Class.*

27   **"The more Bikram came to appreciate the miracle of the heat, the more the thermostat in his studio started sliding up: from 85 degrees F to 95 degrees F one week, to 100 degrees F the next, ultimately climaxing at a scalding 110 degrees F"**: This evolution of the heat has been confirmed by a wide variety of early practitioners. Bonnie Jones Reynolds Jr., Tony Sanchez, L-Like Linda, and Jimmy Barkin all recalled the temperature in Bikram's original studio as a mildly warm 85 degrees F, and all recall it maintained by a few space heaters. By the late 1990s, the temperature had skyrocketed

into the heights of today, kept in place by industrial-strength furnaces. While there is no set temperature, most studio owners I spoke with aimed for 105 degrees F plus or minus ambient humidity. The "climax" I mention in the text of 110 degrees is almost certainly low, as studios that opt for a drier heat have been reported to crank things up into the Death Valley 120-degrees-plus range. All fitting with the attitude I have heard expressed by more than one studio owner: "I asked Bikram about the heat, and he said, 'You cannot get it too high.'"

28   **"Shirley MacLaine took the guru aside and explained . . .":** *Bikram Yoga: The Guru Behind Hot Yoga Shows the Way to Radiant Health and Personal Fulfillment,* 2007.

29   **"By forty, Bikram . . . let a motorcycle ride over his chest on the evening news. . . .":** A stunt repeated multiple times and which did not end well on the final attempt. The motorcycle was driven by the morbidly obese son of Bishnu Ghosh, Bisu Ghosh. Tony Sanchez, who was in attendance, remembers being horrified as his guru was knocked unconscious, head cracked against the pavement, and believes his personality was permanently altered by the incident. Jimmy Barkan remembers that Bikram's back was "full of black holes for months after that." "It was real and he was injured," Barkan says. "Bikram told me he had been in Beverly Hills too long at that point. That he hadn't really prepared and didn't have the concentration."

29   **"By forty-five, he had saved Kareem Abdul-Jabbar's NBA career, rejuvenated John McEnroe's tennis game, collaborated with NASA . . . and massaged a pope. . . .":** All claims repeated by Bikram at Teacher Training Fall 2010 and many, many other places.

29   **"Stashed close to forty Rolls-Royces in its garage . . .":** Clancy Martin, "The Overheated, Oversexed Cult of Bikram Choudhury," *Details,* February 2011.

29   **"In some accounts he started training at three, sometimes at five. . . .":** For differing ages of Bikram milestones, see the websites below (as accessed in March 2012). To underscore the point that I think these discrepancies are less a matter of a sloppy webmaster, and more a matter of Bikram's cavalier attitude when telling or retelling details of his autobiography, I will note that at both Teacher Training Fall 2010 and in his first, now out-of-print book, he repeatedly used the age four for meeting Bishnu Ghosh, an age that differs from the assertion in his most current autobiography that he didn't meet Ghosh until he moved to Calcutta at age six.

> *Bikram Yoga Park Slope:* Starts yoga at three, meets Ghosh at five, wins first championship at eleven, weight lifting accident at twenty (www .bikramyogaparkslope.com/bikram/about-bikram-choudhury/).

BY Encinitas: Starts yoga at four, wins first championship at thirteen, weight lifting accident at seventeen (www.bikramencinitas.com/about_ocn.htm).

BY Charleston: Meets Ghosh at five, wins first championship at twelve (www.bikramcharleston.com/blog/2011/07/remember-bishnu-ghosh).

BY San Jose: Meets Ghosh at three, weight lifting accident at twenty (www.bikramyogasanjose.com/bysj/faq).

Bikram Yoga: The Guru Behind Hot Yoga: Meets Ghosh at age six, wins first championship at thirteen, weight lifting accident at eighteen.

I apply scrutiny to this amazingly minor point only because with inspection, a wide variety of Bikram's claims—the name of a medical conference where his research was presented, the extent of his knee injury, any number of his supposed accomplishments—have a similar slippery feel.

30   **"His famous yoga sequence, the very core of Bikram Yoga, was actually not so much developed or designed by Bikram, but largely excerpted . . . from a longer series of ninety-one postures. . . .":** For more details on the relationship between Bikram's copyrighted twenty-six-posture sequence and the original Ghosh ninety-one-posture series, see Appendix I, online at www.benjaminlorr.com/hellbent.

30   **"Of course, this hasn't stopped the president's library from expressing extreme skepticism that the two ever met.":** From the supremely helpful Jon Roscoe of the Nixon Presidential Library: "This is a question we get consistently and we have yet to be able to confirm any of it. . . . We have almost a minute-by-minute accounting of the president's daily life from 1969–1974 and there is no mention of Mr. Choudhury in any of the records, including trip files for travel in South East Asia and the Pacific. Nor, for that matter, is there mention of yoga instruction by anyone else, named or unnamed."

30   **"NASA has been unable to locate. . . .":** BBC Radio 4, Jolyon Jenkins, "Corporate Karma," London: BBC Radio, January 31, 2011.

30   **"For every Jim Carrey, who has repeatedly and publicly thanked Bikram for his girlfriend's butt . . .":** Staff writer, "Bikram Butt Fan Jim Carrey," www.mElleCanada.com/gossip/bikram-butt-fan-jim-carrey/a/28022.

30   **"Here is Madonna talking about her yoga workouts. . . .":** *Johnjay and Rich in the Morning,* 104.7 KISS FM, December 22, 2008.

30   **"As for the Beatles, Bikram told the BBC he treated them in 1959. . . .":** Exact same claim with impossible date repeated at Teacher Training Fall 2010; BBC Radio 4, Jolyon Jenkins, "Corporate Karma," London: BBC Radio, January 31, 2011.

30   **"It was once common knowledge among students that Bikram won an**

Olympic gold medal. . . .": According to Jimmy Barkan, "Bikram would talk about his gold medal from the 1964 Tokyo Olympics constantly when I first started taking classes. . . . I always was a little suspicious. I mean, if Bikram actually won an Olympic gold medal, do you think he would ever take it off? He would wear it around his waist for the rest of his life!"

30 **"He bragged constantly during the pre-Internet 1970s about the world records he set . . .":** Just in case there is any confusion, according to both James Hilary Evans of SportsReference.com and the Olympic Official Report Records, Bikram Choudhury was not one of the three people selected to represent India in the 1964 Tokyo Olympics for weight lifting, nor did he hold any world records or Olympic records at the time of the 1964 or 1960 Olympics.

31 **Footnote: "A brief sampling of a much lengthier list . . .":**

> *Jabbar:* John Morgan, "Kareem Abdul-Jabbar is hot for yoga," *USA Today,* September 26, 2003.
>
> *Karnazes:* Dean Karnazes, "Dean's Blog: Turning Up the Heat," runnersworld.com, November 23, 2010.
>
> *Murray:* Helen Neill, " 'Hardcore' yoga spurs Murray to victory," BBC News, March 4, 2008.
>
> *Dr. Arnot:* John Morgan, "Kareem Abdul-Jabbar is hot for yoga," *USA Today,* September 26, 2003.
>
> *Aniston:* Admin, "How Hollywood's hottest bodies stay in shape," www.TheGlobeUk.com, June 17, 2011.
>
> *Macpherson:* Staff writer, "Elle MacPherson's Secrets to Staying Fit Over 40," www.CelebrityHealthFitness.com, February 24, 2010.
>
> *McCarthy:* Staff writer, "Best Summer Bodies: Jenny McCarthy," www.MensHealth.com, 2011.

32 **"Right now in America, there are just over 1.1 million men, women, and children who regularly . . .":** No doubt a conservative number, extrapolated from the fact that an estimated 7 percent of all American yoga is Bikram Yoga (Melissa Dribben, "Beverly Hills Yogi: It's a Calcutta-to-California Tale of How a Vigorous Brand of Yoga, Called Bikram, Led to Great Wealth—and Litigation," *Philadelphia Inquirer,* November 23, 2003) and the fact that in 2008, *Yoga Journal* estimated 15.8 million Americans practiced yoga ("Yoga in America Study," *Yoga Journal,* February, 2008).

32 **"He charges just under eleven thousand dollars . . . 1,700 studios open worldwide, filled with over eight thousand instructors . . .":** The state of the Bikram empire in late 2011, it will undoubtedly be even bigger and more expensive by the time this book is published.

33 **"From her office, Dr. Yeargin gives me a crash course in the physiology**

of exercise during extreme heat. . . .": While primarily based on an interview and email follow-up with Susan Yeargin, Ph.D., the following texts and resources were invaluable in filling out this picture of exercise in heat and heat acclimization: Santiago Lorenzo. "Mechanisms of Heat Acclimation and Exercise Performance: A Dissertation." Presented to the Department of Human Physiology, University of Oregon, 2010; Gina Kolata. "To Beat the Heat, Drink a Slushie First." *New York Times,* April 27, 2010; Gina Kolata. "After Heatstroke, When Is It Safe to Exercise?" *New York Times.* June 6, 2010.

37   "Heat is not new to yoga. . . .": The links between *tapas,* yoga, and heat are explored in the following resources: Mircea Eliade, *Yoga: Immortality and Freedom,* Princeton: Princeton University Press, 1958; Georg Feurstein, *Yoga: The Technology of Ecstasy,* New York: St. Martin's Press, 1989; David Gordon White, *The Alchemical Body,* Chicago: University of Chicago Press, 2007.

37   "The world itself is created by the god Prajapati. . . .": *Aitareya Brahmana* as cited in Eliade, *Yoga: Immortality and Freedom,* 1958.

37   "Georg Feurstein notes . . .": Feurstein, *Yoga: The Technology of Ecstasy,* 1989.

37   "Practicing *tapas* gave the gods their immortality. . . .": Feurstein, *Yoga: The Technology of Ecstasy,* 1989.

37   "Through heat the ascetic becomes clairvoyant. . . .": Eliade, *Yoga: Immortality and Freedom,* 1958.

37   "To generate meditative powers, worshippers turn to Agni, the god of fire. . . .": Feurstein, *Yoga: The Technology of Ecstasy,* 1989.

37   "Fasting, withholding respiration, intense concentration, and . . . vigils in front of fire . . .": Eliade, *Yoga: Immortality and Freedom,* 1958.

37   "The ancients describe 'cooking the body in the fire of yoga' to make the body pure. . . .": Examples of the trope of yoga "cooking" or "baking" the body can be found in the *Yoga-Shikha-Upanishad,* the *Yoga-Bija,* and the *Svetasvatara Upanishad.*

39   Footnote: "Reference points from my own practice . . .": All heart rate data collected from a Polar RS800CX, heart rate monitor recording RR heart rate data over the course of two months where I wore said heart rate monitor in class, under my shirt.

46   "Backbenders call it Third-Eye Blowout. . . .": The neurologist I spoke with ascribed the cluster of symptoms I've described as Third-Eye Blowout to a variety of different related causes. The seizures are probably the result of an electrical discharge that comes from overstretching a nerve. The wavy rippling room and slowing of time—similar to the "aura before a migraine"—are likely due to hypersensitivity in the cerebral cortex. The changes in sound and narrowing the field of vision are probably the result of hypoxia, or low blood flow through the tiny capillaries of those organs, brought on by all the previously discussed changes in blood flow due to exercise in heat. My questions about the full-blown hallucinations got a shrug. Acid flashback?

47   "And that's sensible. . . .": Safety? Injuries? While those who backbend regularly will swear there are no long-term injuries associated with it (and to be
sure, I never found any), I would submit that those anecdotals are beside the
point. Backbending—unlike the Beginner Bikram Series—is an extreme en-
deavor, with participants looking to be exposed to an extreme experience.
Risk of injury is not a meaningful way to judge it—even as I feel strongly that,
relatively speaking, when compared to skydiving, free climbing, ultra-
endurance running, participants face far fewer risks. One of the geniuses of
Backbending in particular and Bikram Yoga in general is they take these truly
liminal experiences of pain, exertion, and triumph—the scaling of the peak, the
twenty-sixth mile—and bottle them up into ninety-minute classes available to
a mother of three in the strip mall down the street from her children's day care.

49   "How could you have Macaroni Art before Arturo Boolini invented . . .":
Clarification for people who take things too seriously: There is no Arturo
Boolini, nor did this fictional character invented by my fictional craft-Nazis
invent the real mechanized pasta press in Chicago in 1853 or any other date.

50   "In his book *Yoga in Modern India*, Joseph Alter makes this point. . . .":
Joseph Alter, *Yoga in Modern India: The Body Between Science and Philosophy*,
Princeton: Princeton University Press, 2004.

50   "Yoga is a vast history. . . .": This section and the brief "pop" history that
follows would have been impossible to write without reference to the excel-
lent work by David Gordon White (*Sinister Yogis*, Chicago: University of
Chicago Press, 2009; *The Alchemical Body*, Chicago: University of Chicago
Press, 2007; *Kiss of the Yogini*, Chicago: University of Chicago Press, 2003);
Mark Singleton (*Yoga Body: The Origins of Modern Postural Practice*, Oxford:
Oxford University Press, 2010); Joseph Alter (*Yoga in Modern India: The Body
Between Science and Philosophy*, Princeton: Princeton University Press, 2004);
Elizabeth De Michelis (*A History of Modern Yoga*, New York: Continuum
Press, 2004); Ian Whichler (*The Integrity of the Yoga Darsana*, New York: State
University of New York Press, 1998); Georg Feurstein (*Yoga: The Technology of
Ecstasy*, New York: St. Martin's Press, 1989); Mircea Eliade (*Yoga: Immortality
and Freedom*, Princeton: Princeton University Press, 1958); Gudrun Buhne-
mann (*Eighty-four Asanas in Yoga: A Survey of Traditions*, New Dehli: D.K.
Printworld, 2007); Kenneth Lieberman ("The Reflexivity of the Authenticity
of Hatha Yoga," in *Yoga in the Modern World*, ed. Jean Byrne and Mark Singleton, New York: Routledge, 2008); and Stefanie Syman (*The Subtle Body: The
Story of Yoga in America*, New York: Farrar, Straus, and Giroux, 2010). All
praise to these serious scholars, all errors mine.

50   Footnote: "This penile-straw being *vajroli mudra* . . .": For more information on "urethral suction" see Eliade, *Yoga: Immortality and Freedom* and/or
chapter 3, verses 82 to 89 of the *Hatha Yoga Pradipika*. (*Hathapradipika of Svatmarama*, edited by Swami Digambarji, Poona: Yashavant Mudranalaya, 1970).

51   "The Sanskrit verb *yuj,* from which our noun *yoga* derives, refers to the act of hitching or joining 'a wheeled conveyance to a draft animal'": Quote from White, *Sinister Yogis,* 2009; additional ideas on etymology come from Whichler, *The Integrity of the Yoga Darsana,* 1998, and Feurstein, *Yoga: The Technology of Ecstasy,* 1989.

51   "These proto-Sanskrit speakers were in the midst of a several-century migration. . . .": Feurstein, *Yoga: The Technology of Ecstasy,* 1989.

51   "The earliest of these, the Rig Veda (circa 1500 B.C.E) . . .": If we want to get eager and go way back, approximately five thousand years back, archeologists in the Indus Valley have found stonework depicting various horned men sitting with awkward crossed legs circa 3000 B.C.E. Scholar David Gordon White has done an impressive job surveying these artifacts and points out the eminently reasonable fact that whether or not they constitute evidence of yoga depends largely on imagination. Certainly these were people from the appropriate area of the world sitting in manners that resemble postures taught today as yoga. Certainly there are people who have seized upon this as evidence of yoga's ancient origins. But it is important to remember that these particular postures also resemble sitting. As there is literally zero textual evidence from that time to support interpretation one way or another, the debate becomes fairly existential fairly quickly.

51   "Depicts a yoga largely practiced by warriors . . . or more metaphorically . . . when driving the horses on a holy chariot 'upward through the barrier of the sun'": White, *Sinister Yogis,* 2009.

51   "When the wagoneering proto-Sanskrit invaders rolled into the Indus Valley, they confronted a civilization. . . .": Feurstein, *Yoga: The Technology of Ecstasy,* 1989.

52   "The *yuj/yoga/yoke* conglomeration appears often in their writings in a wide variety of allusions. . . .": Whichler, *The Integrity of the Yoga Darsana,* 1998; White, *Sinister Yogis,* 2009.

52   "Translated into teachings or Upanishads that began to systematically address the major stargazing themes that make up man's quest for knowledge . . .": Literally meaning to "sit down near" a teacher or guru, the two-hundred-plus Upanishads represent some of the most profound meditations on yogic thought recorded in text. They also do an excellent job capturing the waves of authenticity and uncertainty that have shaped yoga over the centuries. In fact, it is safe to say that if you look hard enough, you can find whatever guidance and insight you are looking for within one of the two-hundred-plus Upanishads and associated commentaries. The very oldest are contemporaneous with the Vedas, and indisputably offer ancient knowledge. Many others, however, cannot be dated. Several seem to have been composed in the twentieth century. Cosmologically, the Upanishads vary as well. Some advocate a dualist conception of the universe, others a unitary (aka nondual) framework.

Making things even more difficult is the fact that many of the primary texts are extremely sparse, open to wide interpretation. Much of our current understanding comes from commentaries written after the original text. This is not to undermine the value of these commentaries, simply to undermine the notion that there is one coherent yogic thread running through the centuries.

52   **"Until, finally . . . a text known as the *Katha Upanishad* bursts forth with the first mention of yoga as a spiritual discipline. . . ."**: Singleton, *Yoga Body: The Origins of Modern Postural Practice,* Oxford: Oxford University Press, 2010; Whichler, *The Integrity of the Yoga Darsana,* New York: State University of New York Press, 1998

52   **"In the *Katha Upanishad* . . ."**: The *Katha* tells the fable of Naciketas, a devout young boy impulsively given to Yama, Lord of Death, by his father during a Lear-like tantrum. When Naciketas arrives in the underworld, Yama—ostensibly his host—is absent. In response, the boy waits patiently. When Yama returns, he is so impressed with Naciketas's patience and virtue, he grants the youth three wishes—the third of which Naciketas uses to ask about immortality and thereby unexpectedly extracts yoga from the gods.

53   **"This they consider Yoga / The firm holding back of the senses . . ."**: Translation of the *Katha* primarily from *Eight Upanisads with the Commentary of Sankaracarya,* trans. Swami Gambhirananda, Calcutta: The Modern Press, 1957; supplemented by Eliade, *Yoga: Immortality and Freedom,* 1958.

54   **"As ethnographer Mircea Eliade points out . . ."**: Eliade, *Yoga: Immortality and Freedom,* 1958.

55   **"If consciousness, creativity, memory, emotion . . ."**: The problem of a conscious subjective experience (the "I" we use to describe the objective world or the soprano C we hear when vibrations of 1,046.5 hertz hit our tympanic membrane) has haunted neuroscience for as long as it has been studied. Somehow the raw cellular materials of our brain, the ion channels and chemio-electro circuits, produce the undeniable sensation of first-person experience. Adding to this intrigue, when mapping the brain, this sensation is not linked to any one specific area; instead it appears to occur throughout whenever sensations are experienced. When addressing the topic, neuroscientists have typically followed the lead of Nobel Prize winner Roger Sperry: first shrugging the shoulders at the magnitude of the task, then acknowledging the relative paucity of convincing theories, and finally positing a possible basis whereby the perception of "subjective unity may lie in the way brain process functions as a unity . . . the overall, holistic effect . . ." This concept of holistic emergence is common throughout our universe. To cite an example from neuroscientist David Eagleman: "When you put together a large number of pieces and parts, the whole can become something greater than the sum. None of the individual metal hunks of an airplane have the property of *flight,* but when they are attached together in the right way, the result takes to

the air." Similarly the brain: the interplay of complex material forces that make up our neurons produces our conscious experience; it is an experience present in every part of the system, but located in none. This emergence of mind from complexity, at the very least, leaves the door open for other hyper-complex systems—such as the universe as a whole—to exhibit consciousness as well. Naturally, there is no way to see, understand, or validate this possibility one way or the other, making it entirely outside the realm of science. However, much like the Jamesian notion of pragmatic free will ("my first act of free will shall be to believe in free will"), there seems, to me, to be benefits for choosing it as an ontological outlook. Not only is it rational, materialistic, and compatible with logic and science (certainly including atheism), but viewing our lives as part of a larger consciousness might make humility, morality, and the good green living necessary for the continuation of the human species a little easier.

55   **"In an early attempt to clarify this tangle, Patanjali . . .":** A note here on the ubiquitous Patanjali and his *Yoga Sutras*. By 2011 c.e., the ability to pay occasional lip service to Patanjali has come to serve as the fundamental dividing line between purely athletic postural yoga, and more "serious" forms (i.e., those with spiritual aspirations and antiquity claims), an easy referent for the enthusiastic student who wants more than his gym class can provide: an anchor for every modern teacher, Indian or Indianan, to root their particular teachings. This emphasis overstates both Patanjali's historical importance and his sutras' relevance to modern yoga practice. Patanjali was neither innovator nor endpoint: he was a compiler foremost, a Diderot rather than Rousseu. As such, his *Sutras* represent a curated collection of the yogic ideas of his time period, immensely valuable to anyone seeking to explore the range of ideas that fall under yogic thought. However, the idea that Patanjali informs the specific postures taught in modern yoga studios is the type of deranged claim that belies the existence of libraries. The *Yoga Sutras* mention postures in exactly one line among 196 aphorisms. And that one line consists of only three words: *sthria* ("steadiness" or "focus"), *sukha* ("comfort" or "ease"), and *asana* ("postures"). That's it. To claim that the *Yoga Sutras* can be used to determine whether one postural practice is more authentic than another makes as much sense as saying the New Testament specifies the types of Christmas gifts you should give. It would be laughable if it didn't point to a deeper, more desperate insecurity: the need to cling to false roots in the face of the incredible recency of innovation.

56   **"Approximately one thousand years later, a wholly different yoga emerges from the jungle. . . .":** Eliade, *Yoga: Immortality and Freedom,* 1958; White, *Sinister Yogis,* 2009; *The Alchemical Body,* 2007; *Kiss of the Yogini,* 2003. Singleton, *Yoga Body: The Origins of Modern Postural Practice,* 2010. Feurstein, *Yoga: The Technology of Ecstasy,* 1989.

57   "Prior to the medieval rise of hatha yoga, standing contortive postures simply did not exist. . . . The asana practices described in pre-hatha yogic literature were meditative postures. . . .": Buhnemann, *Eighty-four Asanas in Yoga: A Survey of Traditions*, 2007; Singleton, *Yoga Body: The Origins of Modern Postural Practice*, 2010.

57   "Vyasa the sage says that perfection in the posture occurs 'when efforts disappears. . . .' ": Vyasa's commentary on the *Yoga Sutras*, as quoted in Eliade, *Yoga: Immortality and Freedom*, 1958.

57   "Eliade the ethnographer says: 'refusal to move, to let one be carried along. . . .' ": Eliade, *Yoga: Immortality and Freedom*, 1958.

57   "Their early texts alternate between being refreshing and frightening in their vulgar specificity. . . .": See the *Siva Samhita*, trans., Rai Bahadur Srisa Chandra Vasu, Allahabad: Panini Press, 1914; *Gheranda Samhita*, trans., Rai Bahadur Srisa Chandra Vasu, Allahabad: Panini Press, 1914; *The Hathapradipika of Svatmarama*, edited by Swami Digambarji, Poona: Yashavant Mudranalaya, 1970.

58   "Drinking the middle third of your urine stream will, for instance, destroy diseases of the eyes, grant you clairvoyance . . .": When translated, references to *Amaroli mudra* can be found in chapter 3, verses 94–96 of the *Hatha Yoga Pradipika*. Several benefits touted within the *Pradipika* and many others expanded on in related commentaries.

58   "The Naths became outlawed people. . . . Labled as 'Miscellaneous and Disreputable Vagrants,' their traditional costume and outfits were banned. . . .": Singleton, *Yoga Body: The Origins of Modern Postural Practice*, 2010.

58   "When yoga jumped to America, its different traditions were packaged together for export. . . .": This is obviously a great sweeping historical assertion of a much more nuanced process. I hope I do not too greatly overstate the case in the interest of simplicity. For centuries, yoga, like many things spiritual, was part of a larger cultural exchange between India and the world to its west. Certainly this exchange was not monolithic or neatly packaged for export. However, during the nineteenth century, just as this exchange was kicking into high gear, yoga as an idea was swept up by the great Brahmo reformation movement intent on modernizing and nationalizing Hinduism (and in the process bowdlerizing hatha). It is no understatement to say the vision of yoga offered by these reformers was simplified and trimmed of its "eccentricities" to appeal to a Westernized audience—and that it received a wildly popular reception that has cast a significant legacy. For more information, see De Michelis, *A History of Modern Yoga*, 2004; De Michelis, "Modern Yoga: History and Forms," *Yoga in the Modern World*, 2008; Singleton, *Yoga Body: The Origins of Modern Postural Practice*, 2010.

58   "Instead, its 'queer breathing exercises' and 'gymnastics' were neatly

snipped off. . . .": Both quotes from Swami Vivekananda describing hatha yogis to the *Memphis Commercial* 1894 as quoted in Singleton. For further evidence of his hostility to toward the practice, see his follow-up remarks when pressed about the postures: "What have those things to do with religion? . . . Do they make a man purer? The Satan of your Bible is powerful, but differs from your God in not being pure."

70   **"Until I find a description by neuroscientist Richard Restak of a recovering stroke victim . . .":** Richard M. Restak, *The Modular Brain,* New York: Touchstone Press, 1995.

72   **"Her husband, an ex-marine, now paraplegic, out of his wheelchair on the floor balanced on the remainder of his legs . . .":** "My husband lost his legs in the first Gulf War, and was *not* into yoga. Not before the war, not coming home. It wasn't his style. He was a weights and calisthenics man. But he knew it meant a lot to me, and when I decided to become a teacher, he visited me during my training. . . . And when he came out to visit—this is when I was doing giant amounts of yoga—we sat outside and I would practice my teaching while he listened. One day in the middle of it, he cut me off, 'Whatever it is you are doing, I want it.' Now he comes to the advanced seminars, just gets out of his wheelchair and does the postures along with everyone else."

Part III: The Living Curriculum

77   **"Heartbreak opens . . . /For even breaking is opening . . .":** Dee Rees, *Pariah,* New York: Sundial Pictures, 2011.

83   **"Practitioners who are taught never to push themselves will only rarely push to the point of injury even in the most irregular alignment. . . .":** Hence the modern vinaysa flow class at its most gymnastic, where the teacher calls out a posture with almost no description of alignment beyond feet, knees, hips, and hands and the students en masse bound into it. Although the basic forms students take are similar, the specificities are left to imagination, prior knowledge, or the position of the body directly in front of them.

83   **"Everything in the sequence was within the normal range of motion. . . ."** Compare to how another major hatha guru of the twentieth century handled this potential contradiction: B. K. S. Iyengar also brought yoga postures to the masses and also did so with an unstinting dedication to maintaining the proper alignment. However, Iyengar decided that to spread yoga to the masses, he would use props (like the blocks, straps, and padded blankets ubiquitous in modern studios), which would help ease stiff bodies into alignments they otherwise couldn't reach. Bikram decided that to spread the yoga to the masses, he would teach only very simple postures that stiff bodies could enter correctly without props. Thus, you have one guru teaching advanced postures with assistance from props and another guru teaching basic postures

with no assistance from props, and in between, a million arguments about authenticity.

Part III: Not Dead Yet!

109   "If we take man as he really is, we make him worse. But if we overestimate him . . .": Viktor Frankl, "Man's Search for Meaning," *lecture*, Toronto, 1972.

118   "The English word *pain* comes to us from Poena, a dominatrix goddess responsible for vengeance and atonement. . . ." This section on pain would have been impossible to write without access to the following excellent work by: Patrick Wall (*Pain: The Science of Suffering*, New York: Columbia University Press, 2000); Frank Vertosick Jr. (*Why We Hurt: The Natural History of Pain*. Orlando: Harcourt Press, 2000); V. S. Ramachandran (*Phantoms in the Brain: Probing the Mysteries of the Human Mind*, New York: HarperCollins, 1998); Norman Doidge (*The Brain That Changes Itself: Stories of Personal Triumph from the Frontiers of Brain Science*, New York: Penguin, 2007); Richard Restak (*The Modular Brain*, New York: Touchstone Press, 1995); Melanie Thernstrom (*The Pain Chronicles: Cures, Myths, Mysteries, Prayers, Diaries, Brain Scans, Healing, and the Science of Suffering*, New York: Farrar, Straus, Giroux, 2010). Impossible not to add that much of my curiosity about these interior workings of pain was sparked by a wonderful article read over ten years ago by Atul Gwande ("The Pain Perplex," *The New Yorker*, September 1998) that I could not get out of my brain.

119   "C. S. Lewis called it 'God's megaphone'": C. S. Lewis, *The Problem of Pain*, New York: HarperOne, 2001.

119   "Listen to neurosurgeon Frank Vertosick Jr. talk about pain. . . ." Vertosick Jr., *Why We Hurt: The Natural History of Pain*, 2007.

119   "Writing in 1664, Descartes encapsulated what, for many of us, still feels like an accurate explanation of physical pain. . . .": Rene Descartes, *Treatise of Man*, trans., Thomas Steele Hall, New York: Prometheus Books, 1972.

121   "In experiments where subjects were lucky enough to self-administer pain . . .": Jeffery Dolce, Daniel Doleys, James Raczynski, John Lossie, Lane Poole, and Melanie Smith, "The role of self-efficacy expectations in the prediction of pain tolerance," *Pain*, 1986.

121   "Consider, for example, the fifty-two-year-old machine shop foreman cited by Ronald Melzack and Patrick David Wall. . . .": Wall, *Pain: The Science of Suffering*, 2000.

122   "This was the experience of Dr. Henry Beecher during World War II. . . .": Mark Best and Duncan Neuhauser, "Henry K Beecher: pain, belief and truth at the bedside. The powerful placebo, ethical researcher and anaesthesia safety," *Quality and Safety in Health Care*, 2010.

122   **"Feeling only slight pain at the sight of their massive wounds . . .":** For an extreme modern example, after his 1981 shooting, Ronald Reagan was completely unaware he had been shot through the chest, until he got to the hospital and started coughing up blood from a punctured lung. "I had never been shot before, except in the movies," he said. "Then you always have to act hurt."

122   **"The new theory, known as the gate control theory . . .":** Patrick Wall and Ronald Melzack, *Textbook of Pain,* New York: Churchill Livingstone Press, 2005; Wall, *Pain: The Science of Suffering,* 2000.

123   **"Factors such as emotions, memories, beliefs, mental suggestions are all channeled to the checkpoint, mediating our experience of pain. . . .":** Wall, *Pain: The Science of Suffering,* 2000; Ronald Melzack and Patrick Wall, *The Challenge of Pain,* New York: Penguin, 2004; Fabrizio Benedetti, *Placebo Effects: Understanding the Mechanisms in Health and Disease,* Oxford: Oxford University Press, 2009.

123   **"Finally and most important—actually overthrowing the gate control theory itself—researchers discovered there are pains that exist *only* in the brain. Phantoms . . .":** Wall, *Pain: The Science of Suffering,* 2000; Ramachandran, *Phantoms in the Brain: Probing the Mysteries of the Human Mind,* 1998.

123   **"One of the extremely helpful qualities of neural networks is they get stronger the more often they are activated. . . .":** Doidge, *The Brain That Changes Itself: Stories of Personal Triumph from the Frontiers of Brain Science,* 2007.

124   **"Of the forty-six members who completed the study, only three decided to continue with the surgery. . . .":** B. Nelson, D. Carpenter, T. Dreisinger, M. Mitchell, C. Kelly, and J. Wegner, "Can Spinal Surgery Be Prevented by Aggressive Strengthening Exercises? A Prospective Study of Cervical and Lumbar Patients," *Archives of Physical Medicine and Rehabilitation,* 1999. For more information, see also D. Carpenter and B. Nelson, "Low Back Strengthening for the Prevention and Treatment of Low Back Pain," *Medicine and Science in Sports and Exercise,* 1999; and S. Leggett, V. Mooney, L. Matheson, B. Nelson, T. Dreisinger, J. Van Zytveid, "Restorative Exercise for Clinical Lower Back Pain," *Spine,* 1999.

124   **"But that was because the Physicians Neck & Back Clinic in Minnesota was pioneering a new type of rehab. . . .":** Although Dr. Nelson was a successful orthopedic surgeon, trained at the University of Minnesota, one of the best residencies in the country for orthopedic surgery, few of his ideas on back care came from his training. "Back then, if we didn't operate on someone, we told them to rest," he tells me. "We had some of the most famous spine surgeons in the country, but the actual benefits to patients were extremely limited. . . . Everything I know about exercise physiology comes from one man, Arthur Jones." Jones, an old-fashioned multimillionaire eccentric of the best kind, no doubt worthy of an entire book himself, was a self-taught polymath,

best known to the general public as the man who pushed the precise alignments of Nautilus machines into gyms across America. As a trainer, Jones was
a solid thirty years ahead of his time, recommending exercise until failure
("bicep curls until you puke") at a time when conventional wisdom had elite
weight lifters working slowly but steadily in the gym for seven hours a day.
He used his techniques to produce staggering results (see his pupil, Casey
Viator, putting on a whopping sixty-three pounds of muscle in twenty-eight
days without steroids) and became a force in the professional bodybuilding
world. By the time Dr. Nelson met him, Arthur Jones was in the midst of a
restless retirement living off his Nautilus fortune in Florida, attempting to
grow the world's biggest alligator, and engaging in a self-described project to
revolutionize back care in America. Jones had become steadily disgusted with
the current system, which he believed lucratively rewarded doctors for offering options that produced little relief for patients and then trapping patients
into accepting those options by offering higher disability payments if they
accepted them. When he heard that Dr. Nelson was a young orthopedic surgeon open to hearing unorthodox ideas, he flew him on a private plane to his
retirement compound and proceeded to pitch a thoroughly researched case
for back-pain rehab based on strength training. Dr. Nelson left shaken but
impressed. Their relationship would grow over the years, with many of the
rehab techniques of the Physicians Back & Neck Clinic growing directly out
of the collaboration. Fascinating also to learn that Arthur Jones was another
socially coarse perfectionist, who slept little and possessed a totally domineering self-confidence and truckloads of charisma, a man who was seared with a
conviction that he was giving something to the world, and constantly inse-
curely pitching himself to make up for the fact that his formal education
stopped at the eighth grade, a man prone to calling Dr. Nelson late into the
night to talk exuberantly for hours and hours, much to the exasperation of Dr.
Nelson's wife.

127   "Instead of pain being some exceptional outlier . . . all perception operates within the anti-Cartesian principles of pain and the gate control
theory. . . .": Ramachandran, *Phantoms in the Brain: Probing the Mysteries of the
Human Mind,* 1998; Ramachandran, *The Tell-Tale Brain: Unlocking the Mystery
of Human Nature,* New York: Random House, 2011.

127   "Our consciousness only an interpretation, minimally corresponding to
the stimulus external to our brains. . . .": At the far extreme, we have patients with a type of multiple personality disorder that extends beyond personality into the physiological: where two or more "people" reside in the same
brain, each having slightly different vital signs, allergies, vision (one might be
nearsighted, the other have 20/20 vision), and hormonal profiles. Ramachandran, *Phantoms in the Brain: Probing the Mysteries of the Human Mind,* 1998; Ramachandran, *The Tell-Tale Brain: Unlocking the Mystery of Human Nature,* 2011.

127   "Neuroscientist V. S. Ramachandran talks about the essential dilemma this dichotomy produces in his patients. . . .": Ramachandran, *The Tell-Tale Brain: Unlocking the Mystery of Human Nature,* 2011.

127   "Jill Bolte Taylor took a decidedly less pleasurable route to this same realization . . . In her book, *Stroke of Insight* . . .": Jill Bolte Taylor, *My Stroke of Insight: A Brain Scientist's Personal Journey,* New York: Plume, 2009.

128   "The Human Physiology Department of the University of Oregon published the first scientific paper demonstrating that the benefits of heat acclimation . . .": Santiago Lorenzo, John Halliwill, Michael Sawka, and Christopher Minson, "Heat Acclimation Improves Exercise Performance," *Journal of Applied Physiology,* August 2010.

Part IV: Like Kool-Aid for Water

133   " 'We talked of everything,' he said, quite transported at the recollection. . . .": Joseph Conrad, *Heart of Darkness and the Congo Diary,* New York: Penguin Classics, 2007.

148   "That it was none other than Bhagwan Shri Rajneesh, the proudly deviant, ultimately monstrous force of twentieth-century charismatic wisdom, who famously decreed that 'authenticity is morality' . . .": Bhagwan Rajneesh, *Philosophia Perennis,* Rajneeshpuram: Osho International Foundation, 1981.

149   "That he does not tolerate the color green in his presence . . .": When asked about the interdiction on green, Bikram is clear: "Okay. It's superstition. India has millions of superstitions. If the slipper by the door is upside, things go bad. . . . For my guru, green was superstition, but it was also personal." In 1942, Bishnu Ghosh's son Krishna was trapped in a tent and burnt alive when a fireworks demonstration went awry. He had last been seen wearing a green shirt, and the guru passed down the tradition of forbidding green on his disciples.

154   "And his tea has been brewed. . . .": A lemon, ginger, honey infusion into hot water, no caffeine, designed to soothe the throat of a professional speaker, who may or may not be about to launch into a Castro-like marathon lecture.

155   "Tonight's lecture is on the art of teaching. . . .": As I hope I have conveyed in the text, the lectures at Teacher Training were extremely discursive, and as a participant, my brain was often fairly frayed. All quotes are directly from my transcribed notes, and the themes are ones Bikram referred to repeatedly. And while I am certain meaning is conveyed as Bikram intended it, the exact order of the sentences—often reconstructed from a jumble of page-crawling lines in my notebook—might be shuffled throughout this section.

157   "That he wants to show us a movie. A Bollywood movie!": While some

of these movies are yoga related, most are not. By far the most memorable is a serialized version of the great Indian epic the *Mahabarata* that is so implausibly low budget that I get a contact high every time we hear the opening soundtrack. In this *Mahabarata,* every prop is made of cardboard, every special effect is recycled in at least two or three different scenes, the sound mixing swings wildly with scene changes, beards disappear and reappear during reaction shots, and all weapons clash with the same weird clanging your first-generation computer made when you would press too many keys at the same time. It is interesting to note that Bikram loves this serialized *Mahabarata* with zero irony. He leans into the screen and cackles into his headset microphone, often pausing it to explain the unrelated moments of his life back in India he associates with watching the show as a young man.

159   **"The bushes outside the tent after class always have a least a few people weeping into them. . . ."**: The more modern science looks at sweating, the less evidence it finds for detox. That is just not the way most chemicals exit our bodies. However, the heat-induced suffering in a Bikram class—the sustained effort, the freaky acceleration of heartbeat that comes despite standing stock-still, the fear of pressing up against a physical edge—definitely produces an emotional release. This emotional detox is very real and occurs as kinetic memories—memories stored in association with certain movements or physiological sensations—rise to the surface during the controlled environment of a class. The repeated nature of the series, the safety of the entirely bland surroundings, the anonymity of strangers, the intimacy of the mirror, and the repeatedly psychotically confident assurances of a teacher insisting that everything you experience is not just normal but evidence that you are doing things correctly, provides an ideal framework to work through trauma. Eventually, as with all sensations in the yoga room, you become witness to all that you don't control: sensations from the deep past rise up and wash over your cortex, your eyes in the mirror remain, and unlike whatever heavy metals may or may not be floating through your bloodstream, there is the possibility of true release.

173   **"The dialogue reflects Bikram's genius for teaching a class that successfully gets inside the head of a struggling practitioner. . . ."**: For instance, when going into a certain front stretch, where the legs are four feet apart and the body bends forwards until the forehead touches the ground, weight needs to be pushed to the balls of the feet. The official dialogue calls for "Heels in one line, feet slightly pigeon-toed" because for most people it is only when they try to pigeon-toe their feet that they will actually get them parallel enough to push the weight in the ball of the feet and feel the proper stretch. When, during a seminar in Hawaii, one senior teacher asked Bikram what he meant by "feet slightly pigeon-toed," the guru replied somewhat indignantly, "Pigeon-toed! So the feet become parallel!"

173   **"The need to adhere to Bikram's broken, often counterproductive,**

phrasing . . .": Consider the phrase "Grab your *h-e-e-l* heel," which every trainee must parrot incessantly during training. An essential Bikramism for Bikram because with his thick Indian accent, *heel* sounds almost indistinguishable from *hill* and therefore without it, people grab at all sorts of hill-like body parts and screw up their postures. However, when spoken by someone with any other type of accent, it produces at best quizzical looks from new students, and at least one "I know what a heel is, asshole" from someone clearly slipping right over the brink of exhaustion into rage.

179   **"The demonstration consists of ninety-one postures . . .":** The actual number of postures depends on who's counting and how they count. It varies between 84 and 106, a range that might seem odd, considering it's a static series performed with an identical series of motions every time. But as with most things yogic, certainty and exactitude are unhelpful. In the Advanced Series, many postures contain multiple movements, evolving in discrete stages, while other posed movements have precise instructions for alignment but are not considered "postures," for reasons that probably hint at both the mechanism and practice of innovation within the series. These nonposture postures are referred to as "warm-ups," "openers," or in Bikram's terminology, "masturbation." At the low end, the number eighty-four is considered an auspicious number within Hinduism—historically many of the great yogic texts make mention of the eighty-four asanas—so there is a constant downward effort to conjoin postural movements to make the series conform to that goal. (Buhnemann, *Eighty-four Asanas in Yoga: A Survey of Traditions*, 2007.)

187–88   **"Bikram Choudhury, on the other hand, will adjust a single posture in a thousand ways, or, if the case warrants it, throw the whole thing out. . . .":** For example, consider a woman who tells him that her son always gets a headache when doing Locust pose. Bikram asks, "Always?" And when the woman affirms it, he announces triumphantly, "For him, fuck Locust, better he do Lotus! Better yet, maybe nothing . . . If every time the asana causes pain, why would you do that again and again? That is not the purpose of yoga." The answer, entirely reasonable, feels totally at odds with almost everything we have heard from other senior teachers when confronted with people who describe aches and pains in postures.

188   **"Nice boobs too. I have picture!":** While I have no idea which picture Bikram is referring to, there is a whole series of photographs of Bikram doing Crow on women's chests in his 1970s "Red Book," including a young Emmy Cleaves and an icky Crow-on-chest of a preteen Justine Bateman.

Part VI: Sickness of the Infinitude

193   **"A careful scrutiny of various schools of psychoanalytic psychology . . .":** Robert L. Moore, *Facing the Dragon: Confronting Personal and Spiritual Grandiosity*, Wilmette: Chiron Publications, 2003.

194 "Only the third person Bikram allowed to teach his yoga . . .": It is worth noting that Linda's teaching certificate—which still hangs proudly in her room of yogic hoardings—was not issued from Bikram's Yoga College, but rather by his guru's school in India, and is signed by his guru's son. It took her seven years of daily training to earn, and except for the names, is identical to Bikram's own certificate.

196 "A 1988 study investigating the personality traits of eighteen charismatic leaders . . .": Len Oakes, *Prophetic Charisma: The Psychology of Revolutionary Religious Personalities,* Syracuse: Syracuse University Press, 1997.

196 "The Romans had a similar concept, using the word *facilitas* to describe a hero's ability . . .": As found in Oakes, *Prophetic Charisma: The Psychology of Revolutionary Religious Personalities,* 1997.

197 "The aging, reclusive George Washington was dragged to the Constitutional Convention because the Framers believed his physical presence . . .": Washington oozed this quality his entire life, inspiring the greatest men of his age to fall into weird homoerotic spells when recalling him. We can find Thomas Jefferson waxing poetic on his erect stature on horseback, Gilbert Stuart fawning over his broad nose and deep eyes, the Marquis de Chastellux gushing that his physical proportions matched his moral perfection, and Dr. James Thatcher (practically defining charisma for the modern reader) relating his belief that "no one can stand in [Washington's] presence without feeling the ascendancy of his mind." This was not a simple case of sucking up before power either. At age twenty-five—*after* he resigned his military position—Washington was begged by a group of twenty-seven officers to come back to them. "Your presence only," they explained, "will cause a steady firmness and vigor to actuate in every breast." It is perhaps Washington's greatest credit that he grew steadily distrustful of this effect on others, recognizing its potential for abuse, and repeatedly chose to remove himself from the public sphere to allow democracy to flourish. (Ron Chernow, *Washington: A Life,* New York: Penguin Press, 2010; James Thomas Flexner, *Washington: The Indispensible Man,* New York: Little Brown and Company, 1969; James Thomas Flexner. *George Washington: The Forge Experience,* New York: Little Brown and Company, 1965; "Rediscovering George Washington," PBS.org, 2002.)

197 "We have a mere touch from Bhagwan Rajneesh described as incomparable bliss. . . .": Huge Milne, *Bhagwan: The God That Failed,* London: Caliban, 1986, as quoted in Oakes, *Prophetic Charisma: The Psychology of Revolutionary Religious Personalities,* 1997.

198 "It creates a powerful, almost anti-intellectual instinct toward surrender. . . .": And thus, perhaps, the inevitable reference—definitely not to be misconstrued as comparison—to Von Ribbentrop. In Gustave Gilbert's 1947 profile, he describes the former German Foreign Affairs Minister at his

trial in Nuremberg watching a film of Hitler. In tears, he shouts to the courtroom: "Can't you see how he swept people off their feet? Do you know, even with all I know, if Hitler should come to me now and say 'Do this!'—I would still do it?"

198   **"To Weber, the energy between charismatic and follower was . . .":** Max Weber, *Theory of Social Organization,* trans., A. M. Anderson and Talcott Parsons, New York: The Free Press, 1964; Christopher Adair-Toteff, "Max Weber's Charisma," *Journal of Classical Sociology,* 2005.

198   **"Heinz Kohut did not set out to study charisma. . . .":** Charles B. Strozier, *Heinz Kohut: The Making of a Psychoanalyst,* New York: Other Press, 2004. Oakes, *Prophetic Charisma: The Psychology of Revolutionary Religious Personalities,* 1997.

199   **"But Kohut was struck not by the pathos each patient eventually revealed. He was stuck on their first impressions. . . .":** Heinz Kohut, "Creativeness, Charisma, Group Psychology," in *Freud: The Fusion of Science and Humanism,* edited by John E. Gedo and George Pollock, New York: International Universities Press, 1976. Oakes, *Prophetic Charisma: The Psychology of Revolutionary Religious Personalities,* 1997.

199   **"They glowed. . . .":** Or as Kohut said, they were men and women who "without shame or hesitation, set themselves up as the guides and leaders and gods" of those in need. Kohut, "Creativeness, Charisma, Group Psychology," 1976.

199   **"A link was made clear . . . the professional charismatic can be stripped away to reveal a desperate need for attention. . . .":** It is worth nothing that Kohut was careful to explain that although many charismatic personality types were rooted in a severe disturbance—"some no doubt close to psychosis"—that charismatics "come in all shades and degrees" and a reflexive negative judgment is not warranted, especially as the social effects of these personalities "are not necessarily deleterious."

200   **" 'Remember me! Remember who I am! You think I don't know everything! I know everything!' ":** The drama in these encounters is almost as important as the encounters themselves. Another senior teacher who has been both in and out of the Bikram inner circle described it as feeling "like a movie. It really felt like he was channeling Pacino or something. Bikram had been screaming so long and listing so many crazy threats, it started feeling like we were acting out some scene. At one point my attention broke, and I looked to the side, looking for a director to feed me a line . . . like line, please? How do I get this to end? . . . Bikram didn't even notice I wasn't looking at him anymore. He just kept going."

206   **"And any construction I was involved with used illegal untrained labor.":** Chad elaborates, "Bikram would brag to me about his contractor friends who could circumvent electrical meters and water meters so he could

have free water and electricity. Then he would ask me why I couldn't do the same thing."

206 **"I went through this slow realization that he really and truly does not give a shit about other people. . . .":** More Chad, expressed perhaps more eloquently, and channeling the clinical description of the grandiose narcissist who cannot see others as full humans, but merely extensions to fulfill his own needs: "There is a lot of rhetoric, but watch how he treats people. Bikram does not see his yoga students as 'luminaries of truth,' he sees them as vessels like toilets and trash cans for him to treat as he wishes. He will tell people to their face that they are worthless. He will discard them if they don't do exactly as he wishes. They exist for him only as much as they practice his yoga his way."

206 **"We got over twenty-seven violations from the fire department in a single year. . . .":** Apparently, failure to correct these violations became so acrimonious that Los Angeles City Attorney Rocky Delgadillo held a press conference to announce criminal charges in conjunction with ten of them. (Andrew Blankstein and Jessica Garrison, "City Charges Yoga with Safety Violations," *Los Angeles Times,* June 30, 2006.)

208 **"When we talk, Eleanor begins by addressing these concerns. . . .":** While primarily based on an interview and email follow-up with Eleanor Payson, LMSW, works by the following people were invaluable in filling out this picture of unhealthy narcissism and how it develops in childhood: A. H. Almass (*The Point of Existence: Transformations of Narcissism in Self-Realization,* Boston: Shambhala Press, 1996); Diana Alstad and Joel Kramer (*The Guru Papers: Masks of Authoritarian Power,* Berkeley: North Atlantic Books, 1993); Althea Horner (*Being and Loving: How to Achieve Intimacy with Another Person and Retain One's Own Identity,* Lanham: Rowman and Littlefield Publishing Group, 2005); J. Masterson (*The Narcissistic and Borderline Disorders,* New York: Brunner, 1985); Alice Miller (*The Drama of the Gifted Child: The Search for the True Self* (Revised Edition), New York: Basic Books, 1997); Carol Lynn Mithers (*Therapy Gone Mad: The True Story of Hundreds of Patients and a Generation Betrayed,* New York: Addison Wesley, 1994); Andrew Morrison (*Essential Papers on Narcissism,* New York: New York University Press, 1986); Robert L. Moore (*Facing the Dragon: Confronting Personal and Spiritual Grandiosity,* Wilmette: Chiron Publications, 2003); Eleanor Payson (*The Wizard of Oz and Other Narcissists,* Royal Oak: Julian Day Publications, 2002).

210 **"It turns out, not surprisingly, that people who experience a certain type of wounding in childhood are more vulnerable to the charismatic image. . . .":** Payson, *The Wizard of Oz and Other Narcissists,* 2002; Miller, *The Drama of the Gifted Child: The Search for the True Self* (Revised Edition), 1997; Morrison, *Essential Papers on Narcissism,* New York: New York University Press, 1986.

210   **"Both are children who are not 'seen' for who they actually are. . . .":** In
both, the wounding is passed down, almost as legacy, from a narcissistic caregiver. This does not prevent positive childhood memories with strong displays
of affection. "On the contrary," psychologist Alice Miller writes in her essay
"Depression and Grandiosity," "the mother often loves her child as her self-
object passionately, but not in the way he needs to be loved. Instead, he develops
something which the mother needs." The child learns to fulfill the parent's
warped expectation. Often this includes model behavior: extreme willpower,
cleanliness, academic accomplishment, or expertise in dance, music, or athletics. "But," as Miller continues, no matter how successful the outward reception
of these talents, or how completely the child fulfills his parent's grandiose expectations, his skills will "prevent him throughout life from being himself."
Alice Miller, "Depression and Grandiosity," *Essential Papers on Narcissism,* edited
by Andrew Morrison, New York: New York University Press, 1986.

211   **"One only needs to read the title of Alice Miller's** *Drama of the Gifted
Child* **. . .":** Miller, *The Drama of the Gifted Child: The Search for the True Self*
(Revised Edition), 1997.

214   **"All the easier to discard . . .":** Discard? Did I really write that? Have I
learned nothing? Yoga, with its quest for union, asks for integration—it asks
us to assimilate even the imperfect parts of our existence to create a cohesive
whole. Discarding Bikram the man, our own ego, competition, or even our
former "inadequate" selves simply isn't part of the operation. As Anna, my
friend from Teacher Training with the alcoholic ex-husband and fresh set of
brass balls, says, "My yoga practice integrates. Healing is the idea something
needs to be fixed. Instead, Bikram Yoga integrated me. I am still me—with
all the pathetic parts—only better." So why "discard"? Partly a crutch of language, but partly to impress the idea that to truly see how something fits into
your life, it can be invaluable to step away.

Part VI: All Lies Are Aspirational

217   **"The true opponent, the enfolding boundary, is the player himself. . . .":**
David Foster Wallace, *Infinite Jest: A Novel,* New York: Little Brown and Company, 1996.

218   **Footnote "Love! And a word about its use herewith . . . Oxytocin is a
neuromodulator. . . .":** On Oxytocin and unlearning: Norman Doidge, *The
Brain That Changes Itself: Stories of Personal Triumph from the Frontiers of Brain
Science,* New York: Penguin, 2007; on hormones released by intense exercise:
John J. Ratey, *Spark: The Revolutionary New Science of Exercise and the Brain,*
New York: Little Brown and Company, 2008.

221   **"What my favorite teacher, Courtney Mace, calls 'the battle between
the ego and the soul'":** "People seems to like that phrase, 'the battle between the ego and the soul,' a lot, and I realize I said it so it's out there, but I

hate it. I hated it the moment the words left my mouth," Courtney says. "They simply do not express what I mean. Pitting the 'soul'—a word so ambiguous, I loath to use it—against the 'ego' only serves to strengthen the idea that these two aspects are separate. Worse, it suggests that the ego can be vanquished. That is not my goal in yoga. That is not my goal ever. . . . I'm looking for union, harmony between the ego and the higher self. I hate that I said it's a battle between the two because that is exactly what the lowest part of me would want to think. In battling, the ego thrives. But it doesn't need to be eliminated. It needs balance. . . . We are human. It's not possible or desirable to abolish an essential part of who we are."

Part VII: Finding Balance

254   **"He demanded Tony break up with his girlfriend—soon-to-be-wife—Sandy. . . .":** This was not an unusual request. According to many early teachers, Bikram took great pleasure both in arranging marriages between his students and, when he felt a couple was poorly matched, demanding they stop dating. In this particular case, there were certainly other issues at play. Tony had recently asked Bikram if he could buy him out of the studio. Bikram incorrectly blamed Tony's attempts at independence on his new relationship with Sandy—and threatened by that independence, decided to nip the threat in the bud.

256   **"He did a last interview with a reporter from _Self_ magazine. . . .":** The reporter was calling for comment on the latest yoga sex scandal, celebrity teacher Rodney Yee sleeping with students. A scandal juicy only because Yee was simultaneously publicly exhorting the fact that his yoga practice strengthened his happy marriage. To Tony it was an interview that represented everything he was trying to get away from: the celebrities, the sex, the need to wrap yoga in unrelated wholesome morality, and the hypocrisy that resulted when all those values met in the marketplace.

274   **"When selective serotonin reuptake inhibitors (SSRIs) hit the market . . .":** Although seizing on antidepressants as a potent example of the placebo effect had long been decided as my rhetorical strategy, several publications came out during the writing of this book that helped focus this section immensely. Primarily Irving Kirsch's phenomenal deconstruction of antidepressants— _The Emperor's New Drugs: Exploding the Antidepressant Myth_—and several of the articles written in response to his arguments, in particular Marcia Angell's review in _The New York Review of Books,_ "The Epidemic of Mental Illness: Why?"

275   **"Over the next two decades, that number increased sixfold. . . .":** Or 4.5 million Americans taking antidepressants in 1987, 13.3 million in 1996, and 27 million in 2005. Sharon Begley, "The Depressing News about Anti-Depressants," _Newsweek,_ January 2010.

275   **"So that by 2007, approximately a full 10 percent of Americans over the age of six years old were regularly taking an antidepressant . . .":** Marcia Angell, "The Epidemic of Mental Illness: Why?" *The New York Review of Books,* June 2011.

275   **"The SSRI-driven antidepressant market grew into a 19 billion dollar per year . . .":** Irving Kirsch, *The Emperor's New Drugs: Exploding the Antidepressant Myth,* New York: Basic Books, 2010.

275   **"Doctors long wary of the growing influence of the pharmaceutical industry were won over by the powerful results. . . .":** Marcia Angell, "The Epidemic of Mental Illness: Why?" *The New York Review of Books,* June 2011.

275   **"The Hamilton Rating Scale for Depression rates a patient's mood. . . .":** Kirsch, *The Emperor's New Drugs: Exploding the Antidepressant Myth,* 2010.

275   **"As early as 1995, Guy Sapirstein and Irving Kirsch decided to pool the results of previous studies on antidepressants. What they found shocked them. . . .":** Irving Kirsch and Guy Sapperstein, "Listening to Prozac but Hearing Placebo: A Meta Analysis of Antidepressant Medication," *Prevention and Treatment,* 1998.

276   **"Similarly in nine studies in which active placebos were used . . .":** Kirsch, *The Emperor's New Drugs: Exploding the Antidepressant Myth,* 2010.

276   **"My point here is not to argue one way or another about the usefulness of antidepressants":** Even if extremely marginal, the additional benefit an SSRI provides over a placebo might be a critical percent for many patients. Just as a baby may be a critical 5 percent of the volume of a bathtub, the overwhelming presence of the placebo effect is no reason to throw the antidepressant out with the bathwater just yet.

277   **"The effect is 100 percent real. And it works on people. . . .":** This section on the placebo effect could not have been written without the works of Fabrizio Benedetti (*Placebo Effects: Understanding the Mechanisms in Health and Disease,* Oxford: Oxford University Press, 2009); Grant W. Thompson (*The Placebo Effect and Health: Combining Science and Compassionate Care,* Amherst: Prometheus Books, 2005); Irving Kirsch (*The Emperor's New Drugs: Exploding the Antidepressant Myth,* New York: Basic Books, 2010).

277   **"In 2005, Dr. Jon-Kar Zubieta examined the brain scans of men as they underwent a painful injection in their jaw. . . .":** Jon-Kar Zubieta et al, "Placebo Effects Mediated by Endogenous Opioid Activity on u-Opioid Receptors," *The Journal of Neuroscience,* 2005.

277   **"The effects go far beyond depression and pain. . . .":** Benedetti, *Placebo Effects: Understanding the Mechanisms in Health and Disease,* 2009; the number forty-five in the text comes from an informal canvassing of peer-reviewed studies in the literature. Placebo effect on herpes: Benson, Friedman, "Harnessing the power of the placebo effect and renaming it 'remembered wellness,'" *Annual Review of Medicine,* 1996; placebo effect on Parkinson's: Goetz, Leurgans, Ra-

man, Stebbins, "Objective changes in motor function during placebo treatment in Parkinson's Disease," *Neurology,* 2000; placebo effect on ulcers: Enck and Klosterhalfen, "The placebo response in functional bowel disorders: perspectives and putative mechanisms," *Neurogastroenterology and Motility,* 2005.

277 **"Placebos triggering immune responses"**: Pacheco-Lopez, Engler, Niemi, and Schedlowski, "Expectations and associations that heal: Immunomodulatory placebo effects and its neurobiology," *Brain, Behavior, and Immunity,* 2006.

277 **"Lowering heart rates . . ."**: Bienfenfeld, Frishman, and Glasser, "The placebo effect in cardiovascular disease," *American Heart Journal,* 1996.

277 **"Raising energy levels . . ."**: Beedie, Stuart, Coleman, and Foad, "Placebo effects of caffeine on cycling performance," *Medical Sciences and Sports and Exercise,* 2006.

277 **"Enhancing athletic performance . . ."**: Beedie, Stuart, Coleman, and Foad, "Positive and negative placebo effect resulting from the deceptive administration of an ergogenic aid," *International Journal of Sport Nutrition, Exercise and Metabolism,* 2007.

277 **"Improving sleep . . ."**: Fratello, Curcio, Ferrara, et al, "Can an inert sleeping pill affect sleep? Effects on polysomnographic, behavioral, and subjective measures," *Psychopharmacology,* 2005.

277 **"Boosting sex drive"**: Bradford and Meston, "Correlates of placebo response in the treatment of sexual dysfunction in women: a preliminary report," *Journal of Sex Medicine,* 2007.

278 **"The placebo effect is shown to grow stronger if the placebo given has side effects or the doctors in question treat the patients with more 'attention and confidence'. . . ."**: Benedetti, *Placebo Effects: Understanding the Mechanisms in Health and Disease,* 2009.

279 **"Processes we think of as automatic can be brought under something like conscious control. . . ."**: I have been using the *placebo effect* as a blanket term to describe this ability to link the physical body with willpower/imagination/belief, even though it is an inappropriate use of the term: both because placebo studies typically include statistical phenomenon like regression to the mean, which has nothing to do with unity in mind and body, and because some of the most amazing findings relating to a so-called willpower effect could never be described in terms of placebo. Consider a 1992 study by Guang Yue and Kelly Cole, which found that subjects could strengthen their muscles *just by thinking about them*. In the experiment, subjects were divided into two groups. One group did physical finger exercises, fifteen contractions with a twenty-second rest between each. The second group imagined doing the fifteen contractions and taking the twenty-second rest. At the end of the experiment, subjects who exercised physically had 30 percent gains in strength. The subjects who had only imagined the workout increased their muscular strength 22 percent. They are results simultaneously challenging our notions

of what constitutes a workout, and reinforcing the heretofore exasperating urging of coaches everywhere to focus on intangibles like follow-through and proper form. (Guang Yue and Kelly Cole, "Strength increases from the motor program: Comparison of training with maximal voluntary and imagined muscle contractions," *Journal of Neurophysiology*, 1992.)

280   **"Ernest Shackleton's declamation that he had 'pierced the veneer of outside things . . .'":** Ernest Shackleton, *South: The Endurance Expedition,* New York: Signet Press, 1999.

280   **"Jack LaLanne swimming from Alcatraz in the 60-degree San Francisco harbor . . .":** A feat repeated twice. The second time at age sixty!

281   **"Cycling of the Gunas . . .":** And, of course, my last memory of Bikram, not necessarily chronologically, but more what it all comes down to, the remainder stuck to the frying pan of my brain after I've let it soak out for bit: Bikram excited onstage, eyes lit up, telling us a story about Michael Jackson. It's a story I've heard him tell before, maybe five or six times, and like all things Bikram, I have no idea whether it's true or not, and no idea whether I should let that bother me. But Bikram doesn't care, he is continuing to tell us all about the King of Pop—both how he introduced the entire Jackson 5 to their first talent agent, and then that, unlike Elvis, even he, Bikram, could not have saved Michael. "He asked for private class. But no," Bikram says. "It was impossible. The man was a net. His spirit was cut into pieces. I could see that. Too far gone. It is terrible to see a man so beautiful destroyed." Then, just before I can fall into the somewhat obvious reflection, Bikram does something unexpected. Talking about Michael Jackson has made him want to dance. This instant. And so he yells for the sound guy to put on a disco song he recorded. After some fumbling, a Bollywood-infused techno-disco beat starts thumping, and Bikram's unmistakable voice hits the sound system. The room starts clapping. Bikram nods his head a few times and then starts dancing with surprisingly fluid, surprisingly choreographed moves. The room goes wild, and several of the Scandinavian women stand up on their chairs and start grinding along with him. At some point, we come back to reality, but in my memory at least, it's not until the next morning in his hot tent, my face pressed into a sweaty towel, every cell in my body frantic for oxygen, alive and kicking, trying to make it through the next ninety minutes one more time.

Acknowledgments

A book like this is a record of a moment. Everyone involved in this project was constantly thinking and refining their ideas, and I take it for granted that none of the representations in here can define the breadth of who they are or the depth of what they stand for. My own ideas about yoga have changed tremendously over the course of just the editing period; in fact, when I look back, the only constant in writing this book has been the generosity and kindness of the people I encountered. Accordingly, a few overdue thanks:

Thank you to the teachers who shared their wisdom and time: Tony Sanchez, Lucas M., Sarah Baughn, L-Like Linda, Esak Garcia, Mary Jarvis, Bonnie Jones Reynolds, Jimmy Barkan, Joseph Encinia, Chad Clark, Jeff Renfro, Eleanor Payson, Dr. Brian Nelson, Dr. Susan Yeargin, and Dr. Santiago Lorenzo.

Thank you to the teachers who shared their kindness and support: Hector, Janis, Jenny, Cristin, Shaina, Vinny, Denis, Fiona, Afton, Brett, Lauran, Chaukei, Karla, Lisa, David, Jessica, Johanna, Anna, Angie, Mike, Monica, Hilde, Ainsley from BYHQ, Yanus from Austin, Susan, Nikki, Roseann from Roseann Wang Photography, Gil from SandowPlus, and Sandy Wong-Sanchez from Baja, CA.

Thank you to the teachers who don't want to be named due to the nature of this investigation and their privacy.

Thank you to the teachers whom I just can't thank enough for everything they have done for me: Aiko Nakasone, Troy Meyers, and Courtney Mace. You three defined everything positive about my yoga experience. Everyone should be lucky enough to walk into a studio and find such knowledgeable teachers.

Thank you to Bikram in the cosmic sense of making this all possible.

Thank you to my editor Yaniv Soha, who is graced with almost supernatural levels of patience. To my agent Mike Harriot, who was graced with the persistence to continue reading the query letter for this book even though it was addressed to someone else.

To the whole JJ8 crew. To Ash and Sol. To Mu-shu and Wonton. To Raju and Athas for keeping me drunk. To Dave, Christy, Matt BL, Jon, Joe, Josh, Katie, David A. and David M. To Nad. To secret editor Rachel McKeen. To secret photographer Kenan Halabi. To Josh, Stephen, Scott, Mike, and Matt for making group roadside puking the most enjoyable thing in the world.

Thank you to the staff at the Hudson Diner where I wrote this whole damned thing. To Ramón, Sandra, and Gabi for keeping my coffee warm. To El Patron, Rajiv Choudhury, behind the register. To my little green booth of an office.

To Bushwick Outreach Center. To Bushwick Community High School. For never letting me forget that there is real work to be done in this world with real people. And that, however enjoyable, dithering in a yoga class isn't doing anything to impact them. To Mike Rothman at Eskolta for tolerating me showing up at meetings sweaty and stretched out.

To Victoria, who puts up with me, and put up with this book. And who in the putting up, made us both better (me and the book that is). Who knows that I love her madly even though I show it in really weird ways.

To my sister Sarah, 'cause she's the best.

To my Mom and Dad most of all. You've always had my back, and I've always known it. And that has meant the world.